CLINICAL PEDIATRIC ENDOCRINOLOGY

Clinical Pediatric Endocrinology

WELLINGTON HUNG, M.D., Ph.D.

Professor of Pediatrics
Department of Pediatrics
Georgetown University School of Medicine
Washington, D.C.
Senior Clinical Investigator
Developmental Endocrinology Branch
National Institute of Child Health and Human Development
National Institutes of Health
Bethesda, Maryland
Consultant
Department of Endocrinology and Metabolism
Children's Hospital National Medical Center
Washington, D.C.
Professorial Lecturer in Pediatrics
Department of Pediatrics
George Washington University School of Medicine and Health Sciences
Washington, D.C.

Mosby
Year Book

St. Louis   Baltimore   Boston   Chicago   London   Philadelphia   Sydney   Toronto

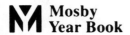

Mosby
Year Book

Dedicated to Publishing Excellence

Sponsoring Editor: Stephanie Manning
Assistant Editor: Jane Petrash
Assistant Managing Editor, Text and Reference: George Mary Gardner
Production Coordinator: Nancy C. Baker
Proofroom Manager: Barbara Kelly

1 2 3 4 5 6 7 8 9 0 GW/MV 96 95 94 93 92

Library of Congress Cataloging-in-Publication Data
Hung, Wellington, 1932-
    Clinical pediatric endocrinology / Wellington Hung.
      p.   cm.
    Includes bibliographical references and index.
    ISBN 0-8016-6266-4
    1. Pediatric endocrinology.   I. Title.
    [DNLM: 1. Endocrine Diseases—in infancy & childhood.
2. Endocrine Glands—physiology.   WS 330 H936c]
RJ418.H8558   1991
618.92'4—dc20   91-27367
DNLM/DLC   CIP
for Library of Congress

Contributors

Val Abbassi, M.D.
Professor of Pediatrics
Chief, Division of Pediatric Endocrinology and
Metabolism
Department of Pediatrics
Georgetown University School of Medicine
Washington, D.C.

Barry B. Bercu, M.D.
Professor of Pharmacology and Therapeutics
Professor of Pediatrics
Department of Pediatrics
University of South Florida College of Medicine
Tampa, Florida

Allen M. Glasgow, M.D.
Professor of Pediatrics
Department of Endocrinology and Metabolism
Children's National Medical Center
George Washington University Medical School
Washington, D.C.

Wellington Hung, M.D., Ph.D.
Professor of Pediatrics
Georgetown University School of Medicine
Washington, D.C.
Senior Clinical Investigator
Developmental Endocrinology Branch
National Institute of Child Health and Human
Development
National Institutes of Health
Bethesda, Maryland

Peter A. Lee, M.D., Ph.D.
Professor of Pediatrics
Department of Pediatrics
University of Pittsburgh School of Medicine
Pittsburgh, Pennsylvania

Allen W. Root, M.D.
Professor of Pediatrics and Biochemistry
Chief, Section of Pediatric Endocrinology
Department of Pediatrics
University of South Florida College of Medicine
Tampa, Florida

I. David Schwartz, M.D.
Pediatric Endocrinologist
Assistant Professor of Pediatrics
Section of Pediatric Endocrinology
University of Missouri, Kansas City School of Medicine
Kansas City, Missouri

Selma F. Siegel, M.D.
Clinical Assistant Professor
Department of Pediatrics
University of Pittsburgh
Pittsburgh, Pennsylvania

Louis St.L. O'Dea, M.B.B.Ch.
Department of Obstetrics and Gynecology
McGill University
Montreal, Canada

W. Douglas Tynan, Ph.D.
Assistant Professor of Psychiatry and Pediatrics
Departments of Psychiatry and Endocrinology
George Washington University Medical Center
Children's National Medical Center
Washington, D.C.

Preface

Our goal in writing this book is to present relatively concise yet comprehensive reviews of physiologic and pathophysiologic principles, with details of practical management of endocrine disorders in pediatric patients. This book is not intended to replace the extensive standard pediatric endocrinology textbooks currently available. Rather, it is designed as a practical guide for the pediatric house officer and the practicing pediatrician and as a preliminary text for beginning fellows in pediatric endocrinology.

Advancements in pediatric endocrinology necessitated that preparation of this book keep pace with current knowledge. My colleagues and I have made every effort to discharge this responsibility. Particular effort has been made to provide extensive recent references. Although every precaution has been taken to avoid error, bias, and prejudice, inevitably some of these become included in the text. The editor assumes full responsibility for these indiscretions.

The editor acknowledges the portions of this work that stem from the Medical Outline Series *Pediatric Endocrinology*, edited by himself in collaboration with Gilbert P. August and Allen M. Glasgow.

The authors hope this book will enable the reader to better understand the function of the endocrine system in the newborn, child, and adolescent, and that it presents a practical plan for diagnosis and treatment.

Wellington Hung, M.D., Ph.D.

Acknowledgments

This book is dedicated to our families, who made it possible; and to our students, residents, fellows, and colleagues who stimulated us to write this book.

We are indebted to Stephanie Manning and her editorial staff, Mosby–Year Book, Inc., who were responsible for editing the book and who were diligent and conscientious in their efforts.

Wellington Hung, M.D., Ph.D.

Contents

Chapter 1

Mechanisms of Hormone Action: General Principles

Allen W. Root

Pediatric endocrinology focuses on disorders of the endocrine system that disrupt normal development, growth, maturation, and metabolism in the infant, child, and adolescent. Endocrinology is a broad science that encompasses the general field of cellular communication, that is, how cells "tell" one another and themselves what to do.[21] Classically, the *endocrine* system has been thought of as the organized "glands of internal secretion" (anterior pituitary, thyroid, parathyroid, adrenal, gonads, pancreas) that synthesize and secrete their products into the circulation for action at a distant target cell. However, there is direct cell-to-cell communication (*paracrine*), autocommunication in which the cell sends a signal to itself (*autocrine*), and even internal communication (*intracrine*)[19,25] (Fig 1–1). Many of the products of the endocrine gland are secreted not only into the bloodstream (*hormones*) but also locally to exert a paracrine effect on adjacent cells (e.g., in the control of pancreatic islet cell function, where cells that secrete insulin, pancreatic polypeptide, somatostatin, and glucagon interact). In addition, other systems (central nervous, gastrointestinal, cardiovascular, genitourinary, immunologic) secrete products that act locally or distally but have not been considered classic endocrine glands. Within the central and peripheral nervous systems are peptides that function as neuromodulators or neurotransmitters. Many of these peptides are also products of peripheral tissues (e.g., calcitonin, somatostatin, endorphins, enkephalins, cholecystokinin, and peptide Y).

Thus the demarcation between the classic endocrine hormone system and other methods of cellular communication has become blurred and indistinct as we envision the body's global information and communication system.

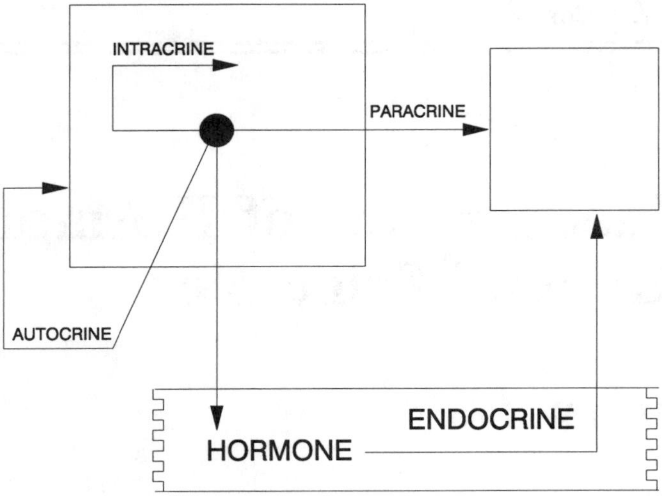

FIG 1–1.
Mechanisms of intercellular and intracellular communication.

PROTEIN HORMONES

Protein hormones are synthesized and secreted by the hypothalamus (the neurohormonal anterior pituitary release-stimulating and release-inhibiting peptides), the posterior pituitary or neurohypophysis (antidiuretic hormone, oxytocin), the anterior pituitary, thyroid and parathyroid glands, thymus, intestines, kidney, heart, and pancreatic islets. They are transported in the circulation, either free or bound to carrier proteins (i.e., growth hormone–binding protein, insulin-like growth factor I [IGF-I]–binding protein) to a target cell. At the plasma membrane of the target cell the hormone encounters a protein receptor to which it binds. This triggers one or more second messenger systems within the cell membrane and cytosol, resulting in phosphorylation of selected cell proteins, which proteins in turn cause the cell to function as intended.

Protein Hormone Synthesis and Secretion

After activation of the structural gene for the protein hormone by an appropriate stimulus, the DNA message is *transcribed* to its complementary messenger RNA (mRNA) in the nucleus by RNA polymerase II bound to a recognition sequence upstream from the gene (Fig 1–2). *Exons*, those sequences of the gene that code for the active protein hormone, are separated from *introns*, intervening sequences of untranslated DNA, by specific enzymes (processing); the exons are then spliced together to form mature mRNA. The pattern of exon splicing from the same gene sequence may vary (e.g., both calcitonin and calcitonin gene–related protein are derived from the same gene by recombination of various exons after transcription of the primary gene). Mature mRNA leaves the nucleus and enters the cytoplasmic ribosomal apparatus, where *translation* of the message into a protein takes place with the aid of ribosomal and transfer RNAs.[15]

The initial, very long-chain protein product (preprohormone) contains a leader sequence of hydrophobic amino acids, which is removed as the protein undergoes *posttranslational processing* within the rough endoplasmic reticulum and Golgi apparatus, where it is cleaved to the prohormone and native hormone(s), glycosylated, its subunits assembled, enclosed within secretory granules, and transported to the inner surface of the plasma membrane to await release. Hormone is secreted both continuously in a nonregulated manner (constitutive secretion) and in a regulated manner by exocytosis in response to a stimulus.[4] Exocytosis is the process wherein the membranes of the secretory granule and cell fuse and the contents of the granule are extruded into the extracellular space. Co-localized within the secretory granule of many endocrine and neuroendocrine cells is chromogranin A (secretory protein I), which is released with the primary hormone. Chromogranin A is a 439 amino acid (mol wt 68 kDa) peptide, containing within it a 49 amino acid peptide, pancreastatin, so named because it was initially identified in pancreatic islets. Pancreastatin inhibits the secretion of insulin, somatostatin, and parathyroid hormone, and may represent an autocrine form of regulation of protein secretion.[3,9]

Protein Hormone Receptors

Receptors for the protein hormones are present on the plasma membrane of the target cell. These receptors are proteins with three segments or domains: extracellular, transmembrane, and intracytoplasmic. Many of the protein hormone receptors are serpentine, long-chain polypeptides with seven transmembrane domains (Fig 1–3), typified by the β-adrenergic receptor, but also characteristic of receptors for acetylcholine, serotonin, thyrotropin, the gonadotropins, adrenocorticotropin, many of the hypothalamic neuropeptides, parathyroid hormone, glucagon, and antidiuretic hormone.[13,23] The hormone binding region of this type of receptor may be found on one

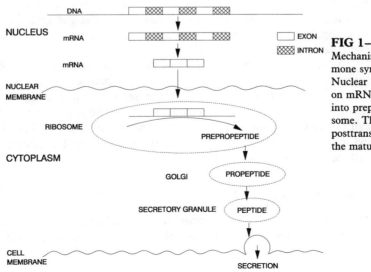

FIG 1–2.
Mechanism of protein hormone synthesis and secretion. Nuclear DNA is transcribed on mRNA, which is translated into prepropeptide in the ribosome. The latter undergoes posttranslational processing to the mature peptide.

FIG 1–3.
Cell membrane receptors for protein hormones. Structures of receptors with G protein–activating and intrinsic tyrosine kinase properties and other mechanisms of action. IGF-I, -II = insulin-like growth factors; EGF = epidermal growth factor; GH = growth hormone, PRL = prolactin.

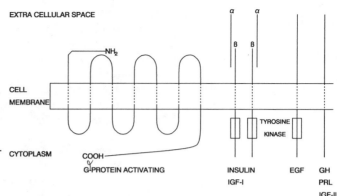

of the extracellular segments or on a transmembrane site, whereas the site for second messenger activation is on an intracellular domain. The C-terminus of the receptor is within the cytoplasm and is the site of reversible phosphorylation, which can activate or inactivate the receptor. These receptors function primarily by activating guanosine triphosphate (GTP)–binding proteins (G proteins), which link the message of the activated receptor to a second messenger system (see below).[12]

Receptors with intrinsic protein kinase activity, such as those for insulin and IGF-I, are composed of two paired alpha and two paired beta subunits, forming a four-subunit structure with the extracellular hormone binding domain present on the alpha subunit, a transmembrane domain, and an intracellular domain with the tyrosine kinase activity intrinsic to the beta subunit (see Fig 1–3). The receptor for epidermal growth factor is a single-chain polypeptide with tyrosine kinase activity on its intracytoplasmic domain.

Receptors for growth hormone (GH), prolactin, and IGF-II–mannose-6-phosphate are straight-chain peptides with three domains (see Fig 1–3). The structure of circulating GH-binding protein is identical to the extracellular domain of the GH receptor, but whether it is derived from the receptor itself or arises by an alternative synthetic pathway from the GH receptor gene is unknown.

After binding of the hormone to its receptor and activation of receptor function, hormone receptor complexes aggregate and form a coated pit, which is then internalized. Once within the cytoplasm the ligand-receptor complex can be catabolized; the ligand can be separated from the receptor and degraded; the ligand and receptor can be separated and both returned to the cell surface; the ligand may associate with cytoplasmic or nuclear receptors; or the ligand-receptor complex may return to the cell surface where the ligand is released.

Second Messengers

After hormone binds to receptor there is a change in the tertiary configuration of this unit, which permits interaction with one or more second messenger systems (Fig 1–4).

Guanosine Binding Proteins

The guanosine (G)-binding proteins serve an intermediary function, carrying the primary message of protein hormone receptor interaction to a second messenger, which eventually effects intracellular protein phosphorylation and cell function.[12,13,24] The receptors usually associated with G-binding proteins are long-chain, folded proteins with seven domains that traverse the cell membrane between the intracellular and extracellular compartments. The C-terminal sequence of these receptors interacts

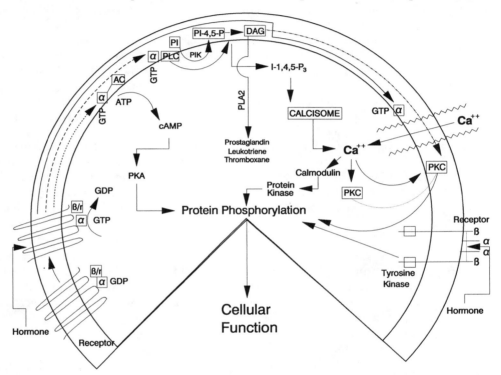

FIG 1–4.
After binding of hormone to a receptor that activates a guanosine-binding protein (G-binding protein), the guanosine diphosphate *(GDP)* on its alpha subunit is replaced by guanosine triphosphate *(GTP)*. The alpha-GTP subunit separates from the beta-gamma subunit complex, and transverses the plasma membrane to activate one or more of the second messenger systems: (1) Adenyl cyclase *(AC)* converts ATP to cyclic adenosine monophosphate *(cAMP)*, which in turn activates protein kinase A *(PKA)*, which enhances intracellular protein phosphorylation. (2) Phospholipase C *(PLC)* converts membrane phosphoinositide *(PI)*, after formation of phosphoinositide-1,4-bisphosphate by phosphoinositide kinase *(PIK)*, to inositol-1,4,5-trisphosphate *(I-1,4,5-P₃)*, and diacyglycerol *(DAG)*. After action by phospholipase A_2 *(PLA2)*, DAG is converted to prostaglandins, leukotrienes and thromboxanes. I-1,4,5-P₃ releases Ca^{2+} from the calcisome storage site. (3) calcium channels are "opened" by the alpha-GTP subunit of the G-binding protein. As the cytosolic concentration of Ca^{2+} increases, protein kinase C *(PKC)* is translocated to the cell membrane, where it is activated by DAG to cause protein phophorylation. Ca^{2+} acts also through association with calmodulin to enhance activity of other protein kinases. Hormones that bind to receptors with intrinsic tyrosine kinase activity also enhance protein formation. These receptors may act through G-binding proteins as well.

with the G-binding protein at an intracellular site immediately adjacent to the inner surface of the cell membrane. The G-binding protein consists of three subunits (alpha, beta, gamma); in the inactive state the hormone receptor-specific alpha subunit is bound to the receptor, to guanosine diphosphate (GDP), and to a combined beta-gamma subunit complex. When the receptor is activated by binding to hormone, a conformational change occurs, as a consequence of which the alpha subunit of the G-binding protein dissociates from the receptor and from the beta-gamma subunit complex, GDP is replaced by guanosine triphosphate (GTP) and the alpha subunit–GTP complex translocates along the cell membrane to the second messenger involved in the cell's response to the primary hormonal stimulus.

There are stimulatory (Gs) and inhibitory (Gi) G-binding proteins. After stimulation or inhibition of the second messenger, GTP is hydrolyzed to GDP and the alpha subunit returns to the inactive heterotrimeric configuration at the receptor site. Some data suggest that it is the beta-gamma subunit complex that exerts an inhibitory effect on the second messenger system, rather than a specific inhibitory form of the alpha-GTP subunit.

G-binding proteins interact with several second messenger systems, including cyclic adenosine monophosphate (cAMP), the membrane phospholipids, and transport channels for calcium, potassium, and other ions. In addition, G-binding proteins may be mediators of receptor function with other configurations (i.e., insulin and IGF-I receptors).

Cyclic Adenosine Monophosphate

Adenyl cyclase, a membrane-bound enzyme, catalyzes the transformation of adenosine triphosphate (ATP) to cAMP, which in turn activates protein kinases that phosphorylate many cellular proteins. Cyclic AMP also stimulates Ca^{2+} release from intracellular storage sites, raising intracellular Ca^{2+} concentrations. In turn, Ca^{2+} activates phosphodiesterase, which degrades cAMP.

Phospholipids

Cell membrane phospholipids are an important source of intracellular second messengers. Activated by the alpha subunit–GTP complex of the G-binding protein, phospholipase C cleaves 1,4,5-phosphatidylinositol bisphosphate (1,4,5-PIP$_2$) into the second messengers diacylglycerol (DAG) and inositol triphosphate (IP$_3$).[6,20] Phospholipase A$_2$, activated also by the G-binding protein, removes arachidonic acid from DAG; arachidonic acid serves as a second messenger and as a precursor for prostaglandins, thromboxanes, and leukotrienes. Inositol trisphosphate increases Ca^{2+} mobilization from intracellular stores.

Ion Flux

Some G-binding proteins and the majority of second messengers affect cellular function by altering the intracellular concentration of Ca^{2+} and other ions (K^+ and Na^+). Intracellular levels of Ca^{2+} may be increased by opening transmembrane Ca^{2+} channels directly by G-binding proteins or second messengers (cAMP) or by mobilizing Ca^{2+} from its intracellular storage sites in membrane-bound calcisomes (cAMP, IP$_3$). After binding to calmodulin, Ca^{2+} and other second messengers activate a number of protein kinases (including protein kinase C), which leads to phosphorylation of specific proteins and thence to cellular function.[16] The steps involved in cell function after protein phosphorylation are not understood at this time. The influx of sodium into the cell cytoplasm and the efflux of potassium from the cell through specific channels are influenced by the cell's second messenger systems and also are involved in cell function in response to the appropriate hormonal stimulus.

Protein Kinase

The final effectors of the second messengers are a family of protein kinases that transfer phosphate from ATP to tyrosine and serine residues on specific proteins, which are then linked to cell function.[11] Some receptors (insulin, IGF-I, epidermal growth factor [EGF]) have intrinsic protein kinase (often tyrosine kinase) activity leading to direct protein phosphorylation. However, there is evidence that these receptors also may act through G-binding proteins and phospholipase C, because there are acute changes in intracellular levels of phosphoinositides (DAG, IP_3) after ligand-receptor interaction in these systems as well.

Transport of Protein Hormones

The concept that protein hormones circulate in the free state is being challenged. A specific GH-binding protein (GH-BP) has been identified, and a family of proteins bind IGF-I and IGF-II; in addition, data suggest that there may be circulating binding proteins for some of the glycoprotein hormones. Serum GH-BP has a structure similar to that of the extracellular domain of the GH receptor, but whether it is derived by posttranslational processing of this peptide or arises as an alternative product of the GH receptor gene is uncertain. The physiologic role of GH-BP is unknown, as more than 50% of circulating GH is not bound to GH-BP, but its absence from serum (as determined by its ability to bind radioiodinated GH) correlates with defects in the GH receptor and with tissue insensitivity to GH. In vitro, GH-BP inhibits the biologic effect of GH.[14]

There are several IGF-binding proteins (IGF-BP-1, -2, -3, -4). IGF-BP-1 (mol wt 25.3 kDa) is a non-GH-dependent protein found in endometrium, placenta, and amniotic fluid; IGF-BP-2 (mol wt 31.5–33 kDa) is a non-GH-dependent protein found in serum and in cerebrospinal fluid; IGF-BP-3 (mol wt 28.7 kDa) is part of the large protein complex that binds the bulk of circulating IGF-I and IGF-II; it is GH-dependent, that is, its synthesis is stimulated by GH. IGF-BP-4 is a glycoprotein of molecular weight 26 kD. The IGF-BPs are not only present in the circulation but also are secreted by many cells locally, where they act in a paracrine or autocrine manner to enhance or inhibit the physiologic effects of IGF on cell division, growth, and function. They also may have intrinsic biologic activity.

STEROID, THYROID, AND VITAMIN D HORMONES

Steroid, thyroid, and vitamin D hormones are enzymatically synthesized from precursor molecules (steroid and vitamin D hormones from cholesterol, thyroid hormones from tyrosine) in specific glands (adrenal, gonads, thyroid) or other organs (skin, liver, kidney). They act primarily at an intracellular locus, through a nuclear-bound receptor, to promote or inhibit gene transcription.

Receptors

After diffusion through the cell membrane, steroid, thyroid, and vitamin D hormones bind to nuclear-associated protein receptors. There also may be cytoplasmic gluco-corticoid receptors, but the physiologically relevant receptors are those within the nucleus. These receptors are large peptides comprised of three regions: the hormone or ligand binding domain at the C-terminal, a midregion DNA-binding domain, and an N-terminal domain necessary for activation of gene transcription and specificity of receptor binding to DNA[2,8] (Fig 1–5). These receptors are synthesized in cyto-plasmic microsomes and enter the nucleus by diffusion through the nuclear membrane or by transport through nuclear membrane pores; protein sequences important for nuclear translocation are present in steroid receptors, localized to the carboxyl side of the DNA binding region. After binding to a specific ligand, a dimer of the hormone-receptor complex binds to its specific DNA hormone response element (HRE) up-stream from the gene whose transcription is to be initiated or repressed. A receptor without its hormone binding domain spontaneously binds to and activates its HRE. Thus the binding domain of the receptor serves to inhibit receptor function prior to hormone binding. In the ligand-unbound, inactive state, steroid receptors are asso-ciated with large proteins, among them a family of heat shock proteins (HSP, mol wt >70–90 kDa), so named because of the association of HSP with the response to a high temperature insult.[18] Two HSPs are associated with one steroid receptor. After ligand binding the steroid receptor sheds the HSPs and is then able to bind with and activate its HRE.

The DNA binding domain is composed of two zinc fingers (Fig 1–6), thought to permit the ligand-receptor complex to interact with its HRE. The similarity of amino acid composition of the zinc fingers has permitted classification of these re-ceptors into three subfamilies (see below). The N-terminal domains of the steroid, thyroid, and vitamin D receptors vary widely, but are thought to be important for activation of transcription and for specificity of activity.

Receptor Subfamilies

The three receptor subfamilies are distinguished by the two–amino acid sequence between the third and fourth cysteine residues of the first zinc finger (see Fig 1–6). In the steroid receptor subfamily, these amino acids are glycine-serine; in the thyroid–

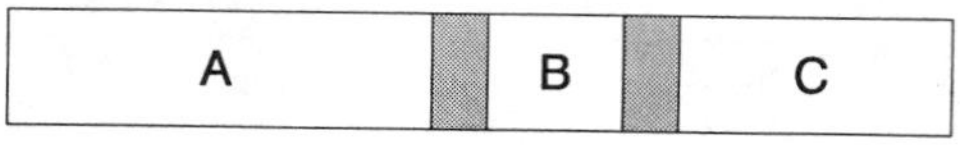

FIG 1–5.
Structure of the nuclear receptor for steroid, thyroid, and vitamin D hormones. **A,** hypervar-iable transcription activating–domain. **B,** DNA-binding domain. **C,** ligand-binding domain. *Shaded areas,* connecting sequences.

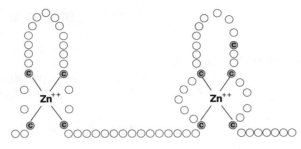

FIG 1–6.
DNA-binding domain of the steroid, thyroid, and vitamin D hormones demonstrating the zinc fingers and critical cysteine (*C*) residues.

TABLE 1–1.

Amino Acid Number and Percent Homology of Steroid, Thyroid, and Vitamin D Receptors Compared with Glucocorticoid Receptor*

| | | Domain (AA/%) | | |
Receptor	Amino Acid	Transcriptional	DNA Binding	Ligand Binding
Glucocorticoid	777	421/100	66/100	250/100
Mineralocorticoid	984	603/<15	66/94	251/57
Progesterone	934	567/<15	67/90	235/55
Androgen	918	556/<15	68/76	253/50
Estrogen	595	185/<15	66/52	241/30
Thyroid-α	410	53/<15	68/47	228/17
Thyroid-β	456	162/<15	68/47	225/17
Vitamin D	427	24/<15	66/41	236/<15
Estrogen-related$_1$	521	176/<15	66/56	227/28
Estrogen-related$_2$	433	103/<15	66/56	222/28

vitamin D receptor subfamily, glutamic acid–glycine; and in the estrogen-related subfamily of receptors, glutamic acid–valine.

Steroid Receptors

The receptors for glucocorticoids (GR), mineralocorticoids (MR), progestins (PR), and androgens (AR) make up one subfamily (Table 1–1); there is considerable sequence homology among these receptors, but by and large the ligand binding domains of these receptors are highly specific. One exception to this is the MR, which binds both glucocorticoids and mineralocorticoids with equal avidity. However, the MR is rendered mineralocorticoid-specific by the copresence of 11β-hydroxysteroid dehydrogenase (11β-HSD). This enzyme, found in mineralocorticoid-responsive tissues such as the renal tubule, metabolizes glucocorticoids to inactive 11-keto analogues (i.e., hydrocortisone $\xrightarrow{\text{11β-HSD}}$ cortisone), thereby permitting the MR to be exposed only to mineralocorticoids.

Estrogen, Thyroid Hormone, and Vitamin D Receptors

The hormone receptors in this subfamily have a common amino acid sequence between cysteines 3 and 4, but otherwise are disparate. There are three receptors for the thyroid hormone, two of which (α and β) are expressed widely, whereas the expression of the third is limited to the anterior pituitary.

Estrogen-related Receptors

Included in this family are receptor proteins with similarities to the estrogen receptor (hence estrogen related) and for several growth factors.

Transport of the Steroid, Thyroid, and Vitamin D Hormones

Unlike the protein hormones, only minute amounts of steroid, thyroid, and vitamin D hormones circulate in the free state.[7,17] The bulk of these hormones are bound to specific and nonspecific (albumin) plasma proteins that serve to transport and distribute these hormones to the appropriate target tissues. In general, these proteins are not absolutely necessary. A deficiency of some of these proteins occurs frequently and apparently is of no clinical consequence (e.g., deficiency of thyroxine-binding globulin); however, others (e.g., vitamin D binding and corticosteroid binding proteins) may be essential for life. The hormone carrier proteins are listed in Table 1–2.

CONCLUSION

The concept of cellular communication has expanded the discipline of endocrinology far beyond its classic confines. Increasing knowledge about the mechanism of action of protein and nonprotein hormones gained through the technology of molecular biology has permitted identification of patients with disorders due to subtle amino

TABLE 1–2.

Transport Proteins for Steroid, Thyroid, and Vitamin D Hormones*

Hormone	% Free	Binding Protein
Thyroxine (T_4)	0.03	T_4-binding globulin (TBG; mol wt 54 kDa) binds 70% of circulating T_4, 40% of T_3
Triiodothyronine (T_3)	0.3	
		T_4-binding prealbumin (TBPA, transthyretin; mol wt 55 kDa) binds 10% of T_4, 35% of T_3
		Albumin binds 20% of T_4, 35% of T_3
Cortisol	3	Corticosteroid binding globulin (CBG, transcortin; mol wt 50 kDa) binds 90% of cortisol
		Albumin binds 7% of cortisol
Testosterone	2.5 (M)	Sex hormone binding globulin (SHBG; testosterone-estradiol binding globulin, TEBG; mol wt 92 kDa):
	1.4 (F)	
Dihydrotestosterone		Adult male: binds 49% of testosterone, 35% of estradiol
Androstenedione		Adult female: binds 76% of testosterone, 66% of estradiol
Estradiol	3 (M)	Albumin:
	1 (F)	Adult male: binds 49% of testosterone, 62% of estradiol
		Adult female: binds 23% of testosterone, 33% of estradiol

*Data from references 1, 5, 10, 22.

acid and DNA base substitutions within hormones and receptors and to abnormalities of protein synthesis and processing, receptor formation and function, and intracellular metabolism.

REFERENCES

1. Bartalena L: Recent achievements in studies on thyroid hormone–binding proteins. *Endocr Rev* 1990; 11:47–64.
2. Carson-Jureco MA, Schrader WT, O'Malley BW: Steroid receptor family: Structure and functions. *Endocr Rev* 1990; 11:201–220.
3. Chromogranin A: Always a bridesmaid, never a bride? (editorial). *Lancet* 1989; 2:542.
4. Chung KN, Walter P, LaPonte GW, et al: Molecular sorting in the secretory pathway. *Science* 1989; 243:192–197.
5. Cooke NE, Haddad JG: Vitamin D binding protein (Gc-globulin). *Endocr Rev* 1989; 10:294–307.
6. Drucker BJ, Mamon JN, Roberts TM: Oncogenes, growth factors, and signal transduction. *N Engl J Med* 1989; 321:1383–1391.
7. Ekins R: Measurement of free hormones in blood. *Endocr Rev* 1990; 11:5–46.
8. Evans RM: The steroid and thyroid hormone receptor superfamily. *Science* 1988; 240:889–895.
9. Fasciotto BH, Gore S-U, Bourdeau AM, et al: Autocrine regulation of parathyroid secretion: Inhibition of secretion by chromogranin A (secretory protein-I) and potentiation of secretion by chromogranin A and pancreastatin antibodies. *Endocrinology* 1990; 127:1329–1335.
10. Hammon GL: Molecular properties of corticosteroid binding globulin and the sex-steroid binding proteins. *Endocr Rev* 1990; 11:65–79.
11. Hanks SK, Quin AM, Hunter T: The protein kinase family: Conserved features and deduced phylogeny of the catalytic domains. *Science* 1988; 241:42–52.
12. Johnson GL, Dhanasekarun N: The G-protein family and their interaction with receptors. *Endocr Rev* 1989; 10:317–331.
13. Levitzki A: From epinephrine to cyclic AMP. *Science* 1988; 241:800–806.
14. Lim L, Spencer EA, McKay P, et al: Regulation of growth hormone (GH) bioactivity by a recombinant human GH-binding protein. *Endocrinology* 1990; 127:1287–1291.
15. Mains RE, Dickerson IM, May V, et al: Cellular and molecular aspects of peptide hormone biosynthesis. *Front Neuroendocrinol* 1990; 11:52–89.
16. Means AR: Molecular mechanism of action of calmodulin. *Recent Prog Horm Res* 1988; 44:223–259.
17. Mendel CM: The free hormone hypothesis: A physiologically based mathematical model. *Endocr Rev* 1989; 10:232–274.
18. O'Malley B: The steroid receptor superfamily: More excitement predicted for the future. *Mol Endocrinol* 1990; 4:363–369.
19. O'Malley BW: Did eucaryotic steroid receptors evolve from intracrine gene regulation? (editorial). *Endocrinology* 1989; 125:119–120.
20. Rhee SG, Sub PG, Ryu SH, et al: Studies of inositol phospholipid–specific phospholipase C. *Science* 1989; 244:546–550.
21. Root AW, Rogol AD: Organization and function of the endocrine system, in Kappy M, Blizzard R, Migeon C (eds): *Wilkins' Endocrinology of Childhood and Adolescence*, ed 4. Springfield, Ill, Charles C Thomas, Publishers, in press.

22. Rosner W: The functions of corticosteroid-binding globulin and sex hormone–binding globulin: Recent advances. *Endocr Rev* 1990; 11:80–91.
23. Sibley DR, Benovic JL, Caron MG, et al: Phosphorylation of cell surface receptors: A mechanism for regulating signal transduction pathways. *Endocr Rev* 1988; 9:38–56.
24. Spiegel AM: Receptor-effector coupling by G proteins: Implications for endocrinology. *Trends Endocrinol Metab* 1989; 1:72–76.
25. Sporn MB, Todara GJ: Autocrine secretion and malignant transformation of cells. *N Engl J Med* 1980; 303:878–880.

Chapter 2

Normal Growth and Development

I. David Schwartz
Barry B. Bercu

Growth is a fundamental parameter in assessing childhood health and development. Disturbances of growth (height, weight, or both) often alert the parent and health professional to underlying disease states or syndromes. This chapter reviews factors that affect fetal growth, normal growth, and development during childhood, growth during puberty, and diagnostic approaches to growth disorders.

FETAL GROWTH

Growth of the fetus is marked by cell replication and cell enlargement. Tissue development and organogenesis occur during early embryogenesis. Intrauterine growth may be divided into three stages[3]: (1) cellular hyperplasia, the initial phase characterized by active mitosis during gestational weeks 1 to 16; (2) cellular hyperplasia and hypertrophy, occurring during weeks 16 to 32 of gestation, marked by a slowing rate of mitosis but progressive increase in cell size; and (3) cellular hypertrophy, occurring from gestational week 32 to term, the final phase of fetal growth, which is characterized by the accumulation of fat, muscle, and connective tissue. The accumulation of fetal protein and fat has been estimated as well; at the end of 13 weeks the accumulation of fetal fat and protein is nominal. During the first portion of the second trimester, accretion of fat is approximately 0.3 g/day, and of protein is 1.0 g/day; by the end of the second trimester the fetus accumulates about 1.2 g/day fat and 1.7 g/day protein. During the last trimester, fat and protein accretion may range from 3.5 to 9.8 g/day and from 3.4 to 6.0 g/day, respectively.[50]

Insults occurring during any phase may lead to growth abnormalities. Disruption of cellular growth during the first stage leads to symmetric growth retardation; insults occurring in the third stage lead to asymmetric growth retardation. An intermediate pattern of growth retardation occurs with fetal insult during the second stage. Prerequisite to understanding appropriate fetal growth are standards used to define normal fetal growth. However, despite widespread descriptions of fetal growth abnormalities, there are no uniform standards for normal growth. The various "standards" derived thus far that provide our "definitions" differ in such important variables as geographic location, maternal parity, infant gender, and ethnic diversity. In addition, the upper and lower limits of normal birth weight are arbitrary points for any given gestational age; these limits have included 2 SD surrounding the mean, the 3rd or 5th and 97th or 95th percentiles of birth weight, and the more commonly used 10th and 90th percentiles.[13,32] Adding confusion is the delineation of intrauterine growth retardation (IUGR) vs. small for gestational age (SGA). IUGR implies a pathologic process that limits normal growth of the developing fetus but infers growth potential, and SGA implies limited growth potential and catch-up growth; but these terms are often used interchangeably. Studies that include premature infants in the "standards" add further confusion. A unified, single national standard to define intrauterine growth retardation has been proposed.[13]

Often used to define normal infant size is the ponderal index (PI). The PI is defined as mass (g) divided by the cubed crown-to-heel length (cm) multiplied by 100

$$\text{Weight (g)}/\text{Length (cm)}^3 \times 100$$

Infants with IUGR have a low PI (<2.32); constitutionally small and otherwise normal infants have PIs of 2.32 to 2.85; the PI of obese or macrosomic infants is greater than 2.85.[25] In one study, 40% of SGA infants were not growth retarded as defined by PI; 53% labeled as growth retarded by the PI had appropriate weight for gestational age.

Pathogenesis of Altered Fetal Growth

A number of factors influence fetal growth (Table 2–1); these variables may have global effects on fetal growth throughout pregnancy or may affect selective developmental periods during gestation.[5,22,34,47,49] It is beyond the scope of this chapter to discuss each in depth. The major influences on fetal growth are parental genetic factors and maternal nutritional status. There is a direct relationship between maternal height and weight and fetal size.[33] Infant gender positively influences growth: male infants are 5% heavier (150–200 g) and 1.2% longer than female infants. This may be due to the effects of testosterone. In general, infants born to multiparous women are larger than those born to primiparous women.[33]

Worldwide, maternal malnutrition is the most common cause of IUGR, yet the fetus is relatively resistant to the effects of maternal malnutrition.[25] Total caloric consumption, rather than protein or fat consumption, appears to be the primary nutritional influence on birth weight. In well-nourished women, overall dietary intake

TABLE 2–1.

Factors That Adversely Affect Fetal Growth

I. **Maternal**
  A. Congenital
    1. Genetic
      a. Ethnic
      b. Age
    2. Malformation (e.g., bicornuate uterus)
  B. Acquired
    1. Inflammation
      a. Autoimmune (e.g., systemic lupus erythematosus)
      b. Infectious
    2. Toxin
      a. Alcohol
      b. Tobacco
      c. Illicit drugs
        (1) Cocaine
        (2) Heroin
      d. Irradiation
    3. Tumor (e.g., uterine leiomyoma)
    4. Health status
      a. Nutritional
      b. Cardiac
      c. Pulmonary
      d. Renal
      e. Endocrine
        (1) Hypertension
        (2) Diabetes
      f. Hematologic
      g. Previous parity
    5. Socioeconomic
    6. Other environmental factors (e.g., high altitude)

II. **Fetal**
  A. Congenital
    1. Genetic
      a. Gender
      b. Multiple gestation
      c. Chromosomal
      d. Other genetic disorders
        (1) Inborn metabolic errors
        (2) Eponymic syndromes
    2. Malformation
      a. Placental abnormalities
      b. Fetal abnormalities
  B. Acquired
    1. Inflammation (infectious)
      a. Viral
        (1) Rubella
        (2) Cytomegalovirus
        (3) Human immunodeficiency virus
      b. Bacterial (e.g., syphilis)
      c. Parasitic
        (1) Toxoplasmosis
        (2) Malaria
    2. Trauma

and energy expenditure per kilogram change very little during the course of pregnancy compared with the nonpregnant state, yet there is weight gain during pregnancy. This appears to be due to differences in the efficiency of energy utilization.[50] Chronically undernourished women give birth to smaller infants, primarily because malnutrition has led to diminished prepregnancy height and weight. However, the placentas of malnourished women have decreased DNA content, consistent with diminished growth during the hyperplastic phase of fetal growth.[20] The effect of acute malnutrition on pregnancy outcome depends on the time of the insult during the pregnancy. A 66% reduction in caloric intake results in only 9% reduction in birth weight.[50] Nutritional supplementation studies in chronically malnourished women have demonstrated minimal changes in fetal weight. On the other hand, macrosomic infants are born to obese women, but this probably reflects maternal prepregnancy body mass.

  The principal cause of asymmetric IUGR is uteroplacental insufficiency secondary to maternal hypertension, diabetes mellitus, and renal and collagen vascular diseases. In hypertensive mothers the placenta demonstrates decreased permeability secondary to arteriolar degeneration, intimal thickening, trophoblastic membrane thickening, and cytotrophoblast hyperplasia. Thus there is diminished fetal oxygenation and nutrient delivery. Certainly, more direct "environmental" factors influence fetal growth: a malformed uterus, uterine fibroid, and multiple gestation pregnancy physically impede normal fetal growth. Maternal consumption of alcohol, use of illicit drugs, and cigarette smoking have been associated with lower birth weight.

Fetal factors affecting growth include chromosomal and genetic conditions. Growth retardation is a significant component to gestations with intrauterine infections and to trisomies 13, 18, and 21. Other conditions with somatic anomalies (Russell-Silver and Seckel syndromes) are associated with IUGR, as are conditions of isolated fetal malformation (anencephaly, cyanotic congenital heart disease). Other conditions associated with increased fetal size are Sotos and Weaver syndromes, congenital hypothyroidism, polycythemia, fetal hydrops, and more commonly, conditions associated with fetal hyperinsulinism, such as infants born of diabetic mothers and the Beckwith-Wiedemann syndrome.

Fetal Endocrinology

Insulin

The major endocrine (and probably paracrine) regulator of fetal growth is insulin, although the effect of insulin may be more "permissive," affecting fetal nutrition, rather than direct. The regulatory role of insulin in fetal growth and "overgrowth" and its complete mechanism of action are still unclear. Data suggest that the human fetus can grow to the size of a 30-week-gestation fetus independent of insulin.[11] Insulin is present in fetal pancreatic tissue by 8 weeks of gestation, and is measurable in plasma by 12 weeks.[29] The placenta was thought impermeable to insulin; however, a recent report disputes this, with the demonstration of antibody-bound insulin in the cord blood of some fetuses born to mothers with type I diabetes.[28] However, the fetal pancreas is still the major source of fetal insulin, and secretes insulin in response to fetal blood glucose levels by 20 weeks of gestation. Chronic fetal hyperglycemia accelerates the maturation of the insulin-secreting mechanism. Such enhanced maturation is not seen in the anencephalic fetus, suggesting a regulatory role of the fetal hypothalamic-pituitary unit in insulin secretion.[11]

In the fetus, insulin receptors on cell membranes can be demonstrated in liver, erythrocytes, monocytes, neural tissue, and placenta, more so on the maternal (syncytiotrophoblast) aspect than on the fetal surface. Placental insulin receptors are subject to downregulation with mild maternal hyperglycemia. In pregnancies associated with growth retardation, the number of placental insulin receptors may be diminished. In the rat model, there is no effect on net fetal hepatic glycogen synthesis by insulin despite an increased number of insulin receptors, suggesting a role of fetal insulin other than glycogen deposition. Insulin is associated with increased fetal glucose and oxygen consumption and lipogenesis. Amino acid uptake seems unaffected by insulin.

Insulin enhances the synthesis and secretion of fetal insulin-like growth factor I

(IGF-I) and may bind to IGF-I receptors, although there is no direct evidence that fetal IGFs regulate fetal growth. IGFs contribute to fetal growth because these peptides regulate cell replication and differentiation; they do not cross the placenta. Serum levels of IGF-I are increased in Beckwith-Wiedemann syndrome and are diminished in Laron-type dwarfism.

As is discussed further in Chapter 3, IGF-I and IGF-II are similar monomeric peptides with structural homology to each other, insulin, relaxin, and nerve growth factor beta. The IGFs circulate bound to several binding proteins (BPs) that act as IGF "reservoirs," reducing the rate of tissue IGF exposure and prolonging the biologic half-life of IGFs. Serum levels of IGF-BP-1 and -3 are elevated in the fetus. IGF-BPs also may have direct cell surface membrane effects by enhancing or inhibiting cellular response to IGFs[6]; IGF-BP-1 may be a primary inhibitor of fetal growth.

In the fetal circulation, serum levels of IGF-II are increased. In addition, there may be a distinct fetal IGF that may be structurally related to IGF-II. IGF-I secretion in the fetus is independent of growth hormone (GH), but may be regulated by placental lactogen, which is related structurally to GH; in humans these compounds share the same gene complex on chromosome 17. In rat fibroblasts, ovine placental lactogen (but not human GH) stimulates IGF-II but not IGF-I secretion. However, in vivo studies indicate that placental lactogen does not have a direct effect on IGF secretion.[4,12] There is a positive correlation between fetal size (weight and length) and serum concentration of IGF-I but not serum IGF-II or "fetal" IGF. Nutritional status is probably the major regulator of fetal IGF secretion, thereby interrelating insulin and IGF action: insulin promotes fetal glucose uptake, and cell replication and differentiation; the IGFs (IGF-I) regulate the latter to aid in somatic growth.

Growth Hormone

Growth hormone does not play a significant role in prenatal growth, despite elevated serum concentration of GH (up to 100 µg/L); the postnatal effects of GH on growth are seen after 6 months of age. Neither pituitary aplasia nor congenital hypopituitarism is associated with diminished fetal birth weight. As noted, a slight reduction in birth weight is seen in anencephalic infants. Hepatic GH receptors are not detected until the second trimester, but infants with Laron-type dwarfism have normal birth weight. GH receptors cannot be demonstrated on other fetal tissues.[6]

Recently, investigators have postulated a role for the GH variant gene (GH-V, GH-2) during pregnancy.[10] This gene is expressed during normal pregnancy. This "human placental GH," differing from pituitary GH by 13 amino acids, can be detected in maternal blood during mid-gestation; concentrations increase near term. This molecule has full somatotropic activity. However, a normal-sized infant was delivered to a mother who was homozygous for GH-2 gene deletion.[6]

Placental Lactogen

The gene encoding human placental lactogen (hPL, chorionic somatomammotropin, CSH-1) is located within the gene complex that codes for pituitary GH and placental GH-2. hPL has less somatotropic activity than GH. However, there are specific hPL receptors present on fetal tissues. The interaction of hPL and IGFs has been discussed.

Thyroid Hormone

Although fetal hypothyroxinemia is associated with fetal growth retardation in some species, such does not occur in humans; the birth weight of such infants may be increased. The placenta is probably less impermeable to maternal thyroid hormone than previously thought; perhaps sufficient thyroid hormone crosses the placenta to sustain fetal growth. On the other hand, severe maternal hyperthyroidism may lead to fetal growth retardation, probably due to the hypermetabolic state and decreased substrate delivered to the fetus.

Other Growth Factors

A number of putative growth factors[17] have been identified and categorized, based on structure and function, into families (Table 2–2). Such factors have complex interactions with tissues and other growth factors and contribute to cell replication and differentiation.

TABLE 2–2.

Families of Growth Factors*

I. Insulin
  A. Proinsulin
  B. Insulin-like growth factors (IGFs)
    1. IGF-I
    2. IGF-II
  C. Relaxin
  D. Nerve growth factor
II. Urogastrone
  A. Epidermal growth factor (EGF)
  B. Transforming growth factor-α (TGF-α)
III. Transforming growth factor-β (TGF-β)
  A. Transforming growth factor-β (TGF-β)
    1. TGF-β 1:1
    2. TGF-β 1:2
    3. TGF-β 2:2
  B. Inhibin
    1. Inhibin A
    2. Inhibin B
    3. Activin
  C. Müllerian inhibiting substance (MIS)
IV. Heparin-adsorbable growth factors
  A. Fibroblast growth factor
  B. Angiogenic growth factor
  C. Endothelial cell growth factor
V. Interferon
  A. Interferon-α and subclasses
  B. Interferon-β and subclasses
  C. Interferon-γ and subclasses
VI. Interleukins
VII. Platelet-derived growth factors

*Adapted from Hollenberg MD: *Am J Med Genet* 1989; 34:35.

GROWTH DURING INFANCY AND CHILDHOOD

Growth Charts and Standards

Many factors discussed in the previous section greatly influence postnatal growth. Again, standards are required so that deviant growth patterns may be discerned. In the United States, growth standards have been compiled by the National Center for Health Statistics (NCHS). The NCHS growth charts depicting length, height, weight, and head circumference are widely available, and demonstrate the statistical range of growth between the 5th and 95th percentiles (± 2 SD) (Fig 2–1). It is important to note that these charts were developed from data derived from single (one time) measurements and hence represent cross-sectionally derived observations. Thus these charts have smoothed curves, especially when depicting growth occurring during adolescence. Longitudinally derived growth data have been compiled by Tanner and colleagues for both British and North American children (Figs 2–2 and 2–3). Such standards offer the advantage of more clearly defining the growth channel and pattern of any individual patient. In addition, these charts depict curves 2.5 SD on either side of the mean, thus encompassing the 3rd and 97th percentiles into the "normal" range, and depict the pubertal growth spurt more accurately than the NCHS charts. One can appropriately use NCHS charts to screen for growth disorders. We use the Tanner charts to individualize the longitudinal growth pattern for any given patient before and during any intervention. Pomerance[35] has developed longitudinal growth charts based on height and weight slope velocities accumulated in the office setting; he believes the slope velocity model allows easy plotting of data and ready separation of normal and abnormal growth patterns.

Growth velocity (growth per year) standards (Fig 2–4) have been derived from longitudinal growth charts. During the first year of life there is rapid growth; the growth rate decelerates fairly rapidly after 2 years of age, then gradually slows to a more constant rate by mid-childhood. By 1 year of age, average length increases by approximately 50%, and weight increases threefold.

From these charts or from data tables, one can derive the height age (HA) and weight age (WA) for an individual, that is, the 50th percentile for a given age. These data, along with an assessment of skeletal maturation (bone age, BA) are instrumental in assessing the child with aberrant growth. For example, the short child whose BA is consistent with chronologic age (CA) but is greater than HA probably has intrinsic short stature. However, if that child's BA is within 75% of CA, then constitutional delay in growth and development (CDGD) would be higher on the differential. Growth retardation characterized by delay in BA more than 75% of CA often signifies more pathologic processes, including systemic disease states and endocrinologic disorders. Disease-specific growth charts have been developed for several disorders associated with poor growth, including gonadal dysgenesis (Turner syndrome), Noonan syndrome, trisomy 21 (Down syndrome), and Williams syndrome.[8,26,30,37,38]

It is important to emphasize the need to obtain accurate data when following up growth disturbances. Height (or length in patients younger than 2 years) is measured without shoes and socks on. The patient is placed with heels and back against a

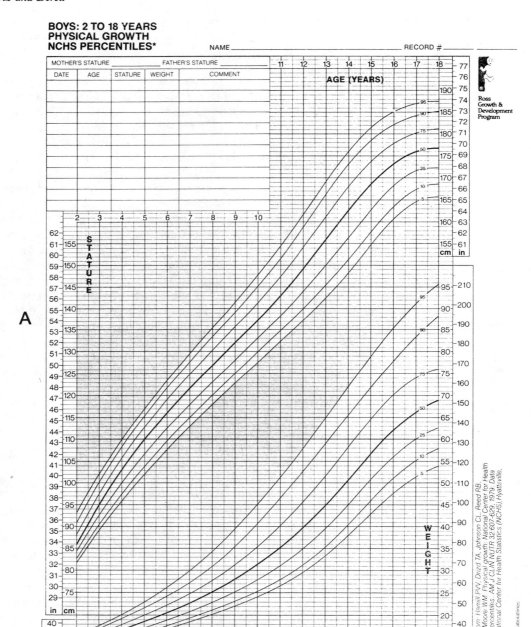

FIG 2-1.
National Center for Health Statistics (NCHS) growth charts for boys (**A**) and girls (**B**) aged 2 to 18 years. Note the gradual increase in slope in stature during adolescence. (From Ross Laboratories, Columbus, Ohio. Used by permission.)

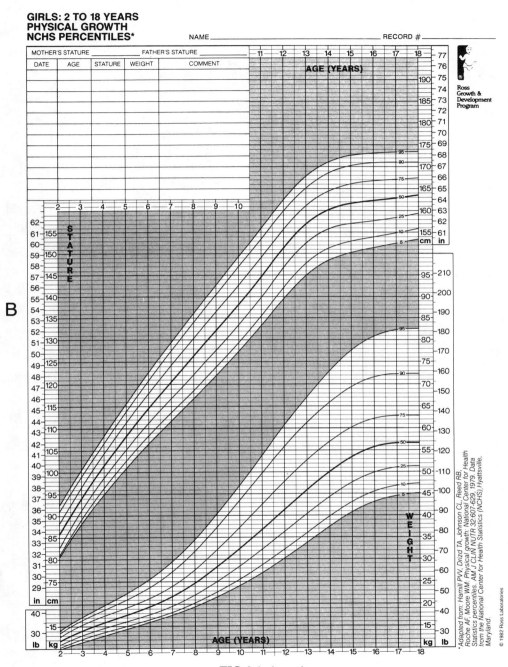

FIG 2-1. (cont.).

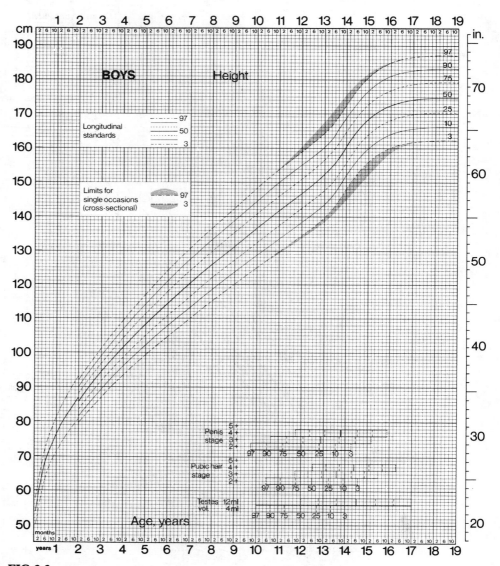

FIG 2-2.
Tanner-Whitehouse longitudinally derived standard height charts for boys (**A**) and girls (**B**). (From Castlemead Publications, Ware, Herts, England.) Used by permission.)

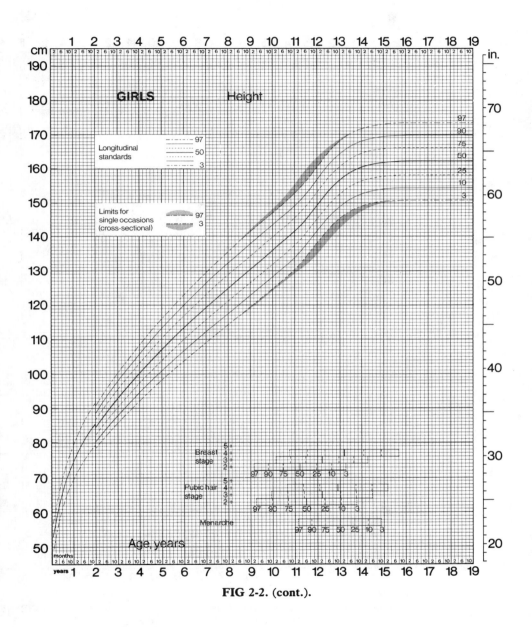

FIG 2-2. (cont.).

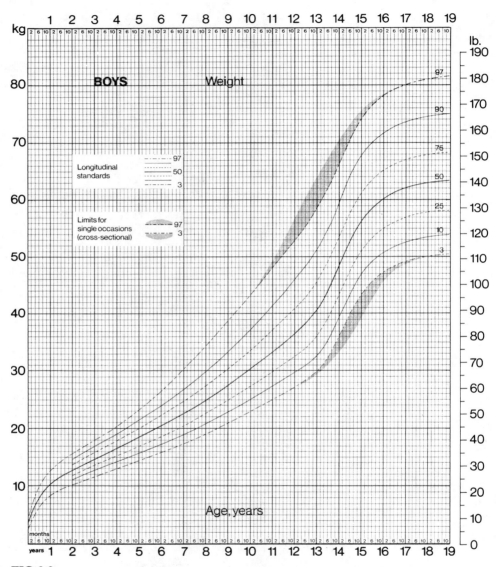

FIG 2-3.
Tanner-Whitehouse longitudinally derived weight charts for boys (**A**) and girls (**B**). (From Castlemead Publications, Ware, Herts, England. Used by permission.)

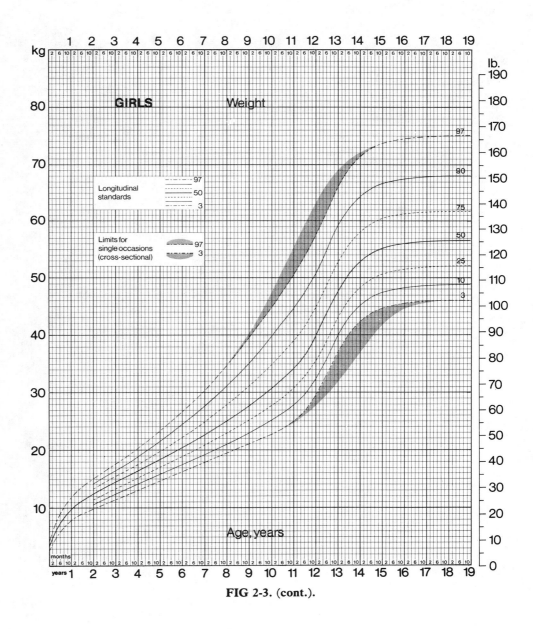

FIG 2-3. (cont.).

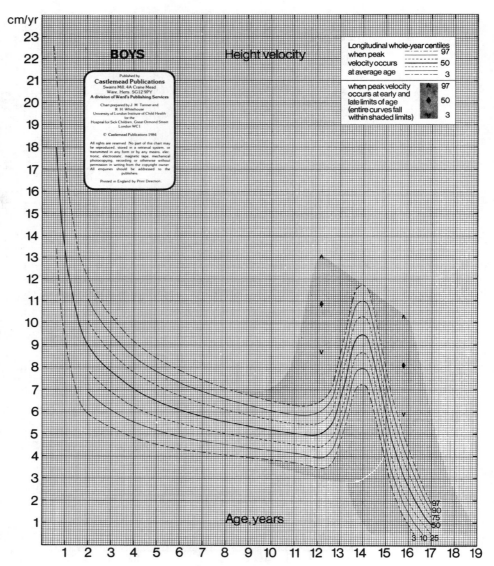

FIG 2-4.
Growth velocity standards in boys (**A**) and girls (**B**). Ideally, such data from an individual patient are derived after 12 months of observation. (From Castlemead Publications, Ware, Herts, England. Used by permission.)

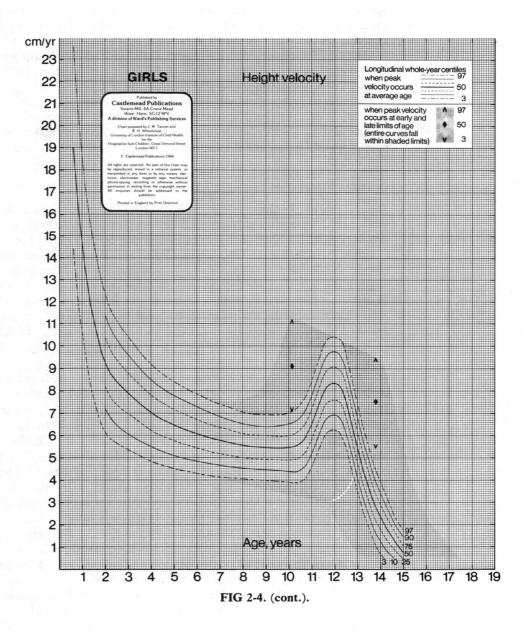

FIG 2-4. (cont.).

measured, calibrated, fixed, vertical support (e.g., a wall). The head is held with gentle upward support such that the outer orbital canthi are horizontally aligned with the external auditory meatuses, thus minimizing subtle slouching or morning-evening variation. A flat board or block is brought down onto the head at 90 degrees to the vertical upright support. A similar horizontal device and technique are used to measure recumbent length in younger children. Such devices, with a counterweighted measuring block, are called *stadiometers*.

Similar to prenatal growth, normal postnatal growth depends on the appropriate interaction of nutritional, genetic, emotional, neuroendocrine, and peripheral response factors. Endocrinologically, during childhood, normal growth and development depends on normal interaction between GH, thyroxine, and probably insulin.

Osseous Maturation

Skeletal maturation proceeds in an orderly fashion that is relatively independent of size, growth rate, and chronologic age; assessment of skeletal maturation, or BA, provides another objective tool to assess normal development. The more popular and common methods are the Greulich and Pyle[15] and Tanner-Whitehouse 2 (TW2) methods. In the Greulich and Pyle method, radiographs of the epiphyses of the digits and wrist of the left hand are compared with those compiled by and based on the Brush Foundation study of normal skeletal maturation in boys and girls.[15] The TW2 method numerically scores the maturation of each epiphysis of the radiograph; summed scores are then given a percentile rank. Boys and girls have a slightly different score for each stage of bone maturation. In children younger than 2 years, a hemiskeletal BA radiograph is obtained.

An imprecise estimate of final adult height may be predicted with these indices of skeletal maturation. Three different methods commonly are used to predict ultimate stature: the Bayley-Pinneau (B-P) method, published in 1952, utilizes CA, the Greulich-Pyle assessed BA, and current stature.[1] The advantage to this method is ease of calculation; disadvantages have to do with the small sample size of patients with markedly delayed or accelerated BA. The TW2 method uses CA, TW2 assessment of BA, current stature, midparental stature, and pubertal status.[45] The Roche-Wainer-Thissen (R-W-T) method utilizes CA, BA as assessed by Greulich and Pyle, recumbent length, weight, and mid-parental stature. Different investigators advocate different methods. None of the methods accurately predicts ultimate height in children with abnormal growth patterns. In our unit, we tend to use B-P height predictions in the mid-pubertal child and only in those children observed for less pronounced growth abnormalities. In a recent study of 22 short children with BA delay and normal serum GH concentrations to provocative stimuli who were given exogenous GH for 1 to 3 years, Shulman and Bercu[43] demonstrated that predicted stature increased 1.0 cm or more in 11 children, decreased 1.0 cm or more in 8 children, and remained unchanged from pretreatment predictions in 3 children by the TW2 method. With the B-P method, predicted stature increased in 14 children, decreased in 1 child, and remained unchanged compared with pretreatment predictions in 2 children. The B-P tables probably "underpredict" growth potential.[43]

Longitudinal bone growth is influenced and regulated primarily by nutritive, genetic, and endocrine factors. Drugs and mechanical forces also regulate chondrocyte activity within the growth plate cartilage.[19,24] This latter disclike structure is located between the epiphysis and metaphysis of long bones. The growth plate chondrocytes are arranged in zones which are spatially perpendicular to the longitudinal axis of the bone. In addition, the chondrocytes are organized into columns which may represent the functional units of bone growth. The zones of the epiphyseal plate are arranged from the epiphysis to the metaphysis as follows: (1) The zone of resting cartilage contains cells that anchor the other zones and support capillaries that nourish the epiphyseal plate. (2) The zone of proliferating chondrocytes contains rapidly dividing chondrocytes and forms a "pool" of cells; the peripheral layer of this zone is sometimes referred to as the zone of Ranvier. (3) The zone of hypertrophying chondrocytes contains large cells that accumulate glycogen and lipid and express increased activities of alkaline phosphatase and carbonic anhydrase. Alkaline phosphatase promotes the calcification of the extracellular matrix. In addition, this zone has diminished amounts of protease inhibitors, proteins, and type II collagen, thereby permitting vascular invasion and angiogenesis. (4) The zone of provisional calcification contains mineralized bone matrix and osteoblasts which deposit bone matrix (Fig 2–5).[7]

Embryologically, the skeleton forms from mesenchymal tissue covered by ecto-

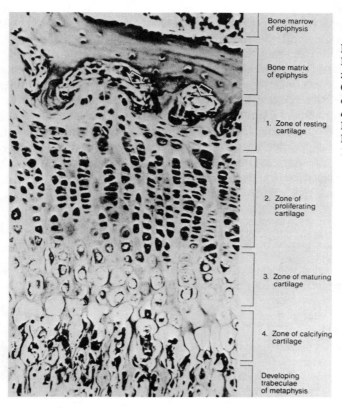

Bone marrow of epiphysis

Bone matrix of epiphysis

1. Zone of resting cartilage

2. Zone of proliferating cartilage

3. Zone of maturing cartilage

4. Zone of calcifying cartilage

Developing trabeculae of metaphysis

FIG 2-5.
Photomicrograph of the four zones of the epiphyseal plate. Capillaries that nourish the chondrocytes are indicated by *arrows*. (From Cormack DH: Bone, in *Ham's Histology*. Philadelphia, JB Lippincott, 1987. Used by permission.)

derm. Cartilage-specific proteins (type II collagen and cartilage proteoglycan core protein) appear early. Chondrogenesis continues with the synthesis and secretion of bone matrix, a composition of these and other proteins including types IX and XI collagen and proteoglycan-linked protein. This process forms the skeletal anlage, or template of the developing skeleton. As the template is transformed to bone, an ossification front forms between the remaining cartilage and the newly formed bone. Chondrocytes within the template synthesize matrix composed of type X collagen, fibronectin, and osteopontin which promote the expression of the hypertrophied chondrocytes in the zone of hypertrophied cartilage. Bone matrix provides a supportive "coat" around the chondrocyte; chondrocytes maintain their volume and shape independently of an internal cytoskeletal system.

Complete regulation of this process is not known. Three types of receptors have been proposed or identified on chondrocytes.[18] The first type includes those that bind peptide growth factors, such as GH, insulin, IGF-I and -II, parathyroid hormone, skeletal growth factor, and other growth factors (see Table 2–2). The second type binds steroid hormones (sex hormones, vitamins A and D). These complexes then bind to specific receptors within the cell nucleus onto DNA binding domains, thus regulating gene transcription. The last type of chondrocyte receptors are extracellular "cell adhesion" receptors that bind collagen and other proteins. They function to autoregulate the chondrocytes; changes in the composition of the matrix regulate chondrocyte activity. Thus chondrogenesis, cartilage hypertrophy, and osteogenesis are modulated by endocrine, paracrine, and autocrine regulators.

Under physiologic conditions and steady growth, there is an increase in the number of cells within the proliferation zone while cell cycle time remains constant. Under conditions of growth acceleration, there is a decrease in the proliferative zone cell fraction but a compensatory decrease in cell cycle time. In the rat model, 20% of prepubertal longitudinal bone growth is due to increased cell height within the hypertrophied zone. Growth deceleration is due to decreased number of proliferating chondrocytes, that is, a diminished height of cells within the hypertrophied zone.[19] In terms of time and energy expenditure, cell hypertrophy is a more efficient means of columnar cell growth than is cell replication alone.[19]

GROWTH AND DEVELOPMENT DURING PUBERTY

Adolescence is a period of physical, emotional, and social growth. Puberty denotes the physical changes that accompany adolescence and marks the stage of complete sexual reproductive capability. The onset of puberty correlates more closely with skeletal maturation than with CA—a BA of approximately 10 years in girls and 11 years in boys. With onset of normal puberty, there is release of central nervous system inhibition on the gonadotropin-releasing hormone [GnRH] "pulse generator," allowing episodic release of GnRH from the hypothalamus. Acting on the pituitary gonadotrophs, GnRH promotes synthesis and release of the gonadotropins: luteinizing hormone (LH) and follicle-stimulating hormone (FSH). The earliest measurable event in puberty, therefore, is an increase in the frequency and amplitude of nocturnal (sleep-associated) bursts of serum LH. As adolescence progresses, LH bursts become more frequent until by late puberty, they occur every 2 hours daily. Increased gonadotropin secretion leads to increased sex hormone production by the gonads, primarily testosterone in boys and estradiol in girls.

Tanner[44] has devised a classification scheme presenting the sequential physical changes of sexual maturation (Fig 2–6, Tables 2–3 and 2–4). In the male, the first

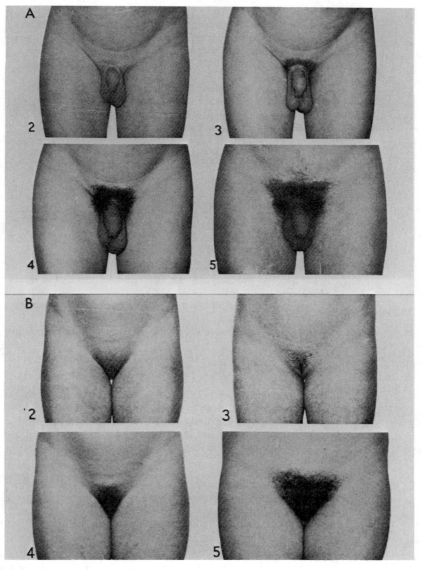

FIG 2-6.
Tanner stages of pubic hair development in boys (**A**) and girls (**B**). Stage I, prepubertal, not shown. (From Tanner JM: Growth and endocrinology of the adolescent, in Gardner LI (ed): *Endocrine and Genetic Diseases of Childhood and Adolescence.* Philadelphia, WB Saunders, 1975, Used by permission.)

TABLE 2–3.

Stages of Pubertal Development in Boys*

Stage	Mean Age (yr)	Range (yr)
Genital growth		
1 Prepubertal		
2 Enlargement of testes and scrotum, thinning and pigmentation of scrotum	11.6	9.0–14.3
3 Phallic enlargement with further enlargement of testes and scrotum	12.9	10.3–15.5
4 Progressive enlargement of genitalia; further pigmentation of scrotum	13.8	11.2–16.3
5 Adult size and shape of genitalia	14.9	12.2–17.7
Pubic hair growth		
1 No sexual hair		
2 Appearance of long, pigmented hair over base of penis	13.4	10.8–16.0
3 Dark, coarse, curled hair spread sparsely over pubis	13.9	11.4–16.5
4 Sexual hair is adult-type, abundant but limited to pubis	14.4	11.7–17.1
5 Spreading of sexual hair to the medial aspects of the thighs	15.2	12.5–17.9

*Adapted from Tanner JM: Growth and endocrinology of the adolescent, in Gardner LI (ed): *Endocrine and Genetic Diseases of Childhood and Adolescence.* Philadelphia, WB Saunders Co, 1975.

TABLE 2–4.

Stages of Pubertal Development in Girls*

Stage	Mean Age (yr)	Range (yr)
Breast growth		
1 Prepubertal		
2 Breast budding, widening of areola with elevation of mound of subareolar tissue, erect papilla	11.2	9.0–13.3
3 Continued enlargement of breast with widening of areola without separation of their contours	12.2	10.0–14.3
4 Secondary mound of areola and papilla above the plane of the enlarging breast	13.1	10.8–15.3
5 Mature breast, areola and breast in the same plane, erect papilla	15.3	11.9–18.8
Pubic hair growth		
1 No sexual hair		
2 Appearance of long, pigmented hair over mons veneris or labia majora	11.7	9.3–14.1
3 Dark, coarse, curled hair spread sparsely over mons veneris	12.4	10.2–14.6
4 Sexual hair is adult-type, abundant but limited to mons veneris	13.0	10.8–15.1
5 Spreading of sexual hair to the medial aspects of the thighs	14.4	12.2–16.7
Menarche	13.5	11.4–15.5

*Adapted from Tanner JM: Growth and endocrinology of the adolescent, in Gardner LI (ed): *Endocrine and Genetic Diseases of Childhood and Adolescence.* Philadelphia, WB Saunders Co, 1975.

sign of puberty is testicular enlargement to >4 mL in volume or >2.5 cm in longitudinal axis, a result mostly of FSH stimulation of the seminiferous tubules. Testicular size may be measured (longitudinal and horizontal axes) or the volume estimated with an orchidometer. Tanner genitalia staging in boys is as follows: testicular size 2.5 cm, stage II; 3.0 cm, stage III; 4.0 cm, stage IV; ≥5.0 cm, stage V. Stage II genitalia development also is characterized by growth and elongation of the penis and thinning of scrotal skin.

Pubarche, the onset of pubic hair, generally begins within 2 years of testis enlargement, and is generally complete within 3 years after onset. Axillary hair appears during stage III genital development, and peak velocity of the adolescent growth spurt is associated with stage IV genital development. Facial hair occurs during stage IV to V, at a median age of 15 years. Commonly, adolescent boys experience voice "cracking" and subareolar gynecomastia in mid-puberty. Spermarche occurs during stage III genital development. Final voice change occurs around stage IV. Growth velocity slows after the peak adolescent growth; final stature is achieved in most boys within 3 years of spermarche.[23,31,41]

The first sign of puberty in girls usually is breast budding (thelarche; Fig 2–7). Thelarche is complete (i.e., adult) within 4 years after onset. Pubarche generally appears after breast budding, but precedes thelarche in 10% of girls. Pubarche is complete about 2½ years after its appearance. Peak velocity of the adolescent growth spurt is associated with Tanner stage III breast development, with axillary hair noted shortly thereafter. Menarche coincides with stage IV breast development in 60% of girls, and generally occurs 2 to 5 years after thelarche. Over the subsequent 1 to 2 years, ovulatory menstrual cycles develop and growth velocity slows. Adult stature generally is attained within 2 years after menarche.[23,31,41]

In both sexes, the adolescent growth spurt is accompanied by increases in secretion of growth hormone and IGF-I; in boys, this has been studied by Martha et al.[27] The adolescent growth spurt also is characterized by increases in muscle cell number and size. In males, there is a 14-fold increase in skeletal muscle number, and a 10-fold increase in females.[41]

GROWTH ABERRANCY

Growth, as a sensitive indicator of health, may be disturbed in a variety of illnesses and conditions. Thus it is emphasized that poor growth is not a disease. Growth disturbances causing growth retardation may be broadly categorized into three major groups: (1) intrinsic short stature, (2) constitutional delay in growth and development, and (3) systemic disease–related growth disorders (Table 2–5).

Intrinsic Short Stature

The most common form of intrinsic short stature has a genetic basis and a positive family history. It is important to note and plot parental and sibling heights; this may help discern the patient with age-appropriate but familial-inappropriate stature. Patients with familial short stature are otherwise normal. Individuals with various forms of intrinsic short stature generally have skeletal maturation commensurate with CA. Other "genetic" forms of growth retardation include a variety of chromosomal abnormalities, most frequently trisomy 21, and gonadal dysgenesis (Turner syndrome; 45,X or variants) in girls. Various types of chondrodystrophies and skeletal diseases are uniformly associated with growth retardation. The chondrodystrophies, typified by achondroplasia, are characterized by abnormal body proportions, that is, short

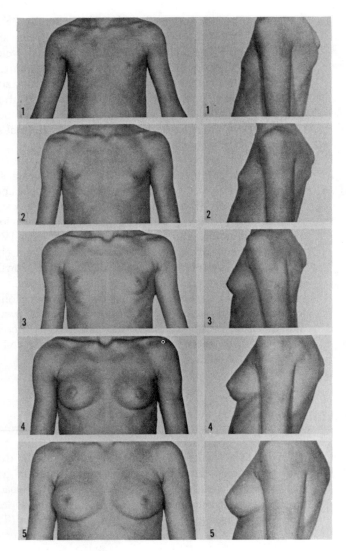

FIG 2-7.
Tanner stages of breast development. (From Tanner JM: Growth and endocrinology of the adolescent, in Gardner LI (ed): *Endocrine and Genetic Diseases of Childhood and Adolescence*. Philadelphia, WB Saunders, 1975, Used by permission.)

limbs and increased upper-lower body ratio. Other examples are given in Table 2–6.[21]

A number of syndromes typified by somatic dysmorphism have been elucidated; many are associated with growth retardation, both of prenatal and postnatal onset.[39] Specific growth charts have been developed that plot the natural growth history of patients with Turner syndrome, trisomy 21, Russell-Silver syndrome, and others. However, these disorders also may have concurrent GH deficiency.[39,42] As discussed

TABLE 2–5.

Causes of Growth Retardation

I. Intrinsic short stature
   A. Genetic
      1. Familial
      2. Chromosomal abnormalities
         a. Trisomies 13, 18, 21
         b. Gonadal dysgenesis (45,X and variants)
      3. Skeletal dysplasias, chondrodystrophies
         a. Achondroplasia (autosomal dominant)
         b. Others (see Table 2–6)
   B. Intrauterine growth retardation associated with other somatic anomalies
      1. Russell-Silver syndrome
      2. Prader-Willi syndrome
      3. Cornelia de Lange syndrome
II. Constitutional delay in growth and development (genetic)
III. Systemic disorders
   A. Psychosocial growth retardation
   B. Nutritional
      1. Kwashiorkor
      2. Marasmus
      3. Zinc/iron deficiency
   C. Gastrointestinal
      1. Malabsorption
         a. Celiac disease
         b. Inflammatory bowel disease
            (1) Regional enteritis
            (2) Ulcerative colitis
         c. Cystic fibrosis
      2. Hepatic
         a. Chronic hepatitis
         b. Glycogen storage disease
   D. Cardiac (e.g., severe congenital heart disease)
   E. Pulmonary (e.g., cystic fibrosis)
   F. Renal
      1. Chronic pyelonephritis
      2. Fanconi's syndrome (and variants)
      3. Chronic renal insufficiency
   G. Endocrine
      1. Hypothyroidism
      2. Hypophosphatemic vitamin D–resistant rickets
      3. Type I diabetes mellitus (poorly controlled)
      4. Pseudohypoparathyroidism
      5. Hypercortisolemia
      6. Precocious puberty
      7. Growth hormone (GH) deficiency
         a. Genetic
            (1) Lack of GH gene
            (2) Associated with immunoglobulin deficiency
            (3) GH unresponsiveness (Laron-type dwarfism)
            (4) Insulin-like Growth Factor I unresponsiveness (African pygmies)
         b. Acquired (see Chapter 3)
   H. Other chronic disease
   I. Drugs (e.g., glucocorticoids)

TABLE 2–6.

Skeletal Dysplasias*

I. Osteochondrodysplasia
  A. Disturbances of long bone or vertebral growth
    1. Achondroplasia (autosomal dominant)
    2. Achondrogenesis
      a. Type IA (autosomal recessive)
      b. Type IB (autosomal recessive)
      c. Type II (autosomal recessive)
    3. Hypochondroplasia (autosomal dominant)
    4. Camptomelic dysplasia (autosomal recessive)
    5. Metaphyseal chondrodysplasia
      a. Schmid type (autosomal dominant)
      b. McKusick type (autosomal recessive)
      c. Jansen type (autosomal dominant)
      d. Schwachman syndrome (?autosomal recessive)
        (1) Neutropenia
        (2) Pancreatic insufficiency
    6. Multiple epiphyseal dysplasia (autosomal dominant)
  B. Defects in diaphyseal or metaphyseal structure
    1. Osteogenesis imperfecta
      a. Type I (autosomal dominant)
      b. Type II (autosomal dominant/autosomal recessive)
      c. Type III (autosomal recessive/autosomal dominant)
      d. Type IV (autosomal dominant)
    2. Osteopetrosis (autosomal recessive/autosomal dominant)
II. Dysostoses affecting:
  A. Face and cranium
  B. Axial skeleton
  C. Extremities (e.g., camptodactyly)

*Adapted from Kaplan SA: Growth and growth hormone: Disorders of the anterior pituitary, in Kaplan SA (ed): *Clinical Pediatric Endocrinology.* Philadelphia, WB Saunders Co, 1990.

previously, fetal growth retardation potentially stems from a variety of factors, including maternal exposure to alcohol and other drugs and nutritional inadequacies.

Constitutional Delay in Growth and Development

Constitutional delay in growth and development (CDGD) describes a condition of modest delay in skeletal maturation and often a delay in pubertal onset in children who are otherwise healthy. There often is a hereditary tendency in this group as well. Although this variation of normal development is diagnosed more often in boys than in girls, girls probably have a similar incidence of CDGD. Often this diagnosis can be made only in retrospect after the exclusion of more serious disorders. Growth in CDGD parallels the Tanner 3rd percentile, and BA delay corresponds to HA. In general, BA is within 75% of CA.

Systemic Disorders

Systemic disorders that lead to growth retardation may be congenital or acquired. For categorical purposes, intrinsic skeletal diseases and chromosomal aberrancies associated with multisystem disease have been previously alluded to. Other congenital disorders include inborn metabolic errors and congenital heart disease. Worldwide, the most common cause of growth failure is malnutrition, usually from inadequate intake but also from infectious and inflammatory bowel diseases and cystic fibrosis leading to malabsorption. Inadequate intake is not limited to developing nations; in the United States, poverty and purposeful and nonintentional parental limitations to food lead to failure to thrive.[36] In humans, unlike the rat, starvation leads to elevations in serum concentration of GH but diminished concentrations of IGF-I. Short stature may be the sole manifestation of occult inflammatory bowel or celiac disease. Celiac disease is more prevalent in Europe and the Middle East than in North America; its diagnosis is problematic. Antigliadin antibodies in serum are an insensitive marker for celiac disease whereas the sensitivity of IgA-class endomysial antibodies for celiac disease approaches 100%.[2,46] Small bowel biopsy remains the gold standard in the diagnosis of celiac disease.

Short stature is also a component of a number of disorders associated with obesity. Simple obesity is usually associated with tall stature and advanced BA. Somatic syndromes associated with obesity include the Laurence-Moon-Bardet-Biedl anomalad,[14] Prader-Willi syndrome (hypogonadism, hypomentia, hypotonicity, growth retardation, and obesity), and Börjeson-Forssman-Lehmann syndrome. Endocrine disorders with short stature and relative or absolute obesity include hypercortisolism, pseudohypoparathyroidism, hypothyroidism, and GH deficiency. These endocrine causes of short stature (see Table 2–5) are discussed elsewhere in this book.

Chronic renal disease leads to growth failure for a variety of reasons, once again including poor nutritional intake. However, abnormalities in vitamin D regulation certainly play an important role. Growth retardation and lack of catch-up growth persists in children receiving dialysis and renal transplantation; immunosuppression with glucocorticoids contributes to the lack of catch-up growth.[9,40]

Tall Stature

Far less often brought to the attention of the health care provider is the child with tall stature. Tall stature, like short stature, is not a disease, but unlike growth retardation, rarely signals an underlying pathologic condition. Disorders associated with tall stature are summarized in Table 2–7. Familial tall stature is the most common diagnosis; appropriate familial heights should also be recorded for purposes of comparison. Children who are inappropriately tall for the family deserve more thorough examination. In general, the conditions listed in Table 2–7 may be distinguished by history and physical examination. Sotos syndrome is associated with macrosomia from birth, prominent coarse facies, and mental retardation. Bone age tends to be advanced, and adolescence may be early. Beckwith-Wiedemann syndrome is associated with hyperinsulinism. Affected infants also have characteristic somatic anomalies including macroglossia, omphalocele, and ear lobe creases. Children with Weaver syndrome have associated hypertonicity, typical facies, camptodactyly, and loose skin. Affected persons have skeletal maturation in advance of CA. Homocystinuria and Marfan syndrome have a similar phenotype. Homocystinuria is distinguished by neurologic findings and mental deficiency. The diagnosis is confirmed by the demonstration of increased excretion of homocysteine and methionine in the urine and decreased plasma

TABLE 2–7.
Differential Diagnosis of Tall Stature

I. Congenital
    A. Intrinsic
        1. Familial
        2. Cerebral gigantism (Sotos syndrome)
        3. Weaver's syndrome
        4. Beckwith-Wiedemann syndrome
    B. Genetic
        1. Marfan syndrome (autosomal dominant)
        2. Homocystinuria (autosomal recessive)
        3. Generalized lipodystrophy (autosomal recessive)
        4. Klinefelter syndrome (47,XXY or variant)
    C. Other
        1. Pituitary mammosomatotroph hyperplasia(?)
        2. Pseudoacromegaly
II. Acquired
    A. Metabolic
        1. Hyperthyroidism
        2. Precocious puberty
           a. Central
           b. Pseudoprecocious
           c. Incomplete
        3. Obesity
        4. Hypersomatotropism

---

concentration of cysteine. The defect is due to diminished or absent activity of cystathionine synthetase. Generalized lipodystrophy is characterized by accelerated growth of limbs, muscle hypertrophy, diminished adipose tissue, hyperlipidemia, hyperinsulinism, phallic enlargement (in boys), and hirsutism, although elevation in serum androgens is not demonstrated. Klinefelter syndrome is discussed elsewhere, as are disorders of GH secretion. Other disorders of tall stature, especially hyperthyroidism and sexual precocity, are evident on physical examination.

EVALUATION

The evaluation of growth aberrancy begins with the history. Details regarding prenatal or perinatal insults should be sought. Birth weight, length, and head circumference should be plotted if available. Old growth records are imperative. A history of lymphedema in an infant girl raises the concern of gonadal dysgenesis. Dietary intake and stool pattern may be clues to the possibility of malabsorptive disorders. There may be a family history of short stature or pubertal delay. The physical examination includes careful measurement of height, weight, and body proportions. Other family members, if available, should be measured. Care should be taken to observe facial dysmorphism as may be seen in several syndromes associated with short or tall stature.

The laboratory evaluation begins with the BA examination. We also screen for occult metabolic or inflammatory disorders with general chemistry panels, complete blood count, sedimentation rate, and urinalysis. Determination of serum thyroxine (T_4) and thyroid-stimulating hormone (TSH) may screen for asymptomatic thyroid disorders. Plasma IGF-I can serve as a screening device for nutritional disorders and for GH secretory abnormalities. Short girls should have a karyotype looking for 45,X gonadal dysgenesis or variants, including mosaicism. If the history or physical examination suggests an intracranial neoplasm, a lateral skull radiograph may reveal an intracranial calcification as well as the size and shape of the sella turcica. However, magnetic resonance imaging or computed tomography provide more detailed anatomy.

In children with aberrant growth, determination of growth velocity is invaluable. A normal growth rate for CA and for BA generally is indicative of a benign process. For patients in whom hypopituitarism is suspected, provocative and endogenous studies of GH secretion may be carried out.

TREATMENT

The treatment of growth retardation depends on correction of the underlying disorder. Exogenous GH therapy is discussed in Chapter 3. Treatment of tall stature is generally not indicated, but involves the administration of gender-appropriate sex hormones to hasten epiphyseal fusion. This is not without risk, which may include metabolic disorders including glucose intolerance, hyperlipidemia, coagulopathy, and acne. Patients with CDGD generally can be reassured of the benign, normal nature of the condition and then observed to verify normal pubertal progression. In boys this is sometimes more difficult. Under special circumstances, when there are significant psychologic concerns, a patient with CDGD may be treated with a short course of low-dose gender-appropriate sex hormone.

Investigations studying intrauterine treatment for the growth-retarded fetus include increased maternal substrate supply and oxygenation. Future directions include in utero treatment of fetuses with congenital infections. Perhaps gene therapy is also on the distant horizon.[16,20,48]

REFERENCES

1. Bayley N, Pinneau SR: Tables for predicting adult height from skeletal age: Revised for use with the Greulich-Pyle hand standards. *J Pediatr* 1952; 40:432.
2. Beutner EH, Kumar V, Chorzelski TP: Screening for celiac disease. *N Engl J Med* 1989; 320:1087.
3. Brar HS, Rutherford SE: Classification of intrauterine growth retardation. *Semin Perinatol* 1988; 12:2.
4. Growne CA, Thorburn GD: Endocrine control of fetal growth. *Biol Neonate* 1989; 55:331.
5. Carlson DE: Maternal diseases associated with intrauterine growth retardation. *Semin Perinatol* 1988; 12:1.
6. Chard T: Hormonal control of growth in the human fetus. *J Endocrinol* 1989; 123:3.
7. Cormack DH: Bone, in *Ham's Histology*. Philadelphia, JB Lippincott Co, 1987.

8. Cronk C, et al: Growth charts for children with Down syndrome: 1 month to 18 years of age. *Pediatrics* 1988; 81:102.

9. Fine RN: Growth after renal transplantation in children. *J Pediatr* 1987; 110:414.

10. Frankenne J, et al: Expression of the growth hormone variant gene in human placenta. *J Clin Endocrinol Metab* 1987; 64:635.

11. Gluckman PD: The role of pituitary hormones, growth factors and insulin in the regulation of fetal growth. *Oxford Rev Reprod Biol* 1986; 8:1.

12. Gluckman PD: Fetal growth: An endocrine perspective. *Acta Paediatr Scand [Suppl]* 1989; 349:21.

13. Goldenberg RL, et al: Intrauterine growth retardation: Standards for diagnosis. *Am J Obstet Gynecol* 1989; 161:271.

14. Green JS, et al: The cardinal manifestations of Bardet-Biedl syndrome, a form of Laurence-Moon-Biedl syndrome. *N Engl J Med* 1989; 321:1002.

15. Greulich WW, Pyle SI: *Radiographic Atlas of Skeletal Development of the Hand and Wrist*, ed 2. Palo Alto, Calif, Stanford University Press, 1959.

16. Harding JE, Charlton V: Treatment of the growth-retarded fetus by augmentation of substrate supply. *Semin Perinatol* 1989; 13:211.

17. Hollenberg MD: Growth factors, their receptors and development. *Am J Med Genet* 1989; 34:35.

18. Horton WA: The biology of bone growth. *Growth Genet Horm* 1990; 6:1.

19. Hunziker EB, Schenk RK: Physiologic mechanisms adopted by chondrocytes in regulating longitudinal bone growth in rats. *J Physiol* 1989; 414:55.

20. Johnson MP, Evans MI: Intrauterine growth retardation: Pathophysiology and possibilities for intrauterine treatment. *Fetal Ther* 1987; 2:109.

21. Kaplan SA: Growth and growth hormone: Disorders of the anterior pituitary, in Kaplan SA (ed): *Clinical Pediatric Endocrinology*. Philadelphia, WB Saunders Co, 1990.

22. Kretchmer N, Schumacher L, Silliman K: Biologic factors affecting intrauterine growth. *Semin Perinatol* 1989; 13:169.

23. Lee PA: Normal ages of pubertal events among American males and females. *J Adolesc Health Care* 1980; 1:26.

24. LeVeau BF, Bernhardt DB: Developmental biomechanics: Effect of forces on the growth, development, and maintenance of the human body. *Phys Ther* 1984; 64:1874.

25. Lockwood CJ, Weiner S: Assessment of fetal growth. *Clin Perinatol* 1986; 13:3.

26. Lyon AJ, Preece MA, Grant DB: Growth curve for girls with Turner syndrome. *Arch Dis Child* 1985; 60:932.

27. Martha PM Jr, et al: Alterations in the pulsatile properties of circulating growth hormone concentrations during puberty in boys. *J Clin Endocrinol Metab* 1989; 69:563.

28. Menon RK, et al: Transplacental passage of insulin in pregnant women with insulin-dependent diabetes mellitus: Its role in fetal macrosomia. *N Engl J Med* 1990; 323:309.

29. Milner RDG, Hill DJ: Fetal growth signals. *Arch Dis Child* 1989; 64:53.

30. Morris CA, et al: Natural history of Williams syndrome: Physical characteristics. *J Pediatr* 1988; 113:318.

31. Nottelmann ED, et al: Developmental processes in early adolescence: Relations among chronologic age, pubertal stage, height, weight, and serum levels of gonadotropins, sex steroids, and adrenal androgens. *J Adolesc Health Care* 1987; 8:246.

32. Ott WJ: The diagnosis of altered fetal growth. *Obstet Gynecol Clin North Am* 1988; 15:237.

33. Ounsted M, Scott A, Moar VA: Constrained and unconstrained fetal growth: Associations with some biological and pathological factors. *Ann Hum Biol* 1988; 15:119.

34. Platt JD: Genetic factors in intrauterine growth retardation. *Semin Perinatol* 1988; 12:11.
35. Pomerance HH: A practical way to assess growth in the office. *Contemp Pediatr* 1990; 7:45.
36. Pugliese MT, et al: Parental health beliefs as a cause of nonorganic failure to thrive. *Pediatrics* 1987; 80:175.
37. Ranke MB: Disease-specific growth charts: Do we need them? *Acta Paediatr Scand [Suppl])* 1989; 356:17.
38. Ranke MB, et al: Noonan syndrome: Growth and clinical manifestations in 144 cases. *Eur J Pediatr* 1988; 148:220.
39. Rimoin DL, Graham JM Jr: Syndromes associated with growth deficiency. *Acta Paediatr Scand [Suppl])* 1989; 349:3.
40. Rizzoni G, et al: Growth retardation in children with chronic renal disease: Scope of the problem. *Am J Kidney Dis* 1986; 7:256.
41. Root AW: Endocrinology of puberty: Normal sexual maturation. *J Pediatr* 1973; 83:1.
42. Schwartz ID, et al: Endocrinopathies in Cornelia de Lange syndrome. *J Pediatr* 1990; 117:920.
43. Shulman DI, Bercu BB: Predicted heights in children with growth retardation and bone age delay following 1 to 3 years of growth hormone therapy. Presented at 72nd Annual Meeting of the Endocrine Society, 1990, abstract 1079, p 294.
44. Tanner JM: Growth and endocrinology of the adolescent, in Gardner LI (ed): *Endocrine and Genetic Diseases of Childhood and Adolescence*. Philadelphia, WB Saunders Co, 1975.
45. Tanner JM, et al: *Assessment of Skeletal Maturity and Prediction of Adult Height (TW2 Method)*. New York, Academic Press, 1975.
46. Tucker NT, et al: Antigliadin antibodies detected by enzyme-linked immunosorbent assay as a marker of childhood celiac disease. *J Pediatr* 1988; 113:286.
47. Warshaw JB: Intrauterine growth retardation. *Pediatr Rev* 1986; 8:107.
48. Weiner CP: Pathogenesis, evaluation, and potential treatments for severe, early onset growth retardation. *Semin Perinatol* 1989; 13:320.
49. Verklan MT: Safe in the womb? Drug and chemical effects on the fetus and neonate. *Neonat Network* 1989; 8:59.
50. Viteri FE, Schumacher L, Silliman K: Maternal malnutrition and the fetus. *Semin Perinatol* 1989; 13:236.

Chapter 3

Anterior and Posterior Pituitary Gland and Pineal Gland

I. David Schwartz
Barry B. Bercu

The axis for the production, secretion, and regulation of many endocrine peptides consists of the hypothalamus and its integration with the pituitary gland. Although these hypothalamic peptides are present in variable amounts throughout the central (CNS) and peripheral nervous systems, they also have been localized to other organ systems, most notably the gastrointestinal tract. These peptides function as neuro-modulators or neurotransmitters, or as both, working to stimulate or inhibit other areas of the nervous or other somatic systems. In this chapter the normal integration of the hypothalamic-pituitary unit is discussed, as is the role of the pineal gland in normal physiology and disease.

HYPOTHALAMUS

Neuroanatomy

The hypothalamus derives embryologically from neuroectodermal tissue of the diencephalon. Bordering the hypothalamus posteriorly are the mamillary bodies and midbrain. The lamina terminalis lies anteriorly; the temporal lobes are located laterally; the hypothalamic sulcus lies superiorly; and the optic chiasm is located inferiorly. The hypothalamus surrounds the inferior portion of the third ventricle (Fig 3–1).[43]

The hypothalamus may be primarily divided into medial, lateral, and basilar portions. The basilar portion is called the *tuber cinereum,* whence emerge the important

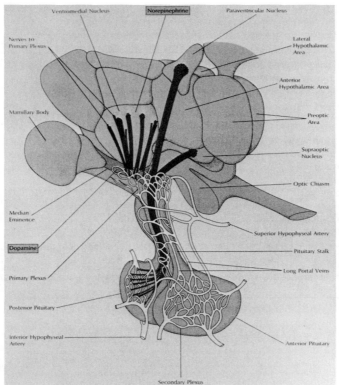

FIG 3–1.
Schematic depiction of the hypothalamic-pituitary portal system and hypothalamic nuclei. (From Frohman LA: Neurotransmitters as regulators of endocrine function, in Krieger DT, Hughes JC (eds): *Neuroendocrinology.* Sunderland, Mass, Sinauer Associates, 1980. Used by permission.)

median eminence and pituitary stalk. The medial portion of the hypothalamus may be further divided into anterior, tuberal, and posterior areas. The lateral portion of the hypothalamus contains the lateral hypothalamic nuclei and the medial forebrain bundle. The periventricular nucleus lies along the base of the third ventricle. The major nuclei of the hypothalamus are shown in Table 3–1 and Figure 3–2.[61]

The median eminence serves as the important final pathway for the secretory products from these various hypothalamic nuclei to the anterior pituitary; the median eminence lies outside of the blood-brain barrier. Three zones constitute the median eminence. The ependymal zone forms the base of the third ventricle and contains ependymal cells and tanycytes. These latter cells allow (or prevent) the passive transfer of median eminence secretory products into the cerebrospinal fluid (CSF) and also may serve as a "skeletal" structure supporting the axons within the median eminence. The internal zone is composed of axons of the hypothalamic-neurohypophyseal axis, which contain neurosecretory granules of vasopressin and oxytocin. The external zone contains axons and axon terminals of the hypothalamic-tuberoinfundibular tract. These axons, which reach the hypothalamic-pituitary long-portal system, contain the hypothalamic peptides that regulate the anterior pituitary.[36,64,82]

The hypothalamus contains two major bundles or tracts containing important functional nuclei. The neurohypophyseal tract contains large neurons that are a part of the paraventricular and the supraoptic nuclei. The majority of these magnocellular

TABLE 3–1.

Major Nuclei of the Hypothalamus*

Nuclei	Function/Product†
Medial group	
Anterior hypothalamic	SRIF
Arcuate	GH-RH, DA, GnRH, SRIF, TRH, β-endorphin, NP-Y
Dorsomedial	NP-Y
Medial preoptic	GnRH, SRIF, NP-Y
Paraventricular	
Magnocellular	ADH
Parvocellular	CRH, TRH, SRIF
Periventricular	SRIF
Suprachiasmatic	
Ventromedial	Satiety, GnRH, GH-RH, TRH, NP-Y
Lateral group	
Lateral hypothalamic	Feeding
Supraoptic	ADH, oxytocin

*Adapted from Frohman LA: Neurotransmitters as regulators of endocrine function, in Krieger DT, Hughes JC (eds): *Neuroendocrinology.* Sunderland, Mass, Sinaver Associates, 1980.
†SRIF = somatostatin; GH-RH = growth hormone–releasing hormone; DA = dopamine; GnRH = gonadotropin-releasing hormone; TRH = thyrotropin-releasing hormone; NP-Y = neuropeptide Y; ADH = antidiuretic hormone (vasopressin); CRH = corticotropin-releasing hormone.

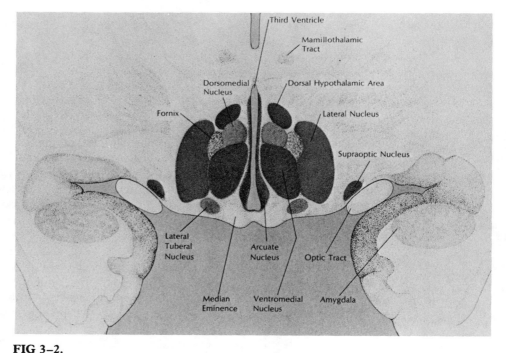

FIG 3–2.

Schematic frontal view of the hypothalamus depicting location of major nuclei. (From Krieger DT: The hypothalamus and neuroendocrinology, in Krieger DT, Hughes JC (eds): *Neuroendocrinology.* Sunderland, Mass, Sinauer Associates, 1980. Used by permission.)

neurons in the supraoptic and paraventricular nuclei secrete vasopressin, although oxytocin is secreted within the more distal aspect of the supraoptic nucleus; oxytocin-secreting neurons also are located in the peripheral aspects of the paraventricular nucleus. Other axons within this tract transport other regulatory peptides including gonadotropin-releasing hormone (GnRH), thyrotropin-releasing hormone (TRH), corticotropin-releasing hormone (CRH), somatotropin release-inhibiting factor (SRIF, somatostatin), and dopamine. The other major nerve bundle of the hypothalamus, the tuberoinfundibular tract, is composed primarily of neurons arising from the periventricular nucleus and the parvocellular division of the paraventricular nucleus. These neurons contain the hypothalamic-pituitary regulatory hormones. Many of these peptides are located within the same nuclei (co-localized) and may contribute to normal physiologic regulation (see Table 3–1).

Hypothalamic Hormones

Corticotropin-Releasing Hormone

Molecular Structure and Genetics.—CRH is a 41-amino acid peptide produced from a larger 196-amino acid precursor molecule encoded by the q13 region of chromosome 8.[74] Synthesized within the medial hypothalamic nuclei, CRH promotes secretion and release of proopiomelanocortin (POMC) and its derivatives from the anterior pituitary. The highest concentration of CRH is within the median eminence where axon terminals from the paraventricular nucleus reach the portal circulation. CRH has been identified also in the cerebral cortex, brainstem, limbic system, and spinal cord; CRH may link the neuroendocrine and visceral autonomic systems and play an important role in integrative learning and behavior. CRH has been isolated outside of the CNS, primarily in the placenta but also in the gastrointestinal system and the adrenal glands.

Secretion and Regulation.—Hypothalamic concentrations of CRH increase during stress and with functional adrenalectomy. In normal adults, plasma concentration of CRH ranges from 2 to 28 pg/mL.[89] There does not appear to be any circadian rhythm or diurnal variation to CRH secretion.[2,67] CRH can cross the placenta; plasma levels increase progressively through pregnancy and peak during parturition. Regulation of CRH is through short-loop inhibition by adrenocorticotropic hormone (ACTH). Ultrashort-loop, or acute autoregulatory inhibition, probably does not occur. Vasopressin (antidiuretic hormone, ADH) inhibits CRH secretion. Glucocorticoids exhibit classic feedback inhibition of CRH secretion.

Function.—CRH promotes pituitary ACTH synthesis and secretion from POMC in a dose-dependent manner. In addition, CRH promotes catecholamine secretion and has an antipyrogenic effect upon the hypothalamus. In vivo studies in rats indicate suppressive effects on pituitary growth hormone (GH, somatotropin) and luteinizing hormone (LH) and on sexual, feeding, and other behaviors.[110]

Mechanism of Action.—CRH promotes pituitary ACTH release by binding to specific receptors on corticotrophs which are coupled to adenylyl cyclase. In addition to cyclic adenosine monophosphate (cAMP), other intracellular messengers mediated by CRH include Ca^{2+} and activated protein kinases.[67,105,110] Extracellular Ca^{2+} and Mg^{2+} are required for the ACTH-releasing effect of CRH. Although regulatory in vitro the physiologic role of prostaglandins in CRH action is uncertain.

Clinical Data.—*Excessive Secretion.*—Elevated levels of CRH may be seen in highly trained athletes and in depressive disorders, anorexia, and alcoholism.[105] These conditions may be associated with hypercortisolism. Hypersecretion of CRH may be seen in isolated ACTH deficiency and in primary adrenal insufficiency, as a result of lack of feedback inhibition. Pituitary-dependent hypercortisolism often is associated with measurable plasma concentrations of CRH. It is unclear whether this represents dysregulation of hypothalamic CRH secretion.[110] Elevated CRH levels may be noted with ectopic CRH secretion from visceral tumors.

Deficient Secretion.—Destructive and functional lesions of the hypothalamus may be associated with diminished CRH secretion and secondary adrenal insufficiency. Low CRH levels also are seen in instances of ACTH-independent hypercortisolism (exogenous glucocorticoids, adrenal tumors) due to feedback inhibition.

End-Organ Insensitivity.—CRH resistance has not been described.

Diagnostic and Clinical Use.—The administration of exogenous CRH may be useful in the differential diagnosis in patients with known Cushing syndrome. Because of a lower metabolic clearance rate, ovine CRH seems to be a superior diagnostic agent than human CRH.[80] Patients with pituitary hypersecretion of ACTH (pituitary ACTH-dependent hypercortisolism, Cushing disease) have a positive ACTH response to exogenous CRH; patients with ectopic ACTH production or non–ACTH-dependent Cushing syndrome generally do not; 93% of patients with Cushing disease may be identified.[80] The CRH test may also distinguish hypothalamic from pituitary causes of central adrenal insufficiency; absence of or a blunted ACTH response to CRH implies primary pituitary disease while an exaggerated ACTH response may be seen in cases of hypothalamic disease. CRH is administered as a bolus intravenous (IV) injection ($1\mu g/kg$) and blood samples are collected at times 0, +1, +5, +10, +15, +30, and +60 minutes.

Gonadotropin-Releasing Hormone

Molecular Structure and Genetics.—GnRH is a decapeptide hormone processed from a larger (91 amino acids) precursor encoded by the p21–q11.2 region of chromosome 8.[74] The amino acid sequence is preserved through all mammalian species. Biologic activity hinges upon the interplay between the N- and C-terminals of the molecule. Residues 2 (histidine) and 3 (tryptophan) are important for binding to pituitary gonadotrophs.[89] The C-terminal region of the precursor peptide is called the GnRH-associated peptide (GAP) and may be involved with inhibition of prolactin (PRL) secretion. GnRH is predominantly located within the median eminence, the arcuate and ventromedial hypothalamic nuclei, and the regions around the third ventricle.

Secretion and Regulation.—The precise mechanisms controlling GnRH synthesis and release are unclear. The so-called GnRH pulse generator is active in both genders during early infancy and is then later "restrained" by uncertain mechanisms. This restraint is removed during late childhood to initiate the biochemical and physical changes associated with puberty. GnRH secretion is episodic and pulsatile. Frequent pulses or continuous infusion leads to gonadotroph desensitization and attenuated gonadotropin release; this is the rationale for the clinical use of GnRH agonist analogues. GnRH release is stimulated by norepinephrine in rats; in humans α-adrenergic blockade leads to diminished GnRH pulses and subsequent decreased pulses of LH. Gonadal steroids, primarily estrogen, inhibit GnRH pulsatility; however, in females, this is menstrual cycle phase–dependent. In the late follicular phase of the menstrual cycle, LH pulse frequency increases as serum concentrations of estradiol increase, presumably reflecting changes in GnRH secretion. Endogenous opioids inhibit GnRH pulsatility.

Function.—Acting specifically on gonadotrophs in the anterior pituitary, GnRH stimulates the release of the gonadotropins, LH, and follicle-stimulating hormone (FSH); these agents influence or are responsible for most (if not all) of the actions of GnRH: normal testicular descent, maturation of the gonads, spermatogenesis, and ovulatory menstrual cycles. GnRH may have a direct inhibitory role in gonadal steroidogenesis.[50]

Mechanism of Action.—The GnRH receptor is a plasma membrane–bound glycoprotein (mol wt ~60 kDa) which probably dimerizes in vivo; ligand receptor binding on the gonadotroph causes receptor cross-linking. The GnRH receptor–ligand complex is then internalized by endocytosis whereby the effector actions of GnRH are carried out by mechanisms that are yet unclear. It is of interest that this internalization of the GnRH-receptor complex is sufficient, but not necessary, for GnRH-stimulated LH release. When cross-linking of receptors is prevented, gonadotropin release by GnRH is unaffected. After internalization, the receptor may be "recycled" to the cell surface.

By whatever specific mechanism, in a given steroid environment, the amplitude and frequency of GnRH can lead to maximal stimulation of GnRH receptors, expression of the LH beta-subunit, and release of LH.[54] The intracellular signal transducers of GnRH involve Ca^{2+} mobilization, phosphatidylinositide metabolism, and protein kinase C activation, but not adenylyl cyclase cAMP generation. However, cAMP secretagogues are able to increase GnRH receptors and stimulate LH glycosylation[78] (Fig 3–3). Again, protein kinase C activation is sufficient, but not necessary, for GnRH-induced LH release.[24,54]

Clinical Data.—Clinical abnormalities in the synthesis, secretion, or action of GnRH are associated primarily with disorders involving the timing, progression, or tempo of pubertal development. Specific disorders of puberty and the regulation of GnRH secretion are discussed in subsequent chapters. GnRH receptors have been identified in breast carcinoma cell lines although the physiologic significance of this is unclear.

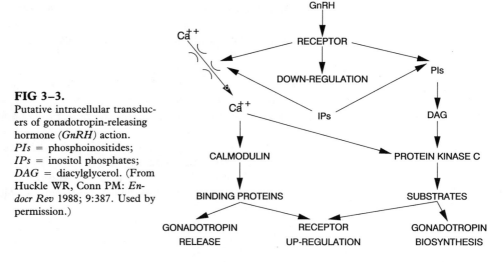

FIG 3–3.
Putative intracellular transducers of gonadotropin-releasing hormone *(GnRH)* action.
PIs = phosphoinositides;
IPs = inositol phosphates;
DAG = diacylglycerol. (From Huckle WR, Conn PM: *Endocr Rev* 1988; 9:387. Used by permission.)

TABLE 3–2.
Gonadotropin Responses Following GnRH Administration*

	Male		Female	
	Basal	Peak	Basal	Peak
Prepubertal				
LH (IU/L)	<5	<21	<5	<21
FSH (IU/L)	<2.5	≤24	<5	>10–50
Pubertal				
LH (IU/L)	3–17	21–75	3–17	21–190
FSH (IU/L)	<1–7	1–22	<1–7	>10–53

*GnRH = gonadotropin-releasing hormone; LH = luteinizing hormone; FSH = follicle-stimulating hormone.

Diagnostic and Clinical Use.—Exogenous GnRH is used primarily as a diagnostic test in the evaluation of disorders in the timing of puberty, i.e., delayed puberty and precocious puberty, although the test is not completely specific. GnRH (100 μg) is administered as an IV bolus. Blood is obtained at times −30, 0, +10, +20, +30, +45, +60, +90, and +120 minutes for determination of serum concentrations of LH and FSH. We also determine sex steroid concentrations (dehydroepiandrosterone [DHEA] sulfate [DHEA-S], and testosterone [in boys] or estradiol [in girls]) at the beginning and end of the study. Gonadotropin responses following GnRH are dependent on gender and degree of sexual maturation. Normal basal and peak stimulated responses to GnRH from our laboratory are shown in Table 3–2. Note that with sexual maturation, while serum LH concentrations rise progressively after GnRH administration, serum FSH concentrations reach a plateau.

Other uses of GnRH include induction of puberty,[101,107,108] and treatment of hypogonadotropin anovulation and cryptorchidism, although in cryptorchidism, results are inconsistent (the rate of success ranges from 0% to 100%). Although in inducing descent of the testes, GnRH probably induces LH to mediate its effect, a recent study showed a superior therapeutic use of human chorionic gonadotropin (hCG) over GnRH.[23] It is evident that the success of GnRH (or hCG) hinges on the degree of testicular maldescent; retractile testes respond to hormonal therapy to induce descent, whereas truly cryptorchid testes do not respond.[23,29]

Synthetic GnRH agonist analogues are available for subcutaneous and intranasal administration and approved for "medical hypophysectomy/orchiectomy" in the treatment of prostatic carcinoma. As noted, these agents work by taking advantage of the downregulation and desensitization of gonadotrophs by continuous (or nonpulse) availability to the GnRH receptor. These agents, some in long-lasting depot preparations, also are used in the treatment of central true and complete isosexual precocious puberty; they may help differentiate constitutional delay in growth and adolescent development from gonadotropin deficiency.[34] GnRH analogues have been utilized, with variable success, in a variety of other conditions influenced by the gonadal steroid milieu. In women, GnRH analogue administration provides short-term contraception, resolution of endometriosis and uterine leiomyomas, adjunctive therapy in polycystic ovarian syndrome, and ovulation induction, but appears to be of no benefit in the treatment of breast carcinoma, especially in postmenopausal women.[24,37,72] In men, GnRH agonists have been used to induce azoospermia both as a proposed contraceptive and as a germ cell protectant during chemotherapy; results to date are without clear benefit.[37] This material has also been used in small trials for the treatment of acute intermittent porphyria and pancreatic carcinoma.[1,48] Spontaneous pituitary and subsequent gonadal activity resumes following discontinuation of GnRH agonists. While GnRH agonists ultimately decrease serum concentrations of LH measured by radioimmunoassay (RIA), fragments of LH (i.e., the alpha subunit) may increase, which may falsely estimate the degree of gonadotroph suppression by cross-reacting in assays. Because they are in fact *agonists*, these GnRH analogues cause transient (1–2 weeks) stimulation of gonadotropins prior to down-regulation. On the horizon are GnRH antagonists which theoretically would cause immediate suppression of the hypothalamic-pituitary-gonadal axis. These agents induce histamine release, however, which has limited their use in clinical trials. Adverse effects common to GnRH analogues relate to their therapeutic effect on hypogonadism: osteoporosis, vaginal dryness, and hot flashes. FSH antagonists have been described in women who have received GnRH antagonists. These "antihormones" appear to be natural biologic products; their role in hypothalamic-pituitary-gonadal regulation is uncertain.[25]

Growth Hormone–Releasing Hormone (GH-RH)

Molecular Structure and Genetics.—The gene for GH-RH has been mapped to chromosome 20 and codes for both a 107 and 108 amino acid GH-RH precursor molecule.[74] Posttranslational processing gives rise to several identified GH-RH peptides containing 29, 37, 40, and 44 amino acids.[44,97] Full biologic activity is contained in the first 29 amino acids.

Secretion and Regulation.—GH-RH is synthesized primarily in the ventromedial and arcuate nuclei of the hypothalamus and released both tonically and with intermittent pulses (every 3–4 hours) throughout the day and night. GH-RH is also identified in gastrointestinal, pancreatic, and adrenal tissues. In vitro studies demonstrate that the fetal pituitary is responsive to GH-RH before complete maturation of the pituitary portal system or the appearance of GH-RH-containing neurons, which suggests that, initially, pituitary GH secretion is hypothalamic GH-RH-independent. The circulating half-lives for GH-RH 1–29, GH-RH 1–40, and GH-RH 1–44 are 10, 50, and 7 minutes, respectively. After a mixed meal, there is biphasic GH-RH release: the first phase, occurring after 60 minutes, probably reflects gastrointestinal release of GH-RH; the second phase occurs after 2 to 3 hours and may be a consequence of hypothalamic GH-RH release. Factors that exert a positive effect on GH-RH release include α_2-adrenergic and dopaminergic stimulation, thyroid hormone, and opioids. GH-RH release is inhibited by somatostatin, and through negative feedback by the hypothalamic-pituitary axis: insulin-like growth factor I (IGF-I) provides classic negative feedback; GH provides short-loop inhibition; GH-RH exerts ultrashort-loop or autoregulatory inhibition. Other small amines influence GH-RH release: galanin and serotonergic and histaminergic agents exert positive release of GH-RH while α-aminobutyric acid (GABA) inhibits GH-RH release.[14,44]

Function.—GH-RH promotes synthesis and release of GH from anterior pituitary somatotrophs; GH-RH is primarily responsible for the pulse amplitude of pituitary GH release.

Mechanism of Action.—GH-RH binds to specific pituitary somatotroph receptors coupled to G proteins activating adenylyl cyclase. GH-RH receptor number is increased by glucocorticoids. In rats, glucocorticoids augment the GH response following GH-RH administration; in humans, glucocorticoids inhibit this response. GH-RH receptors also are influenced by other factors: dopamine and β-adrenergic blockade augment the release of GH following GH-RH stimulation while cholinergic muscarinic blockade inhibits this GH response.[13] Intracellular Ca^{2+} mobilization is also involved with secondary-messenger signal transduction. GH gene transcription is cAMP-dependent, but Ca^{2+}-independent.

Clinical Data.—*Excessive Secretion.*—Hypersecretion of GH-RH increases pituitary GH secretion. Although it is unclear whether excessive GH-RH causes pituitary somatotroph adenoma formation, this agent clearly causes pituitary somatotroph and mammosomatotroph hyperplasia,[76,95] perhaps by paracrine as well as by endocrine effects. Chronic secretion of GH-RH may promote pituitary somatotroph adenoma formation in individuals "primed" or predisposed to tumor formation.[95] GH-RH-secreting tumors are generally gangliocytomas and may originate within the hypothalamus or outside the CNS, usually the gastrointestinal tract, pancreas, or pulmonary system. The mean age of ectopic GH-RH-secreting tumors is 40 years (pancreatic 38.4 years, pulmonary 43.8 years); tumors occur more often in women (22:8 female-to-male ratio).[95] Clinical manifestations include acromegaly and the sequelae of concomitant hormone secretion and mass effect. The mean time lapse between onset of symptoms and diagnosis is 8 years. Medical treatment regimens include the use of dopaminergic agonists, which are largely ineffective, and somatostatin analogues. Surgical excision is the treatment of choice with radiologic and medical modalities as adjunctive therapies.[95] Clinical features of excessive GH secretion are discussed in a subsequent section.

Deficient Secretion.—Hyposecretion of GH-RH is seen in patients who have received an insult to the CNS as in a hypothalamic mass lesion or CNS malformation, toxin exposure (e.g., irradiation), or as a result of inflammation. Clinical manifestations vary with the specific cause but generally consist of those reflecting GH deficiency, most notably growth retardation.

End-Organ Insensitivity.—GH-RH resistance has not been described.

Diagnostic and Clinical Use.—There is a dose-related response in GH release after IV administration of GH-RH. This is detectable within 5 minutes following GH-RH administration with a peak effect after 30 to 60 minutes. Basal conditions are reestablished after 120 to 180 minutes following acute injection of GH-RH. This pattern is present in neonates, children, and young adults and may be used diagnostically in the evaluation of children with short stature. Older persons have a blunted GH response following administration of GH-RH. GH-RH (1 μg/kg) is administered IV and blood samples for GH determination are obtained at times 0, +5, +10, +15, +30, +45, +60, +75, +90, +120, and +150 minutes. We attempt to reduce variability of GH response to GH-RH by first administering somatostatin. Inasmuch as serum GH concentrations may be variable because of the timing of the endogenous GH pulse, somatostatin decreases baseline GH concentrations to a trough level. Exogenous GH-RH administration may differentiate hypothalamic causes of GH deficiency from pituitary causes; the former would have an exaggerated pituitary GH response following GH-RH; the latter would have no or a minimal response. However, this has not been verified in our experience and that of others.[75]

Studies are under way to investigate the use of GH-RH administration in GH-deficient children. Preliminary reports[111] relate that GH-RH can promote GH release in selected populations with resultant short-term acceleration in height velocity. Those children who responded with the most rapid increases in height velocity received 24-hour subcutaneous pulse injections every 3 hours by a pump. GH-RH administration is ineffective in GH-deficient children that lack the GH gene. For GH-RH to replace GH as the treatment of choice for classic GH deficiency, the most cost-effective dose needs to be determined.

Somatotropin Release Inhibiting Factor

Molecular Structure and Genetics.—SRIF (somatostatin) is a tetradecapeptide. The gene for SRIF has been mapped to the q28 region of chromosome 3.[74] The gene encodes for a precursor of 116 amino acids which undergoes posttranslational processing. The disulfide bond that bridges the cysteine residues in positions 3 and 14 of the molecule helps establish optimal biologic activity; endocrine activity is conferred by residues 7–10 of the peptide (Phe-Trp-Lys-Thr).

Secretion and Regulation.—Like GH-RH, there is both pulsatile and tonic secretion of SRIF, which is produced primarily in the anterior hypothalamic, preoptic, and arcuate nuclei of the hypothalamus. Superimposed upon the tonic secretion of SRIF is a pulsatile burst occurring every 3 to 4 hours. Diminution of SRIF tone permits a pulse of GH release from the anterior pituitary somatrophs. SRIF secretion is increased by GH-RH, dopaminergic, and β-adrenergic stimulation, and by GH and IGF-I feedback. Conversely, SRIF secretion is inhibited by arginine, cholinergic, and GABA-ergic stimulation, and through an ultrashort autofeedback loop. The half-life for SRIF is approximately 3 minutes. SRIF is also synthesized in the pancreatic delta cells, and is located in gastrointestinal, renal, and other tissues.

Function.—SRIF has a wide variety of physiologic effects, which are summarized in Table 3–3; SRIF functions primarily as an "endocrine brake" inhibiting the secretion of many other peptides. SRIF inhibits GH release from somatotrophs; it does not diminish GH synthesis. The frequency of diminished SRIF tone determines the frequency and duration of somatotroph GH pulses. In addition, SRIF possesses cell cytoprotective effects,[112] but only when administered prior to tissue damage. Under experimental conditions, pretreatment with SRIF blocks hepatic uptake of toxins and similarly protects adrenal and pulmonary cells. SRIF protects gastric and duodenal mucosa from ulcer formation after induced pancreatitis independent of its effect on gastric acid secretion. Amino acid residues 7–10 of the molecule are sufficient but not required to confer the cytoprotective effects of SRIF. The mechanism by which SRIF exerts cytoprotective effects is uncertain but may involve cell membrane stabilization.

Mechanism of Action.—In the pituitary somatotroph, SRIF binds to specific glycoprotein receptors which couple adenyl cyclase with a regulatory G protein. SRIF receptor number is decreased by glucocorticoids in vitro. In addition, SRIF lowers intracellular Ca^{2+} levels by inhibiting Ca^{2+} flow into cells.

TABLE 3–3.
Physiologic Effects of Somatostatin (SRIF) by Target Organ*

Hypothalamus (inhibitory)	Gastrointestinal (inhibitory)
GH-RH	Gastrin (gastric pyloric G cells)
SRIF	Gastric acid (parietal cells)
TRH	Pepsin
Pituitary (inhibitory)	Secretin (duodenum)
ACTH	Cholecystokinin (duodenum, jejunum)
GH	Motilin (duodenum)
PRL	VIP (jejunum, colon)
TSH	Liver (Glucose production, output)
Pancreas (inhibitory)	Parathyroid (inhibitory)
Endocrine	PTH (chief cells)
Glucagon (alpha cells)	Renal (inhibitory)
Insulin (beta cells)	Renin (juxtaglomerular apparatus)
Pancreatic polypeptide (PP cells)	Free water clearance
Exocrine	Glomerular filtration rate
Amylase	Thyroid (inhibitory)
Bicarbonate	T_4, T_3
Chymotrypsin	Calcitonin (parafollicular C cells)

*GH-RH = growth hormone–releasing hormone; TRH = thyrotropin-releasing hormone; ACTH = adrenocorticotropic hormone; GH = growth hormone; PRL = prolactin; TSH = thyroid-stimulating hormone; VIP = vasoactive intestinal polypeptide; PTH = parathyroid hormone; T_4 = thyroxine; T_3 = triiodothyronine.

Clinical Data.—*Excessive Secretion.*—Increased SRIF tone has been implicated in diminished GH secretion in obese subjects.

Deficient Secretion.—We postulate that in one patient, irradiation damage may have impaired SRIF secretion resulting in elevated basal GH concentrations.[12]

End-organ Insensitivity.—SRIF resistance has not been described.

Diagnostic and Clinical Use.—SRIF is used diagnostically in the evaluation of patients with pituitary hyperplasia or hypersecretion. We use short-term infusions of native SRIF to evaluate more finely the hypothalamic-pituitary (GH) axis in patients with growth retardation. We have also used SRIF to evaluate patients with inappropriate secretion of thyroid-stimulating hormone (TSH) and those with adenomatous secretion of vasoactive intestinal polypeptide (VIP) tumors (vipomas). Clinically, long-acting analogues of SRIF (octreotide) are used in the management of acromegaly, nesidioblastosis, type I diabetes mellitus, inappropriate TSH secretion, estrogen-induced prolactinomas, and vipomas.[63,118] Although SRIF or its analogues have had some benefit in patients with pituitary TSH-secreting adenomas, its effect in patients with resistance to TSH has, in our experience and that of others, been disappointing.[10] Our experience with the long-term management of a child with hypersecretion of VIP has also been disappointing. Octreotide is 45 times more potent in inhibiting GH-RH release, 11 times more active in inhibiting glucagon release, and 1.3 times more potent in inhibiting insulin release than native SRIF.[63] This agonist has an estimated half-life of 113 minutes and does not cause rebound hypersecretion of GH following its administration and biologic effect. Adverse effects of long-term SRIF (or analogue) administration are often transient and include malabsorption, abdominal pain, bloating, and flatulence. Cholelithiasis, glucose intolerance, and water retention with hyponatremia have been reported.[49,63]

Thyrotropin-Releasing Hormone
Molecular Structure and Genetics.—TRH is a tripeptide with a sequence Glu-His-Pro derived from a precursor composed of 123 amino acids. The gene encoding TRH has not yet been elucidated.

Secretion and Regulation.—TRH is identified primarily in the arcuate, paraventricular, and ventromedial nuclei, and the median eminence of the hypothalamus. TRH secretion may be evoked by serotonergic and β_1-adrenergic stimulation, as well as by low serum concentrations of thyroxine (T_4) and triiodothyronine (T_3) through feedback loops regulating the hypothalamic-pituitary-thyroid axis. TRH secretion is inhibited by dopamine, SRIF, elevated thyroid hormones, and possibly cortisol.

Function.—TRH is the only known physiologic stimulator of pituitary TSH secretion. TRH in pharmacologic doses increases PRL secretion. Under conditions of elevated serum basal GH concentrations, TRH causes a paradoxical increase in GH release. The neuroendocrine basis for this phenomenon is unknown.

Mechanism of Action.—TRH exerts its effect on the pituitary thyrotrope by binding to the G protein–coupled TRH receptor. The nature of the TRH receptor has not been completely elucidated but it may be a glycoprotein.[52] Receptor number is inversely related to available TRH for binding (downregulation) and T_4. Estrogens increase TRH receptor levels. Activation of the TRH receptor stimulates phosphoinositide metabolism leading to increased diacylglycerol and inositol-1,4,5-triphosphate (IP_3-3). There is a biphasic TSH response: the first occurs immediately and is associated with increased intracellular Ca^{2+} secondary to IP_3-3; the second occurs upon activation of protein kinase C. It is unclear precisely how TRH promotes PRL secretion but the process may involve protein kinase C activation as well.[52]

Clinical Data.—The role of TRH in conditions associated with isolated TRH excess, deficiency, or resistance states is uncertain. Hypothalamic dysregulation of TRH secretion may cause clinically mild, hypothalamic hypothyroidism.

Diagnostic and Clinical Use.—TRH is used in the evaluation of the hypothalamic-pituitary-thyroid unit. TRH (7 μg/kg) is administered as an IV bolus and blood samples are obtained for determination of TSH and PRL at times 0, +30, +60, and +120 minutes. After TRH administration, serum concentrations of GH may be inappropriately increased in patients with chronic renal failure or those with suspected acromegaly, or other causes of GH excess. In primary hyperthyroidism (e.g., autoimmune Graves disease), the TSH response to TRH is absent. In cases of hyperthyroidism caused by inappropriate TSH secretion, the pattern varies according to the cause of the disorder: in tumoral production of TSH, the TSH response following TRH is suppressed whereas in cases of thyroid hormone resistance, the TSH response to TRH is intact.

The TRH test may also differentiate the level of the defect in hypothyroidism. In primary hypothyroidism, TSH response following TRH is exaggerated; in pituitary (secondary) hypothyroidism, the TSH response to TRH is absent; in hypothalamic hypothyroidism, the TSH response following TRH is prolonged.

Other Hypothalamic Factors

Neuropeptide Y
Molecular Structure and Genetics.—Neuropeptide Y (NP-Y), named for the one-letter tyrosine residues at either end of the molecule, consists of 36 amino acids.

Secretion and Regulation.—NP-Y is identified in the arcuate, paraventricular, ventromedial, dorsomedial, and medial preoptic nuclei of the hypothalamus as well as in the cerebral cortex, basal ganglia, and limbic system.[118] It co-localizes with catecholamines in the CNS suggesting that both transmitters are released with sympathetic stimulation.

Function.—NP-Y is a very potent stimulant of appetite. NP-Y seems to cause selective craving for carbohydrate-rich foods. In animal studies, this food-seeking behavior predominates over other behaviors, including sexual activity. NP-Y inhibits anterior pituitary secretion of GH, TSH, PRL, and LH in males. Its role in diabetes mellitus, obesity, bulimina, and anorexia nervosa are topics of future investigations.

Other hypothalamic factors include bombesin, cholecystokinin, galanin, GABA, neurotensin, substance P, and VIP.

PITUITARY

Neuroanatomy

The pituitary gland is composed of the adenohypophysis, the neurohypophysis, and the intermediate lobe, which in human children and adults is rudimentary. The pituitary is located within the sella turcica, a recess within the anterior cranial fossa of the sphenoid bone. The sella is bounded anteriorly by the tuberculum sellae, posteriorly by the dorsum sellae, superiorly by the optic chiasm, and inferiorly by the sphenoid sinus. The anterior lobe, the adenohypophysis, which makes up about 75% of the gland, derives embryologically from a diverticulum arising from the oral cavity: Rathke's pouch. The adenohypophysis is divided into the pars tuberalis and the pars distalis. The intermediate lobe (pars intermedia) is poorly defined anatomically. The posterior lobe of the pituitary, the neurohypophysis, is comprised of the pars nervosa and the infundibulum (pituitary stalk). The neurohypophysis, a direct extension of the CNS, derives embryologically from an evagination of the third ventricle.

The anterior pituitary is composed of columnar secretory cells, which surround a vascular network, and folliculostellate cells, which do not have secretory capacity. Classically, the secretory cells of the adenohypophysis have been differentiated by the affinities of their secretory granules for various stains. Although stains tend to identify specific types of secretory cells (i.e., corticotrophs and somatotrophs), overlap exists, especially in cases of neoplasia. Hematoxylin-eosin (H&E) identifies cells that stain pink (acidophils), dark (basophils), and nonstaining cells (chromophobes). Periodic acid–Schiff (PAS) staining detects secretory granules containing carbohydrates, and thus identifies glycoproteins. By means of immunocytochemical staining and ultrastructure identification, the cell types listed in Table 3–4 have been identified[8,64]; however, mixed populations also have been identified that reflect progenitor cell populations. The anterior pituitary is innervated by postganglionic sympathetic fibers.

The neurohypophysis, being a direct extension of the brain, has no direct innervation, but is composed of unmyelinated axons and axon terminals that contain secretory granules, glial cells (pituicytes), and a capillary network. The neurohypophysis transmits very intense signals when imaged by magnetic resonance techniques (Fig 3–4).[90] The signals are probably related to intracytoplasmic lipid concentrations in pituicytes.

Vascular Anatomy

The hypothalamic-pituitary unit lies outside the blood-brain barrier. The vascular system of this unit is comprised of the pituitary portal system (see Fig 3–1).[43] The

TABLE 3–4.

Cells of the Anterior Pituitary*

Cell Type (% of Total Cell Population)	Major Products†
Corticotroph (15%)	POMC
	ACTH
	β-LPH
	MSH
Gonadotroph (10%)	FSH
	LH
Lactotroph (15%)	PRL
Somatotroph (50%)	GH
Thyrotroph (10%)	TSH

*Adapted from Frohman LA: Neurotransmitters as regulators of endocrine function, in Krieger DT, Hughes JC (eds): *Neuroendocrinology.* Sunderland, Mass, Sinaver Associates, 1980.

†POMC = proopiomelanocortin; ACTH = adrenocorticotropin; β-LPH = β-lipotropin; MSH = melanocyte-stimulating hormone; FSH = follicle-stimulating hormone; LH = luteinizing hormone; PRL = prolactin; GH = growth hormone; TSH = thyroid-stimulating hormone (thyrotropin).

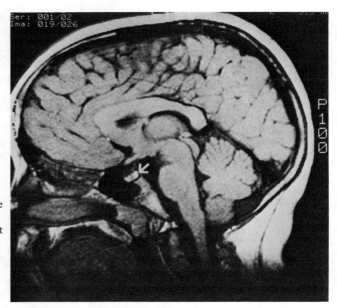

FIG 3–4.
T₁-weighted magnetic resonance image (MRI) of the brain. The *arrow* indicates the high-intensity signal of the neurohypophysis. (From Root AW, et al: *Am J Dis Child* 1989; 143:366. Used by permission.)

internal carotid arteries supply the pituitary with three smaller branches (1) The superior hypophysial artery supplies the infundibulum of the neurohypophysis and the median eminence of the hypothalamus, and divides into the primary and secondary capillary plexuses. The capillary bed of the former abuts the axons from the ventromedial, arcuate, and suprachiasmatic nuclei of the hypothalamus, and the tanycytes of the median eminence which relay material to the third ventricle. This network forms the long-portal vessels, and crosses the exterior of the pituitary stalk to enter the capillary system of the anterior pituitary. (2) The middle hypophysial artery supplies the posterior aspect of the adenohypophysis and the stem of the pituitary stalk. (3) The inferior hypophysial artery forms a capillary bed within the posterior pituitary to form the short-portal vessels.

The blood flow within the hypothalamic-pituitary unit is bidirectional, providing a channel for products of the anterior pituitary to influence the hypothalamus and CNS. There are relatively few venous channels draining the adenohypophysis into the cavernous sinus; more vessels drain the neurohypophysis into this structure. Because of the bidirectional blood flow, some authors have suggested that the major venous drainage of the adenohypophysis is through the short-portal vessels into the venous drainage system of the neurohypophysis.[36]

Posterior Pituitary Hormones

Vasopressin

Molecular Structure and Genetics.—Vasopressin (antidiuretic hormone, ADH) is a cyclic peptide containing nine amino acids. The gene for its precursor molecule, propressophysin, is located on chromosome 20.[74] Propressophysin undergoes posttranslational processing to form vasopressin, the vasopressin carrier protein (neurophysin II), and a C-terminal glycoprotein of uncertain function.

Secretion and Regulation.—Vasopressin is secreted primarily from the magnocellular neurons within the paraventricular and supraoptic nuclei of the hypothalamus. These cells are very responsive to even minor alterations in blood osmolality; a 1% increase in osmolality ($\sim$3 mOsm/kgH$_2$O) stimulates secretion of vasopressin. Normal serum osmolality is about 285 mOsm/kgH$_2$O. Thirst mechanisms are activated at serum osmolality > 290 mOsm/kgH$_2$O. These cells also respond to changes in blood volume, but to a lesser degree. Vasopressin secretion is diurnal with increased nighttime (sleep-associated) serum concentrations. Many factors influence vasopressin secretion (see Table 3–5). The plasma half-life is 10 minutes.

Function.—In addition to its effect on osmoregulation and fluid status, vasopressin has been implicated in hemostasis although the vascular pressor effects probably are of little physiologic importance in humans. In rats, and possibly in humans, vasopressin may also play a role in attention, learning, and short- and long-term memory, although the studies are inconclusive.[65,85] Vasopressin, along with CRH with which it co-localizes, also helps mediate the stress release of ACTH[46].

Mechanism of Action.—Vasopressin acts on two different but specific receptors: V$_1$ and V$_2$ receptors. The V$_1$ receptor, located primarily in smooth muscle of the vascular system, mediates vasopressor effects of vasopressin through phosphatidylinositide metabolism, prostaglandins, and intracellular Ca^{2+} fluxes. The V$_2$ receptors are located primarily in the distal convoluted tubule and collecting ducts of the nephron. In this system, the water retention effects of vasopressin are mediated through activation of adenylyl cyclase. A third receptor, V$_3$, has been putatively identified in the adenohypophysis. It may comediate the release of ACTH by vasopressin and CRH.[85]

TABLE 3–5.

Vasopressin (ADH) Regulation: Factors Influencing Secretion

Decreased ADH Secretion	Increased ADH Secretion
Malformation	Inflammation
Septo-optic dysplasia	Infection (meningoencephalitis)
Encephalocele	Viral
Ectopic posterior pituitary	Bacterial
Congenital cysts	Fungal
Empty sella syndrome(?)	Tubercular
Wolfram (DIDMOAD) syndrome*	Autoimmune (e.g., hypophysitis)
Congenital absence of ADH (X-linked recessive or	Infiltration
autosomal dominant)	Histiocytosis
Inflammation	Granulomas
Infection (meningoencephalitis)	Toxins
Viral	Cholinergics
Bacterial	Carbamazepine (Tegretol)
Fungal	Demeclocycline
Tubercular	Lithium
Autoimmune	Nicotine
Hypophysitis	Opioids
Empty sella syndrome(?)	Tricyclic antidepressants
Infiltration	Trauma
Histiocytosis	Vascular
Granulomas	Surgical (transient)
Lymphoma	Tumors (e.g., pulmonary neoplasms)
Toxins	Other
Irradiation	Adrenal insufficiency
Drugs	Hypothyroidism
Alcohol	Pulmonary disease
Anticholinergics	
Trauma	
Vascular	
Surgical	
Tumors	
Craniopharyngioma	
Germinoma	
Optic glioma	

*DIDMOAD = *d*iabetes *i*nsipidus, *d*iabetes *m*ellitus, *o*ptic *a*trophy, *d*eafness.

Clinical Data: *Excessive Secretion.* —Some conditions associated with hypersecretion of vasopressin are shown in Table 3–5. Excessive secretion results in euvolemic hyponatremia and is often referred to as the syndrome of inappropriate secretion of ADH (SIADH). In children, this most often occurs with CNS insults or following administration of pharmacologic agents, but it is also seen with pulmonary lesions and malignant conditions. The continued antidiuretic effects coupled with abnormal thirst or slightly increased fluid intake results in free water accumulation and dilutional hyponatremia. Contributing to the hyponatremia is a sodium diuresis (natriuresis) that ensues as compensatory mechanisms attempt to prevent the hypervolemic state; increased extracellular fluid volume leads to increased glomerular filtration which leads to decreased proximal tubular reabsorption of Na^+. The roles of aldosterone and atrial natriuretic factor in this phenomenon are uncertain. Thus, the hyponatremia of SIADH is associated with increased urinary concentration of Na^+. Urine osmolality is generally greater than 100 $mOsm/kgH_2O$. Clinically, patients present with nonspecific symptoms of hyponatremia (defined as serum Na^+ <130 mmol/L): anorexia, weakness, lethargy, and in severe cases, obtundity or convulsions. By definition, signs of diminished intravascular volume, edema, hypothyroidism, adrenal insufficiency, and renal disease are absent.

The evaluation of hyponatremia requires the exclusion of states of hyperproteinemia, hyperlipidemia, and hyperglycemia that may falsely lower the measurement of serum Na^+ by flame-emission spectrophotometry or indirect-reading potentiometry of diluted serum. Pseudohyponatremia results when the proportion of water in serum (normally 93% of serum volume) is displaced by nonaqueous components. Since Na^+ is found only in the aqueous component of serum, increased mass of the nonaqueous fraction by lipids or proteins is accompanied by a proportional decrease in the water mass; thus, estimations of Na^+ will be lower by the two methods mentioned above.[117] Hyperglycemia and IV administration of mannitol or glyceride similarly lead to hyponatremia, but, in addition, cause an osmotic movement of water from the intracellular to the extracellular space. Artifactually low measurements of Na^+ can be obviated by employing direct-reading potentiometry using a Na^+-selective electrode in undiluted samples.[117] A select population of patients with hyponatremia have an unusual mechanism for controlling vasopressin; it is presumed these patients have a "reset osmostat" that may suppress vasopressin secretion only in the face of very low serum osmolality.[115]

Severe hyponatremia requires rapid treatment but not rapid correction. This may be accomplished with a slow infusion of 3% hypertonic saline solution (0.1 mL/kg/min) sufficient to increase serum Na^+ to 125 mmol/L. More rapid correction of hyponatremia has been associated with central pontine myelinolysis. Milder cases are treated with fluid restriction. Chronic SIADH may be treated by the administration of lithium or demeclocycline but this is not recommended in children. Vasopressin antagonists may be useful in the future.

Deficient Secretion. —*Diabetes insipidus* (DI) is the term for relative or absolute deficiency of neurogenic vasopressin or cases of functional deficiency (i.e., end organ resistance). Irrespective of the level of the defect, patients have hypotonic polyuria (urine osmolality <300 $mOsm/kgH_2O$) during unlimited fluid intake despite increases in serum Na^+ and osmolality. In children, pronounced neurogenic DI is seen most often following insult to the supraoptic nuclei or supraoptic-hypophyseal tract preventing synthesis or release of vasopressin. Less pronounced DI occurs with lesions of the median eminence or pituitary stalk transection. Idiopathic and familial cases occur. Vasopressin-sensitive DI is also seen in pregnancy attributed to increased catabolism of vasopressin by the enzyme vasopressinase. Of special interest is the triphasic pattern of vasopressin secretion, often, but not always, seen following neurosurgical procedures interfering with the supraoptic-hypophyseal tract:

Phase I: Immediate DI, lasting up to 5 days after interruption of this axis.

Phase II (the interphase): Antidiuresis, lasting several days, secondary to release of prestored vasopressin from damaged neurons.

Phase III: Complete recovery of vasopressin regulation or permanent neurogenic DI.

The salient features of neurogenic DI are polyuria and polydipsia. Nocturia and enuresis may recur in the previously dry child. Often, a preference for cold water is manifested. Signs and symptoms suggestive of a central lesion include visual changes and diminished growth rate. Polyuria may lead to bladder distention and hydronephrosis. Left untreated, hypernatremia (with convulsions) may develop. The differential diagnosis of neurogenic DI from other disorders of polyuria and polydipsia includes vasopressin-resistant (nephrogenic) DI (*see below*), disorders associated with increased renal solute excretion (e.g., diabetes mellitus, hypercalcemia from a variety of causes), and primary polydipsia. Patients with primary polydipsia have either a primary psychiatric illness or an abnormality in the thirst mechanism. Thus the evaluation includes a good history and physical examination, general chemistry screen, and urinalysis with determination of urine Na$^+$ and osmolality. A lateral skull radiograph may reveal a craniopharyngioma. However, the diagnosis of DI may be established by the use of plasma vasopressin concentration in conjunction with serum or urine osmolality (Fig 3–5) or by means of a 7-hour water-deprivation test.[42] For the latter, we study patients at 8:00 AM; they need not have fasted. At baseline, after

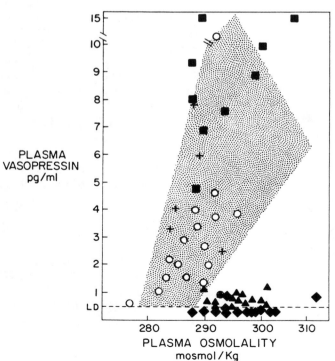

FIG 3–5.
Nomogram differentiating vasopressin-sensitive vs. resistant form of diabetes insipidus (DI). *Shaded area* = normal range; + = normal subjects; *open circles* = primary polydipsia; *solid squares* = nephrogenic DI; *solid triangles* = partial neurogenic DI; *solid diamonds* = severe neurogenic DI. (From Vokes TJ, Robertson GL: *Endocrinol Metab Clin North Am* 1988; 17:281. Used by permission.)

TABLE 3–6.

Water Deprivation and Disorders of Vasopressin (ADH)*

	Response to Thirsting		
	Urine Osmality	Urine Volume	Plasma ADH
Normal	Increased	Decreased	Normal increase
Hypernatremia			
Neurogenic DI	Decreased	Increased	Absent/low
Nephrogenic DI	Decreased	Increased	Very high
Primary hypodipsia	Increased	Decreased	Normal increase
Essential hyperna-tremia	Increased	Decreased	Normal increase
Hyponatremia			
SIADH	Increased	Decreased	Increased
Primary polydipsia	Increased	Decreased	Increased

*DI = diabetes insipidus; SIADH = syndrome of inappropriate antidiuretic hormone secretion.

emptying the bladder, urinalysis and osmolality are determined. Patients are weighed and blood is obtained for Na^+, osmolality, and vasopressin concentration. If hypernatremia (>145 mmol/L) or hyperosmolality (>295 mOsm/kgH$_2$O) is present despite dilute urine (<300 mOsm/L), then DI is established and the second phase of the study may proceed. However, most patients require a period of water deprivation. Patients are weighed and urine is collected hourly. Serum Na^+ and osmolality and urine osmolality are determined every 2 hours. Normal individuals have diminished, but concentrated, urine output while maintaining serum osmolality; after 7 hours of thirsting, the urine-serum osmolality ratio is >1.5. The test may be terminated in such cases or earlier in those who more rapidly show diagnostic criteria of DI such as hypernatremia, polyuria, or 5% weight loss. The second phase of the study, a diagnostic and therapeutic challenge with the vasopressin analogue desmopressin (1-desamino-8-D-arginine vasopressin, DDAVP) is then performed. After obtaining blood for vasopressin determination, 2.5 μg of desmopressin is administered intranasally and the test proceeds as before for an additional 1 to 2 hours. In vasopressin-sensitive (neurogenic) DI, administration of desmopressin results in almost immediate decline in urine output and increase in urine osmolality. Patients with nephrogenic DI will not respond to this agent, and endogenous serum concentrations of vasopressin are very elevated, reflecting the hormone-resistant state. The dehydration study may also differentiate the psychogenic water drinker (Table 3–6). One caveat: Patients must be supervised closely for the duration of the study to prevent surreptitious water drinking. It is important to note that abnormalities in vasopressin secretion are often associated with abnormalities in thirst regulation. The treatment of choice for neurogenic DI is desmopressin (see below).

End Organ Insensitivity.—The syndrome of resistance to vasopressin results in functional vasopressin deficiency and is termed *nephrogenic diabetes insipidus*. Although this condition may occur sporadically, familial cases, transmitted as an X-linked recessive trait, occur more commonly; the gene for this disorder has been mapped to the q28 region of the X chromosome.[74] These patients seem to have an isolated deficiency of V_2 receptors. Other causes of nephrogenic DI include intrinsic renal disease secondary to chronic inflammation or infection, vascular insult, or exposure to toxins (lithium, demeclocycline). The clinical presentation is similar to that of neurogenic DI: often male infants will present in the first weeks of life with constipation, intermittent fever, irritability, polydipsia, and failure to thrive. Undiagnosed, hypernatremia will result. Maternal pregnancies of affected infants are often associated with polyhydramnios. Older children may have learning difficulties, presumably due to subtle neurologic injury from unrecognized or overt hypernatremia during infancy. Treatment for nephrogenic DI involves thiazide diuretics in combination with either prostaglandin synthesis inhibitors (indomethacin) or with potassium-sparing diuretics (amiloride). Thiazides promote Na^+ excretion by interfering with Na^+ reabsorption in the distal tubule of the nephron and altering inner medullary osmolality; the former promotes increased proximal tubule reabsorption of Na^+ and the latter leads to increased free water absorption from the collecting duct. The mechanism of the additive effect of prostaglandin synthesis inhibitors is unknown. Potassium-sparing diuretics inhibit Na^+ reabsorption in the collecting duct; the synergistic effect of thiazide and potassium-sparing diuretics promotes a greater natriuresis without inducing kaliuresis,[58] an adverse effect of thiazides requiring K^+ supplementation. Prostaglandin inhibitors may adversely affect the gastrointestinal, renal, hematopoietic, and nervous systems. Adverse effects of potassium-sparing diuretics are uncommon, but include gynecomastia.

Diagnostic and Clinical Use.—Synthetic vasopressin is available for clinical use in an aqueous form and in an oil suspension (Pitressin). This material has been used with success for postoperative DI and for inducing hemostasis in patients with active bleeding or those with von Willebrand's disease.[85] Patients with von Willebrand's disease lack factor VIII coagulation activity (VIII:C) and the associated von Willebrand factor (VIII:vWF). Vasopressin (or analogues) increases these factors 4 to 6 times and acts on platelet-derived V_2 receptors. Pharmacologic doses of vasopressin act on V_1 receptors in the treatment of hemorrhage in patients undergoing surgical procedures. The treatment of choice for neurogenic DI is desmopressin (DDAVP).[87] These structural modifications in the molecule enhance the antidiuretic effect 2,000- to 3,000-fold and prolong the half-life 3 to 5 times. The duration of action is similarly increased, lasting up to 20 hours. There is, however, an abrupt onset of urine flow ("breakthrough") following full metabolism of desmopressin. DDAVP, usually given intranasally, has been given orally but with limited success. The IV form may be given when the nasal route is inaccessible. However, since IV desmopressin is approximately 10 times more potent than intranasal desmopressin, the dose is one-tenth the usual intranasal dose. Intranasal DDAVP may be diluted with normal saline and given safely to infants without adverse affects (0.14–0.52 μg/ kg/day).[98] Older patients generally respond to 2.5 to 10 μg administered once or twice daily. In general, the drug is initiated at night to diminish the inconvenience of needing to awaken to drink or void. In untreated patients with an intact thirst mechanism and full access to water, hypernatremia is rarely a problem. Large doses (20–40 μg) at night have been used to relieve bed-wetting in otherwise normal patients.

The major risks of desmopressin administration are water intoxication and hyponatremia. It is wise to allow breakthrough urination to begin when individualizing the dose. The dose may require modification following swimming or during upper respiratory illness. Antibody formation may occur in patients who lack the vasopressin gene; allergic reactions have occurred following administration of Pitressin (8-argininevasopressin), but these may be related to contamination by the vehicle or by neurophysin. Finally, the drug is expensive.

Oxytocin

Molecular Structure and Genetics.—Oxytocin, like vasopressin, is a cyclic nonapeptide derived from a larger molecule, prooxyphysin, coded on chromosome 20.[74] Similar to propressophysin, prooxyphysin contains the oxytocin carrier protein neurophysin I; the C-terminal glycoprotein is not integral to the prooxyphysin molecule. The amino acid sequence differs from vasopressin in positions 3 (isoleucine substituted for phenylalanine) and 8 (leucine substituted for arginine).

Secretion and Regulation.—Oxytocin is secreted episodically throughout the day from the magnocellular neurons of the supraoptic and paraventricular nuclei within the hypothalamus. Serum levels are generally low in males and nonpregnant females and are measurable in fetal pituitary tissue at 14 weeks of gestation. The fetal pituitary releases oxytocin and vasopressin during parturition. The greatest serum concentration of oxytocin is found during vaginal deliveries; oxytocin is very low in cesarean section deliveries without labor. The half-life is 3 to 17 minutes.[22] Estrogen stimulates oxytocin synthesis and secretion; oxytocin concentrations increase at midcycle of the menstrual period and during pregnancy; secretion probably increases in a pulselike fashion during labor because intermittent release has a greater effect on uterine contractility than does a continuous infusion.[22] Oxytocin release is stimulated by changes in osmolality,[28] by dopamine, by various intestinal peptides such as cholecystokinin, and by prostaglandins. Two well-described reflexes elicit oxytocin release: (1) nipple stimulation (primarily suckling) and (2) Ferguson's reflex—the activation of stretch receptors in the lower genital tract. Alcohol and opioids inhibit oxytocin release. Relaxin, a polypeptide secreted by the corpora lutea, may prevent preterm labor by activating opioid receptors.[32]

Function.—Like vasopressin, oxytocin comediates stress release of ACTH; in the rat model, oxytocin increases ACTH secretion, whereas in the primate, the effect of oxytocin on ACTH is inhibitory. Preliminary studies indicate that this is true in humans as well.[46] The effect of oxytocin on CRH release is uncertain; it may augment placental CRH secretion. Oxytocin may play a larger role during emotional, rather than physical, stress. In contrast to studies involving vasopressin, oxytocin seems to have an amnestic effect.[28] The antidiuretic effect of oxytocin is minimal. Oxytocin stimulates PRL release and blunts TSH release following TRH; this may be important in nursing.

Oxytocin causes milk ejection by increasing intramammary pressure causing contraction of myoepithelial cells that surround the mammary alveoli. Although oxytocin levels increase during labor, stimulating uterine contractility, milk expression is not usually evident, perhaps due to the inhibitory effect of prostaglandins and catecholamines on mammary tissue.

Mechanism of Action.—Plasma membrane–bound oxytocin receptors have been identified in mammary myoepithelium, myometrium, and oviducts. Specific CNS receptors have not been defined; putative oxytocin receptors of both high- and low-affinity binding have been localized in greatest concentrations in the olfactory nucleus and amygdala. Estrogen and divalent cations increase receptor affinity and number.[28] Activation of the receptor may be adenyl cyclase–independent.

Clinical Data.—Excessive, deficient, or resistant states of oxytocin secretion are not recognized clinically although lactation does not occur in the absence of oxytocin.

Diagnostic and Clinical Use.—Currently, oxytocin (Pitocin) is widely used to stimulate labor, and to assess placental function and reserve and, indirectly, fetal well-being antepartum. Adverse effects are rare but may include tonic uterine contraction leading to hemorrhage, cardiac dysrhythmias, and water retention.

Anterior Pituitary Hormones

ACTH and Related Hormones
Molecular Structure and Genetics.—ACTH is a 39-amino-acid peptide whose biologic activity is located within residues 1–29. It is derived from a larger precursor glycoprotein molecule proopiomelanocortin (POMC), which is also the precursor for α-melanocyte-stimulating hormone (α-MSH) β-MSH, γ-MSH, corticotropin-like intermediate lobe peptide (CLIP), β-lipoprotein (β-LPH), and the endorphins[35] (Fig 3–6). The gene for POMC is located at the p25 region of chromosome 2.[74] A comprehensive review of the posttranslational events of POMC is available.[104]

Secretion and Regulation.—ACTH is found primarily in the arcuate and ventrolateral nuclei of the hypothalamus and the corticotrophs of the anterior pituitary which are mildly basophilic or chromophobic to H&E staining. Immunoreactive ACTH is identified in the fetal pituitary at 8 weeks of gestation. The corticotroph is the first identifiable secretory cell type in the fetal pituitary.[3] ACTH is present in plasma by 12 weeks of gestation. ACTH is secreted in pulses throughout the day; there is a diurnal pattern with increased secretion occurring in the very early morning. Glucocorticoids and adrenal androgens are entrained with the diurnal release of ACTH. However, this pattern may not be apparent in the infant until several years of age. ACTH secretion is stimulated by CRH, vasopressin, and stress. ACTH secretion is inhibited through a long-feedback loop by glucocorticoids (cortisol) acting both at the level of the pituitary and of the hypothalamus. There is no evidence supporting ultrashort (auto) feedback of ACTH regulation.

Function.—ACTH preferentially stimulates steroidogenesis by the adrenal gland. It maintains the adrenal and stimulates growth of the zonae fasciculata and reticularis. After hypophysectomy, ACTH can maintain normal adrenal weight but

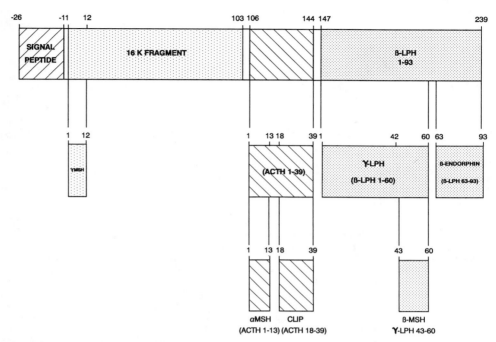

FIG 3–6.
Proopiomelanocortin and derivatives. *LPH* = lipotropin; *ACTH* = adrenocorticotropin;
MSH = melanocyte-stimulating hormone; *CLIP* = corticotropin-like intermediate lobe peptide.

at larger doses than are required to promote steroidogenesis,[89] implying that an additional pituitary factor mediates adrenal growth. ACTH mildly stimulates the zona glomerulosa synthesis of aldosterone; the secretion of mineralocorticoid is under primary control by the serum potassium concentration and the renin-angiotensin system. Up to 20% of available adrenal androgens (DHEA, DHEA-S, androstenedione) are unrelated to ACTH secretion. Adrenal androgens may be regulated by a glycoprotein, cortical androgen-stimulating hormone (CASH) (mol wt 60 kDa).[83]

The hypothalamic-pituitary axis is also intricately involved with the immune system (Fig 3–7). Interleukin-1 and other lymphokines promote CRH release.[6,96] Extrapituitary ACTH is synthesized in leukocytes[6] and may promote autocrine or paracrine effects upon the immune system. Macrophages and neutrophils produce transforming growth factor-β (TGF-β) and a peptide (mol wt 10 kDa) which inhibit ACTH effects in vitro but which are of uncertain physiologic significance.[6] ACTH also inhibits interferon synthesis while stimulating B lymphocytes and immunoglobulin production.

Mechanism of Action.—ACTH activates specific receptors located on the adrenal gland, monocytes, and splenocytes. In the first, the ACTH receptor is coupled to G-binding adenyl cyclase and phosphatidylinositide messengers. Preliminary investigations demonstrate that the ACTH receptor is a tetramer.[20]

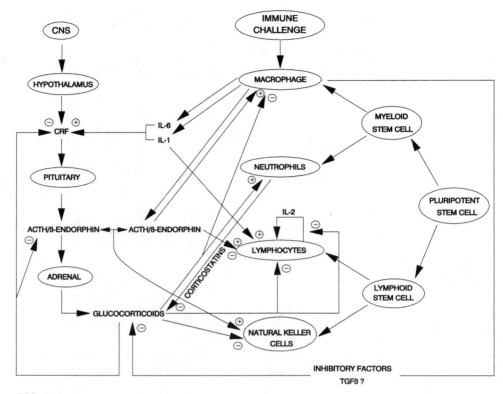

FIG 3–7.
Putative interactions between the hypothalamic-pituitary-adrenal axis and the immune system. *CRF* = corticotropin-releasing hormone; *ACTH* = adrenocorticotropin; *IL* = interleukin; *TGF* = transforming growth factor. (Adapted from Bateman A, et al: *Endocr Rev* 1989; 10:92. Used by permission.)

Clinical Data.—Excessive Secretion.—Hypersecretion of ACTH may be seen in states of primary adrenal insufficiency (Addison disease, congenital adrenal hyperplasia, familial insensitivity to ACTH, and X-linked adrenoleukodystrophy) or may accompany pituitary adenomas or ectopic production of ACTH by neoplasms. These latter processes produce ACTH-dependent hypercortisolism (Cushing disease). A complete discussion and differential diagnosis of Cushing syndrome are presented in Chapter 6. In patients with Cushing disease, there often is loss of diurnal ACTH and cortisol secretion. Salient features include plethora with polycythemia, eosinopenia, behavioral changes, round facies, central obesity, growth retardation, hypertension, hypertrichosis, hair thinning, and generalized hyperpigmentation, especially over pressure-sensitive areas (knuckles), areolae, and gingival and buccal mucosa— the consequence of very elevated levels of ACTH and α-MSH on melanocytes. Cyclic and seasonal manifestations of Cushing syndrome have been described.[47]

The evaluation of Cushing disease hinges on the demonstration of the hypercortisolemic state. This is best accomplished with a 24-hour urine collection for the determination of free cortisol and 17-hydroxycorticosteroids. Loss of diurnal rhythm may be evaluated by determining 8 A.M. and 8 P.M. serum cortisol (and ACTH) levels. The 8:00 A.M. serum cortisol level after 20 μg/kg dexamethasone (overnight dexamethasone) is not suppressed in patients with Cushing syndrome. High-dose dexamethasone 3.75 mg/m²/day in four doses for 2 days, will not suppress cortisol in ACTH-independent Cushing syndrome (adrenal tumor) or ectopic ACTH syndrome, but generally will suppress ACTH and cortisol in pituitary ACTH-dependent Cushing disease. Phenytoin and phenobarbital increase dexamethasone catabolism. Other adrenal androgens may be elevated in Cushing syndrome. Once ACTH-dependent hypercortisolism is confirmed, the source of ACTH may be discerned by use of the CRH stimulation test with inferior petrosal sinus sampling and appropriate imaging studies.[80] The cause of excess ACTH determines the appropriate therapy. Primary adrenal insufficiency requires physiologic replacement of hydrocortisone. Surgical excision is required for pituitary adenomas and ectopic ACTH production. Many ACTH-secreting pituitary adenomas are microadenomas which are difficult to image; such patients may require exploratory transsphenoidal surgery. Prior to such surgery or tumor excision, patients require preoperative and postoperative glucocorticoids.

Deficient Secretion.—Hyposecretion of ACTH may be congenital or acquired and associated with multiple pituitary hormone deficiency. Congenital adrenal hypoplasia from ACTH deficiency occurs (1) sporadically, (2) in an autosomal recessive form, (3) in an X-linked recessive form associated with hypogonadotropic hypogonadism, (4) in an X-linked recessive form associated with glycerol kinase deficiency and associated somatic anomalies,[120] and (5) in an autosomal recessive form with glycerol kinase deficiency and LH deficiency.[21] Neonatal manifestations of congenital adrenal insufficiency include lethargy, somnolence, jitteriness, and seizures consequent to hypoglycemia. Manifestations of acquired ACTH-deficient adrenal insufficiency in older children include lethargy, weakness, anorexia, and weight loss. Unlike patients with primary adrenal insufficiency, hyperpigmentation is absent. Hyponatremia may be present; cortisol is required to facilitate excretion of free water. Because the renin-angiotensin system is intact, mineralocorticoid synthesis and release is intact.

In the neonate, the most common cause of adrenal insufficiency is 21-hydroxylase-deficient congenital adrenal hyperplasia. This may be assessed by determining the serum concentration of 17-hydroxyprogesterone (see Chapter 6 for a discussion of inborn errors of cortisol biosynthesis). ACTH-deficient adrenal insufficiency is confirmed by the absence of serum ACTH during times of adrenal insufficiency (e.g., insulin-induced hypoglycemia). ACTH deficiency may be suspected in the patient with deficiency of other anterior pituitary hormones when random morning serum cortisol concentrations are low. Elevation of serum triglycerides is a salient feature of glycerol kinase deficiency. Treatment of ACTH-deficient adrenal failure requires hydrocortisone replacement (7–15 mg/m²/day in two divided doses).

End Organ Insensitivity.—Resistance to ACTH has been reported both sporadically and as familial X-linked and autosomal recessive disorders. Again, because the zona glomerulosa is essentially ACTH-independent, mineralocorticoid secretion is intact. One report describes ACTH insensitivity with familial vitamin D–resistant hypophosphatemic rickets.[100] Although the phenotype may vary, associated symptoms have included alacrima and achalasia and may reflect a receptor or postreceptor defect; in such patients, adrenal cortisol production has increased transiently after maneuvers to increase intracellular cAMP and Ca^{2+}.[45] The diagnosis is established by demonstrating low serum cortisol and elevated serum ACTH concentrations and an absent glucocorticoid response following exogenous ACTH administration in the absence of other primary or inflammatory adrenal disease. X-linked adrenoleukodystrophy must be excluded by the demonstration of normal plasma concentrations of very long-chain fatty acids.

Diagnostic and Clinical Use.—ACTH is used in the evaluation of adrenal function and reserve. Serum cortisol concentration remains low in patients with adrenal insufficiency. In patients with enzymatic defects of cortisol biosynthesis, ACTH is used to demonstrate the level of the defect. This is discussed more completely in Chapter 6. ACTH often is used empirically in patients with infantile spasms and hypsarrhythmia. Adverse effects to short-term ACTH infusion are minimal; long-term administration can result in hypercortisolism.

Melanocyte-Stimulating Hormone

α-, β-, and γ-MSH also derive from POMC. α-MSH, a 13-amino-acid-peptide — the first 13 residues of ACTH — is located primarily in the intermediate lobe of the fetal pituitary, as is β-MSH, a 17-amino acid peptide derived from the lipotropin portion of POMC. β-MSH may not occur physiologically; its isolation may be artifactual. α-MSH is a 12-amino-acid peptide found primarily in the anterior pituitary and in ACTH-secreting tumors. While α- and β-MSH may stimulate endocrine pancreas secretion in mice and rabbits,[59] γ-MSH may potentiate the effects of ACTH.

Corticotropin-like Intermediate Lobe Peptide

CLIP is composed of the 22 N-terminal amino acid residues of ACTH. Found primarily in the fetal intermediate lobe of the pituitary, CLIP may support the fetal adrenal.

Lipotropin

This subfamily of POMC-derived peptides includes β- and γ-lipotropin and β-MSH. β-LPH is composed of the 93 N-terminal amino acids of POMC. It is further processed to α-LPH (β-LPH 1–60) and to β-endorphin (β-LPH 63–93) which in turn gives rise to α- and γ- endorphin and γ-LPH. The last molecule is the precursor of β-MSH. The *endorphins* possess *end*ogenous *morphine*like or opioid activity. β-endorphin is present in the anterior pituitary and the arcuate and ventromedial nuclei of the hypothalamus, and throughout the cerebrum and brainstem. Related structurally and functionally to the endorphins are the enkephalins which share the N-terminal 5 amino acids of β-endorphin. The two identified enkephalins, met-enkephalin (methionine) and leu-enkephalin (leucine), differ in the moiety occupying the fifth residue. The enkephalins are not thought to derive directly from endorphin because their distribution within the brain differs; no endorphin precursor has been identified in neurons containing enkephalin.

ACTH Fragment 4–10

This fragment of ACTH 1–39 recently has been shown to inhibit the consumption of alcohol in rats and may play a role in the relationship between stress and alcohol consumption in humans[62,79] (and RP Maickel, personal communication).

Growth Hormone

Molecular Structure and Genetics.—GH is a 191-amino-acid polypeptide related in structure and function to PRL and chorionic somatomammotropin and is derived from a 217-amino-acid precursor. The GH gene complex is composed of five genes which have been mapped to the q22–24 region of chromosome 17. Reading 5′ to 3′ the genes include (1) GH-1 (GH normal), (2) CSHP-1 (chorionic somatotropic hormone pseudogene), (3) CSH-1 (chorionic somatotropin-1), (4) GH-2 (formerly thought to be a variant or pseudogene but which may code for a placental GH that is active during pregnancy), and (5) CSH-2.[41,74,77] CS-1 and CS-2 are also termed *placental lactogens*. GH-1 codes for pituitary somatotroph–derived GH which is usually a monomer; dimeric and polymeric forms also have been isolated. The GH isomers vary in regard to biologic activity (i.e., growth-promoting and anti-insulin effects). The former activity lies in the intact molecule; diabetogenic properties derive from the C-7 terminal and midregion. It is of interest that the N-terminal has insulin-like effects.

Secretion and Regulation.—GH has been identified in fetal pituitary tissue at 10 to 11 weeks of gestation; at 12 weeks of gestation, mammosomatotrophs are demonstrated, and distinct somatotrophs may be seen at 15 weeks.[3] The half-life of GH is estimated between 3.5 and 51 minutes but is probably closer to 9 minutes.[51] GH is secreted in a pulsatile fashion throughout the day (approximately six or seven pulses every 24 hours[106]) and is sleep-entrained. GH secretion is regulated primarily by hypothalamic secretion of GH-RH and SRIF.[30,88] GH-RH contributes to the peak amplitude of any GH pulse; SRIF regulates tonic GH secretion and the timing and frequency of GH bursts. A pulse of GH thus requires a coordinated concert of diminished SRIF tone and increased GH-RH. Functional lack of SRIF results in increased basilar GH concentration but with continued pulses of GH secretion. Functional lack of GH-RH causes cessation of pulsatile GH secretion without effect on basal GH tone.

Agents that influence GH secretion do so primarily by altering the relative secretion of either GH-RH or SRIF. Factors that increase GH-RH (thus increasing GH release) include α_2-adrenergic agonists (clonidine), dopaminergic agonists (levodopa), and exercise. Factors that diminish SRIF (thus increasing GH release) include insulin hypoglycemia,[113] arginine, and cholinergic agents. Conversely, inhibition of GH secretion occurs by agents which promote SRIF or diminish GH-RH secretion. The former includes norepinephrine, IGF-I, GH, and GH-RH; GH secretion is depressed in obesity due to decreased cholinergic tone leading to increased SRIF. IGF-I, GH, SRIF, and GH-RH inhibit GH-RH secretion, the last via an ultrashort-feedback loop. In addition, serotonergic and histaminergic stimulation promote GH release by uncertain mechanisms.

Optimal GH secretion requires the appropriate thyroid and sex hormone milieu.

GH secretion increases during early puberty in girls and mid- to late puberty in boys and is reflected by the adolescent growth spurt.[73]

Function.—GH is an anabolic agent promoting protein synthesis and cell replication. Its effect on longitudinal skeletal growth is through its effector agent, IGF-I, which stimulates chondrocytes (see below). GH has dichotomous effects upon carbohydrate metabolism; blood glucose concentrations decrease transiently following GH administration, the physiologic significance of which is uncertain. Better understood is the anti-insulin effect of GH. Patients with excessive secretion of GH may have carbohydrate intolerance and insulin resistance. The anti-insulin effect may contribute to the dawn phenomenon, the early-morning hyperglycemia observed in persons with diabetes. GH increases lipolysis and serum-free fatty acids by mechanisms that are unclear. GH promotes calciuria and (perhaps indirectly) hyperphosphatemia. In humans, GH possesses lactogenic activity.

A broadening field of GH investigation involves immunology. GH may function as a cytokine; GH enhances killer T and NK lymphocyte response, promotes immunoglobulin and thymulin synthesis,[26] and primes macrophages for production of the superoxide radical.[33]

Mechanism of Action.—The effect of GH is primarily through hepatic synthesis of IGF-I. GH binds to specific somatotropic receptors which, in man, are encoded by the p13.1–12 region of chromosome 5[5] and consist of a cytosolic and extracellular region. After binding to the receptor, the receptor-ligand complex is internalized; the specific intracellular mechanisms and messengers that transduce this signal are uncertain but may involve phophatidylinosotide metabolism. Up to 90% of circulating GH may be bound by two GH-binding glycoproteins (GH-BP), the extracellular component of the GH receptor. The GH-BPs have different affinities for binding GH; the major GH-BP has high-affinity, low-capacity GH binding.[7]

The activity of both GH-BPs is lowest in neonates but increases by 1 year of age and remains stable until late adulthood.[7, 103] The low-affinity, high-capacity GH-BP may be sex hormone–dependent.[7] GH-BPs may function as GH reservoirs and prolong the GH half-life. GH-BP is not detectable in the plasma of patients with Laron-type dwarfism (functional lack of GH receptors)[9] and is in low concentrations in African pygmies[8] and in non–GH-deficient short children.[68]

IGF-I and IGF-II share sequence homology with each other, with proinsulin, and with relaxin. The gene for IGF-I has been mapped to the q22-24.1 region of chromosome 12,[74] which codes for two different IGF-I precursor molecules that share the first 134 amino acids: IGF-IA contains 153 amino acids while IGF-IB contains 195 amino acids. IGF-I circulates bound to three different binding proteins: IGF-BP-1, IGF-BP-2, and IGF-BP-3. IGF-BP-1 is GH-independent and is regulated by serum glucose concentration independent of insulin.[66] The physiologic significance of IGF-BP-2 is uncertain.[92] IGF-BP-3, is the only IGF-binding protein that is glycosylated. Both IGF-BP-2 and IGF-BP-3 are GH-dependent proteins.

Serum concentrations of IGF-I increase throughout childhood and depend heavily upon nutritional status, sex hormone (estrogen), and thyroid hormone. During adolescence, serum IGF-I concentrations increase markedly and correlate better with pubertal stage and bone age rather than chronologic age. The effect of IGF-I on skeletal epiphyses is probably a paracrine effect. IGF-I levels are diminished in states of GH deficiency, hepatic disease, malnutrition, and psychosocial dwarfism. IGF-I levels are elevated in states of hypersomatotropism.[4]

IGF-II is a 67-amino-acid peptide coded on the p15.5 region of chromosome 11.[74] IGF-II has 70% sequence homology with IGF-I. Precise regulation of IGF-II is not known; levels are elevated in fetal compared to more mature tissues. The receptor for IGF-I is encoded by chromosome 15q25–26 while the IGF-II receptor is encoded by the q25–27 region of chromosome 6 and is linked to mannose-6-phosphate.[74] The IGF-I receptor is composed of two extracellular, glycosylated, disulfide bond–linked α chains and two transmembrane β chains with protein kinase activity. IGF-II can bind weakly to the IGF-I receptor. The IGF-II receptor is a single polypeptide consisting of extracellular, transmembranous, and intracellular regions.

Clinical Data.—*Excessive Secretion.*—Hypersomatotropism may be due to primary pituitary disease (pituitary somatotroph adenoma, hyperplasia, or mammosomatotroph hyperplasia[53, 76]) or to increased GH-RH either at the hypothalamic level or from ectopic tumor secretion. Accelerated growth rate in childhood before epiphyseal closure leads to gigantism and may be congenital.[17, 76] Other signs of gigantism and acromegaly include soft tissue growth causing coarsening of facial features and enlarged hands and feet, kyphosis and organomegaly, thickened skin, hypertrichosis, galactorrhea, and delayed puberty. Symptoms include headache, visual and other neurologic disturbances, carpal tunnel syndrome, hyperhidrosis, cold intolerance, polyuria and polydipsia, amenorrhea, and impotence.[75]

Laboratory findings that support the diagnosis of hypersomatotropism in the clinically suspect patient include elevation in serum concentrations of IGF-I and GH[4] (Fig 3–8). Secretion of GH increases paradoxically or cannot be suppressed during hyperglycemia. In addition, serum GH concentrations increase following stimuli that usually have little effect on GH secretion (e.g., TRH and GnRH). Basal GH secretion is often increased in patients with malnutrition, anorexia nervosa, depression, and

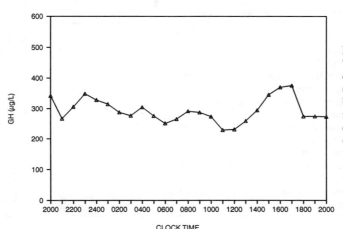

FIG 3–8.
Twenty-four-hour nocturnal endogenous growth hormone (GH) pattern of a 12-year-old boy with a mixed GH-prolactin–secreting tumor. Note the elevation in baseline serum GH concentration.

chronic renal failure. In pediatrics, the standard oral glucose tolerance test consists of administration of 1.75 g of glucose (maximum 75 g) with blood obtained for GH determination every 30 minutes for 4 hours. Normally, serum GH concentration decreases to less than 2 μg/L during the glucose tolerance test.[75] Serum PRL levels may be elevated in patients with pituitary adenomas. Such tumors may be mixed mammosomatotrophs which may be persistent fetal remnants.[3,53,76] Thorough neurologic and ophthalmologic examinations and CNS studies with magnetic resonance imaging (MRI) or computed tomography (CT) is required.

The clinical differential diagnosis of tall stature includes the conditions listed in Table 3–7: cerebral gigantism and homocystinuria have mental deficiency, typical facies, and somatic anomalies; Marfan syndrome has a typical body habitus and normal mentation. Hyperthyroidism and sexual precocity are evident from physical examination.

The etiology of GH hypersecretion determines the treatment program. Pituitary tumors are excised if possible, preferably by the transphenoidal route. Dopamine agonists (bromocriptine), which bind to somatotroph dopamine receptors and "inappropriately" suppress GH secretion, are the mainstay of medical management of GH-secreting pituitary tumors. A review of 514 patients with acromegaly treated with bromocriptine demonstrated lowering of GH to less than 5 μg/L in 20%, reduced tumor mass in less than 20%, and yet clinical improvement in 70% of patients.[75] Effective daily dosage may approach 20 mg. Adverse effects include nausea, vomiting, nasal congestion, and transient postural hypotension.

Long-acting somatostatin analogues (e.g., octreotide) are very effective in suppressing GH release from pituitary adenomas; the clinical response correlates positively with the number of SRIF receptors available on the tumor. Most patients have required 600 μg/day divided into three doses to fully suppress GH secretion. Clinical responses included improvement in symptoms and shrinkage of tumor mass; however, octreotide is not cytotoxic and tumors regrow when the medication is discontinued. The disadvantages of SRIF are the subcutaneous route of administration and the

TABLE 3–7.

Differential Diagnosis of Excessive Growth

Congenital	Acquired
Intrinsic	Metabolic
Familial	Hyperthyroidism
Cerebral gigantism (Sotos syndrome)	Precocious puberty
Weaver syndrome	Central
Beckwith-Wiedemann syndrome	Pseudoprecocious
Genetic	Incomplete
Marfan syndrome (autosomal dominant)	Obesity
Homocystinuria (autosomal recessive)	Hypersomatotropism
Generalized lipodystrophy (autosomal recessive)	
Klinefelter syndrome (47,XXY or variant)	
Other	
Pituitary mammosomatotroph hyperplasia(?)	
Pseudoacromegaly	

TABLE 3–8.

Etiology of Growth Hormone (GH) Deficiency and Hypopituitarism

Congenital	Acquired
Malformation	Inflammation
Anencephaly	Autoimmune (e.g., empty sella syndrome[?])
Holoprosencephaly, schizencephaly	Infection (meningoencephalitis)
Septo-optic dysplasia	Viral
Empty sella syndrome(?)	Bacterial
Hydrocephalus	Fungal
Hypoplasia	Tubercular
Absence of GH gene; other heritable causes	Infiltration
Inflammation	Histiocytosis
Autoimmune (e.g., empty sella syndrome[?])	Granulomas
Infection	Lymphoma
Viral (e.g., rubella)	Toxins (e.g., irradiation)
Toxins	Trauma
Trauma	Vascular
Hypoxemia	Surgical
Intracranial bleeding	Tumor (e.g., glioma)
Tumor	
Craniopharyngioma	
Subarachnoid cyst	
Aneurysm	
Other	
Associated with hypogammaglobulinemia	
GH neurosecretory dysfunction (GHND)	

expense. Adverse effects include those of chronic exposure to SRIF: diarrhea, non-specific gastrointestinal complaints, and cholelithiasis.

CNS irradiation probably is best reserved as adjunctive therapy in medical and surgical treatment plans. Although radiation therapy is cytotoxic, its duration of onset is long and up to 50% of patients develop long-term complications such as hypopituitarism, visual disturbances, and learning impairment.

Deficient Secretion. —The causes of GH deficiency are shown in Table 3–8. GH deficiency is the most commonly recognized abnormality of anterior pituitary function, occurring in approximately 1 in 7,000 children and in 14% of patients referred for short stature.[89] In the majority of cases, the cause is not determined; however, the diagnostic application of GH-RH has demonstrated that cases previously labeled as "idiopathic" were actually cases of hypothalamic GH-RH dysfunction. The male-to-female ratio of GH deficiency is 4:1. GH deficiency may be an isolated finding or part of a more global deficiency in pituitary function. GH deficiency may accompany a number of syndromes.[86] Several genetically linked disorders with GH deficiency are described: I-A:autosomal recessive deletion of the GH-1 gene; I-B:autosomal recessive transmission with normal GH-1 gene; II:autosomal dominant; III:X-linked recessive.[55] Septo-optic dysplasia (SOD) follows idiopathic GH deficiency and craniopharyngioma as the most common causes of GH deficiency. SOD is the triad of optic nerve hypoplasia, absence of the septum pellucidum, and GH (with or without multiple pituitary hormone) deficiency.

Clinical presentation of GH deficiency is somewhat age-specific. The neonate with congenital hyposomatotropism may have recurrent hypoglycemia; birth weight and length are normal. Affected males often have microphallus or cryptorchidism, or both. Often there is prolonged direct hyperbilirubinemia associated with giant cell hepatitis with elevation in hepatic transaminases. Infants with SOD have wandering nystagmus. In older children, GH deficiency manifests as growth retardation and growth velocity deceleration. Generally there is "proportional" short stature. Classically, patients have relative truncal obesity, immature facies (poorly defined nasal bridge, prominent frontal bone), delicate skin, poor body and facial hair growth, high-pitched voice, and a childlike upper-to-lower body ratio (>1). Skeletal maturation is delayed; older subjects may have delay in pubertal onset. When GH deficiency is a component of an intracranial neoplasm, symptoms and signs of increased intracranial pressure may dominate.

There are a number of studies used clinically to assess GH secretion and pituitary GH reserve. Controversy exists as to the precise laboratory definition of GH deficiency. In the appropriate clinical setting, the patient with short stature, slow growth velocity, bone age delay, and peak serum concentration of GH less than 7 μg/L following two or more provocative tests has classic GH deficiency. However, the value of 7 μg/L is arbitrary. Many investigators use 10 μg/L; patients whose peak serum GH concentration lies between 7 and 10 μg/L may be said to have "partial" GH deficiency. Adding further fuel to this fire are the studies of the role of endogenous GH secretion.[15, 91] Provocative testing may not accurately reflect the "daily" ability of the pituitary to synthesize or release GH; this is best exemplified in those patients who have received CNS irradiation and have dysregulation of GH release, perhaps due to defects in higher neurotransmitter secretion or function.[106] Such patients are said to have GH neurosecretory dysfunction (GHND).

Methods we usually employ to provoke GH secretion include exercise, insulin-induced hypoglycemia (0.05–0.1 unit/kg IV), arginine (0.5 g/kg to a maximum of 30 g IV), levodopa (250–500 mg orally), and clonidine (0.1 mg/m^2 orally). Less often, we use glucagon (0.3 mg/kg to a maximum of 1 mg IV or intramuscularly). Some centers "prime" patients with sex hormones prior to testing. Each test has its limitations, but each generally influences GH secretion by modifying the effects of GH-RH or SRIF on GH. Insulin hypoglycemia is a particularly useful study as the hypothalamic-pituitary-adrenal axis may be studied concurrently; patients with hypopituitarism may have profound hypoglycemia following insulin administration. The remainder of the hypothalamic-pituitary unit may be assessed concurrently by the simultaneous administration of TRH and GnRH together with the appropriate blood studies (Table 3–9). In addition, we also investigate the endogenous release of GH by obtaining blood samples throughout the day or night. The reproducibility of such studies has been questioned.[31] Other studies obtained in evaluating the short child include IGF-I levels, CNS imaging, determination of levels of other pituitary hormones, a general chemistry panel to identify occult metabolic derangements, and a karyotype (in girls) to identify 45,X (or variant) gonadal dysgenesis.

TABLE 3–9.

Combined Insulin Tolerance-TRH-GnRH Stimulation Study*

I. Water only after midnight
II. Insert IV normal saline solution at "to keep open" rate
III. Protocol:

Time	GLU	GH	PRL	LH/FSH	TSH	T₃ RIA	F	E₂/T/DHEA-S†	T₄	T₃ RU
− 30 min	X	X	X	X	X	X	X	X	X	X
0	X	X	X	X						

Regular insulin	0.05–0.1 unit/kg IV
TRH	7 μg/kg IV (maximum 500 μg)
GnRH	100 μg IV

Time	GLU	GH	PRL	LH/FSH	TSH	T₃ RIA	F	E₂/T/DHEA-S†	T₄	T₃ RU
+ 10 min	X	X	X	X						
+ 20	X	X	X	X						
+ 30	X	X	X	X	X					
+ 40	X	X	X	X						
+ 60	X	X	X	X	X		X			
+ 90	X	X	X	X						
+120	X	X	X	X	X	X		X		

*TRH = thyrotropin-releasing hormone; GnRH = gonadotropin-releasing hormone; GLU = glucose; GH = growth hormone; PRL = prolactin; LH = luteinizing hormone; FSH = follicle-stimulating hormone; TSH = thyrotropin; T₃ RIA = total triiodothyronine radioimmunoassay; F = cortisol; E₂ = estradiol; T = testosterone; DHEA-S = dehydroepiandrosterone sulfate; T₄ = thyroxine; T₃RU = T₃ resin uptake.
†Gender-appropriate gonadal steroid.

End Organ Insensitivity.—Functional GH deficiency occurs in states of GH resistance characterized by diminished binding of GH to its receptor, as described by Laron. Such patients have somatic features typical of GH deficiency, but basal and provoked levels of GH are normal or elevated. Serum concentrations of IGF-I and GH-BP are low. Such patients fail to demonstrate growth acceleration or increased serum IGF-I levels after exogenous GH administration, but may respond to exogenous IGF-I. Both genders are affected equally; most families described are of Mediterranean descent.

Diagnostic and Clinical Use.—With recombinant DNA engineering, there is virtually an unlimited supply of GH available. Clearly, GH is effective in augmenting growth velocity and increasing adult height in patients with classic GH deficiency utilizing thrice-weekly doses of 0.3 U/kg/wk. There is now evidence that daily injections employing doses of 0.6 U/kg/wk lead to greater gains. Increased final height (over predicted) has been demonstrated in girls with gonadal dysgenesis treated with 0.75 U/kg/wk of GH. (The biologic activity of recombinant human GH is 2.6 IU/mg). This points to another controversy: the role of GH in the treatment of short non–GH-deficient children, in patients with renal failure, and in wound management. In the first, we and others have observed an inverse correlation between the increase in height velocity and the pretreatment height velocity, endogenous GH secretion, and peak GH response to provocative stimuli during 1 year of GH treatment.[99] This latter observation has not been confirmed by others.

In general, advancement in skeletal maturation equals the incremental increase in height as reflected by height age during GH therapy. However, it is also clear that although "standard" doses of exogenous GH (0.3 U/kg/wk increase absolute height (over predicted) in GH-deficient children, the genetic potential (estimated from target height) is not always attained. It is discouraging to note that Kaplan and Grumbach have shown that only 13% (3/24) of "short-normal" patients treated with exogenous GH over several years experienced an increase greater than 2.5 cm in final height over predicted.[56] Thus, in such patients, GH may increase short-term height velocity, but not ultimate height. Further studies are required.

Adverse effects of GH therapy include the development of antibodies to the GH molecule, especially in patients lacking the GH gene. Generally, this antibody formation does not attenuate the effect of GH. Large amounts of GH may alter carbohydrate metabolism and lead to glucose intolerance. Exogenous GH has led to hypothyrotropinemia, perhaps by increasing central SRIF tone or by increasing conversion of T_4 to T_3 with consequent inhibition of the thyrotroph. Contaminated lots of cadaveric human pituitary GH have been linked to the development of Creutzfeldt-Jakob disease (CJD) in patients with GH deficiency. This tragic situation is thought to be a random event; however, the requisite incubation period for the development of CJD has not yet been attained in the majority of exposed patients.[40] Although a cluster of patients treated with GH have developed leukemia, epidemiologic studies have not verified a specific link between them.[27,38,116] Recent work has examined the role of GH as a therapeutic agent in obesity, aging, and wound repair.[71,93,94]

Prolactin

Molecular Structure and Genetics.—PRL is a 198 amino acid monomer that probably derived from the same ancestral gene as GH and which retains 16% sequence homology to GH. The gene encoding PRL has been mapped to the p22.1–q21.3 region of chromosome 6.[74]

Secretion and Regulation.—PRL is detectable in the fetal pituitary at 12 weeks in mammosomatotrophs; characteristic lactotrophs, in the lateral portions of the pituitary, are identified after 23 weeks[3] and fetal serum levels of PRL are detectable shortly thereafter and peak in the third trimester of pregnancy. PRL secretion is similar to that of GH and is sleep-entrained. Hypothalamic dopamine exerts tonic inhibition upon PRL release by activating adenyl cyclase. Secretion of PRL is increased in response to estrogen, glucocorticoids, stress, and TRH, although TRH probably is not physiologically important in this regard.

Function.—PRL promotes mammary gland growth and lactogenesis, but only synergistically with estrogen. Although the role of PRL in promoting longitudinal growth has been questioned, the contribution of PRL to growth under normal physiologic conditions is probably minimal.[17]

PRL receptors on lymphocytes imply a role for this hormone in regulation of the immune system. PRL increases thymic thymulin production, stimulates T cell proliferation, activates macrophages, and promotes interferon-γ production and graft-vs.-host reactions.[16,26,114]

PRL affects the hypothalamic-pituitary-gonadal axis by suppressing GnRH and gonadotropin release; however, hyperprolactinemia may enhance the LH response following GnRH administration. PRL may have a direct effect on the ovary by inducing gonadotropin resistance and decreasing progesterone synthesis.[18] PRL working synergistically with testosterone has positive effects on the development of the male reproductive system; PRL acts as a catalyst for the effects of LH on Leydig cells[18] and may influence 5α-reductase action as well.

Mechanism of Action.—PRL binds to specific receptors, 292 amino acid glycoproteins. The mechanism by which this interaction signals intracellular function is uncertain but may involve protein kinase C. The receptor number is upregulated by estrogen and PRL.

Clinical Data.—*Excessive Secretion.*—Physiologic hyperprolactinemia occurs during stress, pregnancy, parturition, and breast stimulation. Pathologic conditions of excessive PRL secretion are listed in Table 3–10. Hyperprolactinemia occurs more often in females. Hyperprolactinemia can cause galactorrhea but alone usually contributes little to breast growth. Hyperprolactinemia leads to pubertal delay and sexual dysfunction in males and amenorrhea in females by suppressing GnRH release. Hyperprolactinemia caused by CNS tumors may also present with signs of increased intracranial pressure: headache, visual disturbances, and other neurologic manifestations. In adults, prolactinomas may be asymptomatic and discovered only incidentally at autopsy. Hyperprolactinemia is present when the serum concentration of PRL is consistently above 20 μg/L. Levels between 150 and 200 μg/L are indicative of a pituitary macro- or microadenoma. In cases of prolactinoma, PRL response following TRH administration is blunted. CNS imaging and other hypothalamic-pituitary evaluation is required, especially in cases of disturbed sexual maturation.

Medical management for hyperprolactinemia includes the use of dopaminergic

TABLE 3–10.

Causes of Hyperprolactinemia

Malformation (e.g., empty sella syndrome[?])	Trauma (e.g., pituitary stalk transection)
Inflammation	Surgical
Autoimmune (empty sella syndrome[?])	Nonsurgical
Infection (meningoencephalitis)	Tumor
Infiltration	Craniopharyngioma
Histiocytosis	Prolactinoma
Sarcoidosis	Pituitary
Toxin	Ectopic (pulmonary, ovarian)
Irradiation	Pseudotumor cerebri
Drugs	Other
Phenothiazine	Hypothyroidism
Reserpine	
Methyldopa	
Oral contraceptives (estrogen)	

agonists. Bromocriptine in doses up to 20 mg/day is effective in reducing tumor mass in cases of prolactinoma. Sexually active women should be cautioned about renewed fertility and pregnancy with the return of ovulatory menstrual periods. If neurosurgical excision is contemplated, the transsphenoidal route is preferred.

Deficient Secretion. — Hypoprolactinemia usually occurs as a manifestation of hypopituitarism. Except for the inability to lactate, patients are generally asymptomatic and no definitive therapy is required. Hypoprolactinemia has also been associated with pseudohypoparathyroidism, perhaps reflecting a generalized abnormality in adenyl cyclase–coupled receptors.

End Organ Insensitivity. — PRL resistance has not been described; however, asymptomatic prolactin-secreting microadenomas may define this entity.

Luteinizing Hormone and Follicle-Stimulating Hormone

Molecular Structure and Genetics. — LH and FSH are glycoproteins with very similar structural homology to each other, to chorionic gonadotropin (CG), and to thyrotropin. Each is composed of two noncovalently linked peptide chains. The alpha subunit is identical in all these glycoproteins; the beta subunit assigns immunologic and biologic specificity. However, biologic activity requires an intact alpha-beta dimer. The alpha subunit is encoded on the q21.1–23 region of chromosome 6.[74] The genes for the LH and CG beta subunits are located on chromosome 19q13.32; the gene for the FSH beta subunit has been mapped to chromosome 11p13.[74]

Secretion and Regulation. — Gonadotropin-containing cells may be identified in the fetal pituitary by 15 to 20 weeks of gestation.[3] Synthesis and secretion of LH and FSH are regulated by GnRH, sex steroids, and nonsteroidal gonadal peptides throughout fetal life, infancy, childhood, and adulthood. Thus, gonadotropin regulation is influenced by gender, pubertal stage, and, in women, the phase of the menstrual cycle. Gonadotropin secretion begins in midgestation by the fetal pituitary. In boys, increased secretion of gonadotropins leads to elevation in serum testosterone levels in very early infancy. Then, with the onset of central restraint of GnRH, gonadotropin levels decline during childhood, remaining quiescent until puberty. In infant girls, gonadotropin levels may remain elevated for the first 2 years of life, the levels declining later than in boys and increasing earlier at puberty. With the attainment of skeletal maturation (bone age ~10 years in girls and ~11 years in boys), there is loss of central restraint upon GnRH secretion; the first manifestation of such is nocturnal (sleep-associated) secretion of LH. The amplitude and frequency of these pulses increase as puberty progresses, occurring approximately every 2 hours by late puberty. FSH concentrations increase in early puberty and then plateau. In females, this pulsatility leads to gonadal maturation; the rhythmicity of LH and FSH secretion leads to regulation of the ovulatory menstrual cycle.

Because LH secretion is stimulated by GnRH, factors that positively influence GnRH synthesis and release positively contribute to LH secretion. GnRH influences FSH secretion as well; an additional specific FSH-releasing factor has been postulated but not identified.

Several standards and commercial kits have been developed to measure immunoreactive LH and FSH (LHi, FSHi). Presently, serum concentrations of LH and FSH are expressed as international units per liter of the Second International Reference Preparation–Human Menopausal Gonadotropin (2nd IRP-HMG). At puberty, the glycosylation patterns of the gonadotropin molecules are modified slightly, which may render them structurally unrecognizable by RIA. However, the biologic activity (b) of the molecules may increase. Thus the b/i ratio increases at puberty.[81]

Gonadotropin secretion is inhibited by sex hormones. In addition, the gonadal peptide inhibin selectively inhibits FSH secretion. Inhibin is composed of two subunits: the intact molecule is an alpha-beta dimer. Interestingly, a homodimeric beta-beta molecule has the opposite effects on FSH secretion. Such molecules have been termed *activins*. It is of interest that FSH antagonistic peptides have been demonstrated in patients that have received GnRH antagonists. The regulatory role of such peptides in gonadotropin secretion is uncertain.[25]

Function.—LH promotes androgen (testosterone) secretion in the Leydig cells of the testes and the ovarian thecal cells (androstenedione). In girls, FSH secretion promotes granulosa cell proliferation and inhibin synthesis and is required for aromatase activity to synthesize estrogen (estradiol) from androstenedione. In the late follicular phase, LH and FSH, in concert, promote progesterone secretion. FSH induces LH receptors in the granulosa cells. These luteinized granulosa cells further augment estradiol and progesterone secretion. At midcycle, ovulation is mediated by a pulse of LH. In males, FSH stimulates Sertoli cells to synthesize inhibin and to support the maturation and development of spermatozoa.

Mechanism of Action.—The gonadotropins act upon specific receptors. The LH-CG receptor is a 689-amino-acid glycoprotein that is coupled to a G protein and adenyl cyclase. A similar structure for the FSH receptor is proposed. The precise intracellular mechanism of signal transduction is uncertain.

Clinical Data.—Disorders of LH and FSH secretion are best discussed in relation to disorders of gonadal development and function and are therefore discussed fully in Chapters 7 and 8.

Thyrotropin

Molecular Structure and Genetics.—TSH is a 206-amino-acid dimeric (alpha and beta subunits) glycoprotein that is structurally related to the gonadotropins and to CG. The alpha subunit is shared by all these proteins. The unique TSH beta subunit is encoded by chromosome 1 p22.[74] The separately synthesized α and β chains bind within the pituitary thyrotrope. The interested reader is referred to a complete description of TSH biosynthesis.[70]

Secretion and Regulation.—Glycoprotein-containing cells appear in the fetal pituitary by 12 to 15 weeks of gestation; TSH has been identified at 15 weeks. Fetal serum TSH levels begin to increase shortly afterward stimulating the fetal thyroid.

TSH levels plateau by late gestation. However, during parturition and immediately after birth, there is a large surge of TSH release, probably in response to a rapid decrease in fetal body temperature. By 48 to 72 hours post partum, basal TSH levels are again attained, which underlines the importance of the timing of blood samples obtained for newborn thyroid screening programs. This postnatal TSH pulse is attenuated in preterm, small-for-gestational-age, and sick full-term infants.

TSH secretion is regulated by hypothalamic TRH secretion. TSH secretion is circadian; there is increased nocturnal (sleep-associated) TSH release. Estrogen promotes TSH synthesis. TSH secretion is inhibited by T_3 (negative feedback), SRIF, dopamine, and glucocorticoids.

Function and Mechanism of Action.—TSH acts on specific receptors: 744-amino-acid structures that couple a G-binding protein and adenyl cyclase. The gene for the TSH receptor is located on the q11–13 region of chromosome 22.[74] The action of the pituitary-thyroid axis is discussed in Chapter 5.

Clinical Data.—*Excessive Secretion.*—Hyperthyrotropinemia is the usual hallmark of primary thyroid insufficiency. The various etiologies of this entity are discussed in Chapter 5. Of special interest are syndromes of inappropriate TSH secretion. Such patients generally have TSH-secreting tumors or a manifestation of thyroid hormone resistance.

Deficient Secretion.—Hypothyrotropinemia either reflects pituitary suppression of TSH by a hyperfunctioning thyroid gland, or is a manifestation of hypopituitarism.

End Organ Insensitivity.—TSH resistance has not been described definitively.

Empty Sella Syndrome

Empty-sella syndrome (ESS) develops when the sella turcica is partially filled with CSF. This condition may occur as a primary event when the subarachnoid space herniates through the sellar diaphragm superiorly, or secondarily with diminution of intrasellar contents following pituitary insult such as trauma (e.g., surgery), toxin (e.g., irradiation), vascular accident, or possibly, inflammation; autoimmune disease has been implicated.[60] The incidence of ESS is approximately 24% in children with disorders of the hypothalamic-pituitary unit including documented or suspected GH deficiency, DI, delayed or precocious puberty, and hyperprolactinemia.[102] On the other hand, the incidence of ESS in normal children is unknown. However, only 1% of pediatric patients with radiographic ESS have pituitary dysfunction. ESS in adults occurs most often in obese, hypertensive, middle-aged, multiparous women; in children with primary ESS in whom an enlarged sella is not identified, the gender ratio is equal with no preponderance of obesity. The diagnosis is confirmed by CT scan or MRI.

PINEAL GLAND

Neuroanatomy

Lying outside the blood-brain barrier, the pineal gland is attached to the diencephalon by the pineal stalk into which extends the third ventricle. The pineal is separated from the Sylvian aqueduct by the tectal plate. Embryologically, the pineal develops from a diverticulum of the diencephalon during the second month of gestation. It is composed of pineocytes, glial cells, neurons, connective tissue, Pastori's ganglion, and acervuli (calcified areas that develop during infancy but which usually do not image radiographically until puberty).

The pineal innervation is from the suprachiasmatic nucleus, through the medial forebrain bundle and the lateral columns of the spinal cord, thence back to the superior cervical ganglion of the sympathetic chain.

Pineal Hormones

Melatonin

Biochemistry.—Although the pineal contains many small neuropeptides and neurogenic amines, the primary secretory products are indolamines, agents derived from tryptophan metabolism. Melatonin is the primary and best-studied indolamine. The synthesis of melatonin from tryptophan involves four enzymatic steps. The rate-limiting step appears to be the third enzyme in the pathway: serotonin N-acetyltransferase which converts serotonin to N-acetylserotonin.[39] The most important enzymatic step, however, is the fifth enzyme, hydroxyindole-O-methyltransferase (HIOMT), which converts N-acetylserotonin to melatonin. HIOMT is found almost exclusively in the pineal and to a smaller amount in the retina. The enzymes involved with metatonin biosynthesis are regulated by this substrate as well as by α_1- and β-adrenergic mechanisms, VIP, NP-Y, and possibly GABA, pentagastrin, and acetylcholine.[109]

Secretion and Regulation.—Melatonin synthesis and secretion is primarily regulated by photoirradiation, as the suprachiasmatic nucleus is innervated by the retina. Pineal melatonin levels are lowest at noon and reach greatest concentration at night. Electromagnetic field exposure decreases pineal melatonin synthesis. Melatonin diffuses into the bloodstream as pineal levels increase. However, despite this photoperiodicity, a circadian rhythm of melatonin synthesis can be demonstrated. Melatonin receptors have been identified in the suprachiasmatic nuclei.[84] Alterations in the length of daytime cause changes in the duration and amplitude of melatonin secretion. A schematic of pineal regulation is shown in Figure 3–9.

Function.—The precise roles of melatonin are uncertain. There is evidence for its function as an internal "timekeeper"[84] and therefore its role in the regulation of puberty has been investigated. Melatonin probably affects the reproductive system; low gonadotropin levels and delayed puberty have been noted in blind boys[11] while precocious puberty has been described in children with destructive lesions and neo-

FIG 3–9.
Pineal gland regulation.
GnRH = gonadotropin-releasing hormone; *TRH* =
thyrotropin-releasing hormone;
FSH = follicle-stimulating
hormone; *LH* = luteinizing
hormone; *TSH* = thyroid-
stimulating hormone;
ACTH = adrenocorticotropin;
PRL = prolactin;
MSH = melanocyte-
stimulating hormone;
GH = growth hormone;
T₃ = thyroxine;
T₄ = triiodothyronine.
(Adapted from Foley PB,
Cairncross KD, Foldes A:
Neurosci Behav Rev 1986;
10:273. Used by permission.)

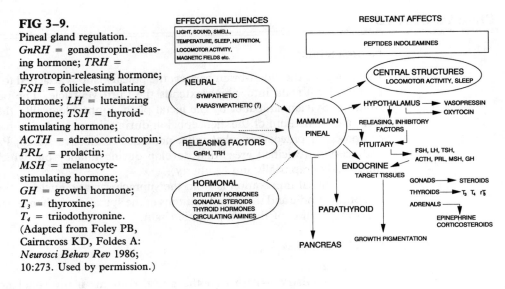

TABLE 3–11.
Tumors of the Pineal Gland

Germ cell tumors	Other
Germinoma	Meningioma
Embryonal cell carcinoma	Melanoma
Endodermal sinus tumor	Paraganglioma
Choriocarcinoma	Craniopharyngioma
Teratoma	Cysts
Pineocytomas	Arachnoid cyst
Ganglioglioma	Epidermoid cyst
Pinealoblastoma	Infectious cyst
Glial cell tumors	Parasitic
Astrocytoma	Abscess
Ependymoma	Granuloma
Choroid plexus papilloma	

plasms of the pineal.[19] The relation between the pineal and carcinogenesis has been investigated.[119]

Clinical Data.—Definitive pathologic conditions of the pineal gland involve neoplastic formation. Pineal tumors make up 1% of intracranial neoplasms.[57, 69] Known tumors of the pineal are listed in Table 3–11. Such tumors present with symptoms and signs of increased intracranial pressure owing to obstruction at either the aqueduct of Sylvius or the third ventricle or with motor ataxia resulting from tumor extension onto the cerebellum. Pineal tumors occur more often in men and there is a higher incidence among Oriental populations.[69] Therapy involves surgical and radioablative measures. Chemotherapies are largely ineffective.[69]

REFERENCES

1. Anderson KE, et al: Prevention of cyclical attacks of acute intermittent porphyria with a long-acting agonist of luteinizing hormone-releasing hormone. *N Engl J Med* 1984; 311:643.
2. Antoni FA: Hypothalamic control of adrenocorticotropin secretion: Advances since the discovery of 41-residue corticotropin-releasing factor. *Endocr Rev* 1986; 7:351.
3. Asa SL, et al: Human fetal adenohypophysis: Electron microscopic and ultrastructural immunocytochemical analysis. *Neuroendocrinology* 1988; 48:423.
4. Barkan AL, Beitins IZ, Kelch RP: Plasma insulin-like growth factor-I/somatomedin-C in acromegaly: Correlation with the degree of growth hormone hypersecretion. *J Clin Endocrinol Metab* 1988; 67:69.
5. Barton DE, et al: Chromosome mapping of the growth hormone receptor gene in man and mouse. *Cytogenet Cell Genet* 1989; 50:137.
6. Bateman A, et al: The immune-hypothalamic-pituitary-adrenal axis. *Endocri Rev* 1989; 10:92.
7. Baumann G, Shaw MA, Amburn K: Regulation of plasma growth hormone–binding proteins in health and disease. *Metabolism* 1989; 38:683.
8. Baumann G, Shaw MA, Merimee TJ: Low levels of high-affinity growth hormone-binding protein in African pygmies. *N Engl J Med* 1989; 320:1705.
9. Baumann G, Shaw MA, Winter RJ: Absence of the plasma growth hormone–binding protein in Laron-type dwarfism. *J Clin Endocrinol Metab* 1987; 65:814.
10. Beck-Peccoz P, et al: Treatment of hyperthyroidism due to inappropriate secretion of thyrotropin with the somatostatin analog SMS 201-995. *J Clin Endocrinol Metab* 1989; 68:208.
11. Bellastella A, et al: Influence of blindness on plasma luteinizing hormone, follicle-stimulating hormone, prolactin, and testosterone levels in prepubertal boys. *J Clin Endocrinol Metab* 1987; 64:862.
12. Bercu BB: Growth hormone neurosecretory dysfunction: Update, in Bercu BB (ed): *Basic and Clinical Aspects of Growth Hormone.* New York, Plenum Press, 1988.
13. Bercu BB, Diamond F: A determinant of stature: Regulation of growth hormone secretion, in Barness L (ed): *Advances in Pediatrics.* Chicago, Year Book Medical Publishers, 1986.
14. Bercu BB, Diamond F: Growth hormone neurosecretory dysfunction. *Clin Endocrinol Metab* 1986; 15:537.
15. Bercu BB, et al: Growth hormone provocative testing frequently does not reflect endogenous GH secretion. *J Clin Endocrinol Metab* 1986; 63:709.
16. Bernton EW, Meltzer MS, Holaday JW: Suppression of macrophage activation and T-lymphocyte function in hypoprolactinemic mice. *Science* 1988; 239:401.
17. Blumberg DL, et al: Acromegaly in an infant. *Pediatrics* 1989; 83:998.
18. Bongiovanni AM: Prolactin: A review with pediatric clinical implications. *Adv Pediatr* 1985; 32:439.
19. Brzezinski A, Wurtman RJ: The pineal gland: Its possible roles in human reproduction. *Obstet Gynecol Surv* 1988; 43:197.
20. Bost KL, Blalock JE: Molecular characterization of a corticotropin (ACTH) receptor. *Mol Cell Endocrinol* 1986; 44:1,
21. Burke BA, et al: Congenital adrenal hypoplasia and selective absence of pituitary luteinizing hormone: A new autosomal recessive syndrome. *Am J Med Genet* 1988; 31:75.

22. Chard T: Fetal and maternal oxytocin in human parturition. *Am J Perinatol* 1989; 6:145.

23. Christiansen P, et al: Treatment of cryptorchidism with human chorionic gonadotropin or gonadotropin releasing hormone: A double-blind controlled study of 243 boys. *Horm Res* 1988; 30:187.

24. Clayton RN: Gonadotrophin-releasing hormone: Its actions and receptors. *J Endocrinol* 1989; 120:11.

25. Dahl KD, Bicsak TA, Hsueh AJW: Naturally occurring antihormones: Secretion of FSH antagonists by women treated with a GnRH analog. *Science* 1988; 239:72.

26. Dardenne M, et al: Neuroendocrine control of thymic hormonal production: I. Prolactin stimulates *in vivo* and *in vitro* the production of thymulin by human and murine thymic epithelial cells. *Endocrinology* 1989; 125:3.

27. Delemarre-Van de Waal HA, et al: Leukemia in patients treated with growth hormone. *Lancet* 1988; 1:1159.

28. Demitrack MA, Gold PW: Oxytocin: Neurobiologic considerations and their implications for affective illness. *Prog Neuropsychopharmagol Biol Psychiatry* 1988; 12:S23.

29. De Muinck Keizer-Schrama SMPF: Hormonal treatment of cryptorchidism. *Horm Res* 1988; 30:178.

30. Dieguez C, Page MD, Scanlon MF: Growth hormone neuroregulation and its alteration in disease states. *Clin Endocrinol* 1988; 28:109.

31. Donaldson DL, et al: Growth hormone secretory profiles: Variation on consecutive nights. *J Pediatr* 1989; 115:51.

32. Dyer RG: Oxytocin and parturition: New complications. *J Endocrinol* 1988;116:167.

33. Edwards CK III, et al: A newly defined property of somatotropin: Priming of macrophages for production of superoxide anion, *Science* 1988; 239:769.

34. Ehrmann DA, et al: A new test of combined pituitary-testicular function using the gonadotropin-releasing hormone agonist nafarelin in the differentiation of gonadotropin deficiency from delayed puberty: Pilot studies, *J Clin Endocrinol Metab* 1989; 69:693.

35. Eipper BA, Mains RE: Structure and biosynthesis of proadrenocorticotropin/endorphin and related peptides. *Endocr Rev* 1980; 1:1.

36. Everitt BJ, Hokfelt T: Neuroendocrine anatomy of the hypothalamus, *Acta Neurochir [suppl] (Wien)* 1990; 47:1.

37. Filicori M, Flamigni C: GnRH agonists and antagonists: current clinical status. *Drugs* 1988; 35:63.

38. Fisher DA, et al: Leukemia in patients treated with growth hormone. *Lancet* 1988; 1:1159.

39. Foley PB, Cairncross KD, Foldes A: Pineal indoles: Significance and measurement. *Neurosci Behav Rev* 1986; 10:273.

40. Fradkin JE, et al: Creutzfeldt-Jakob disease in pituitary growth hormone recipients in the United States. Presented at 72nd Annual Meeting of the Endocrine Society, 1990, abstract 1301, p 350.

41. Frankenne F, et al: Expression of the growth hormone variant gene in human placenta. *J Clin Endocrinol Metab* 1987; 64:635.

42. Frasier SD, et al: A water deprivation test for the diagnosis of diabetes insipidus in children. *Am J Dis Child* 1967; 114:157.

43. Frohman LA: Neurotransmitters as regulators of endocrine function, in Krieger DT, Hughes JC (eds): *Neuroendocrinology.* Sunderland, Mass, Sinauer Associates, 1980.

44. Frohman LA: The role of hypothalamic hormones in the control of growth hormone secretion and growth, *Acta Paediatr Scand [suppl]* 1988;343:3.

45. Geffner ME, et al: Selective ACTH insensitivity, achalasia, and alacrima: A multisystem disorder presenting in childhood. *Pediatr Res* 1983; 17:532.
46. Gibbs DM: Vasopressin and oxytocin: Hypothalamic modulators of the stress response: A review. *Psychoneuroendocrinology* 1986; 11:131.
47. Gomez-Muguruza MT, Chrousos GP: Periodic Cushing syndrome in a short boy: Usefulness of the ovine corticotropin releasing hormone test. *J Pediatr* 1989; 115:270.
48. Gonzalez-Barcena D, et al: Response to D-Trp-6-LH-RH in advanced adenocarcinoma of pancreas. *Lancet* 1984; 1:154.
49. Halma C, et al: Life-threatening water intoxication during somatostatin therapy. *Ann Intern Med* 1987; 107:518.
50. Hazum E, Conn PM: Molecular mechanism of gonadotropin releasing hormone (GnRH) action: I. The GnRH receptor, *Endocr Rev* 1988; 9:379.
51. Hindmarsh PC, et al: The half-life of exogenous growth hormone after suppression of endogenous growth hormone secretion with somatostatin. *Clin Endocrinol* 1989; 30:443.
52. Hinkle PM: Pituitary TRH receptors, *Ann NY Acad Sci* 1989; 553:176.
53. Horvath E: Pituitary hyperplasia. *Pathol Res Pract* 1988; 183:623.
54. Huckle WR, Conn PM: Molecular mechanism of gonadotropin releasing hormone action: II. The effector system. *Endocr Rev* 1988; 9:387.
55. Kaplan SA: Growth and growth hormone: Disorders of the anterior pituitary, in Kaplan SA (ed): *Clinical Pediatric Endocrinology*. Philadelphia, WB Saunders Co, 1990.
56. Kaplan SL, Grumbach MM: Final height of non-growth hormone deficient children with short stature treated with hGH. Presented at Genentech National Cooperative Growth Study Symposium IV, 1989; abstract 9.
57. Klein P, Rubinstein LJ: Benign symptomatic glial cysts of the pineal gland: A report of seven cases and review of the literature. *J Neurol Neurosurg Psychiatry* 1989; 52:991.
58. Knoers N, Monnens LAH: Amiloride-hydrochlorothiazide versus indomethacin-hydrochlorothiazide in the treatment of nephrogenic diabetes insipidus. *J Pediatr* 1990; 117:499.
59. Knudtzon J: Effects of pro-opiomelanocortin-derived peptides of plasma levels of glucagon, insulin and glucose. *Horm Metab Res* 1986; 18:579.
60. Komatsu M, et al: Antipituitary antibodies in patients with the primary empty sella syndrome. *J Clin Endocrinol Metab* 1988; 67:633.
61. Krieger DT: The hypothalamus and neuroendocrinology, in Krieger DT, Hughes JC (eds): *Neuroendocrinology*. Sunderland, Mass, Sinauer Associates, 1980.
62. Krishnan S, Maickel RP: Stress, ACTH and free-choice ethanol consumption in rats. Presented at 21st Congress of the International Society of Psychoneuroendocrinology, Buffalo, NY, 1990.
63. Lamberts SWJ: The role of somatostatin in the regulation of anterior pituitary hormone secretion and the use of its analogs in the treatment of human pituitary tumors. *Endocr Rev* 1988; 9:417.
64. Lechan RM: Neuroendocrinology of pituitary hormone regulation. *Endocrinol Metab Clin* 1987; 16:475.
65. Legros J-J, Timsit-Berthier M: Vasopressin and vasopressin analogues for treatment of memory disorders in clinical practice. *Prog Neuropsychopharmacol Biol Psychiatry* 1988; 12:S71.
66. Lewitt MS, Baxter RC: Inhibitors of glucose uptake stimulate the production of insulin-like growth factor–binding protein (IGFBP-1) by human fetal liver. *Endocrinology* 1990; 126:1527.

67. Linton EA, Lowry RJ: Corticotrophin releasing factor in man and its measurement: A review. *Clin Endocrinol* 1989; 31:225.

68. Lynch JL, Gavin JR III: Growth hormone binding proteins in short children with normal neurosecretory growth hormone regulation. Presented at 71st Annual Meeting of the Endocrine Society, 1989, abstract 1672, p 440.

69. Macfarlane R, Marks PV: Tumours of the pineal region. *Br J Hosp Med* 1989; 41:548.

70. Magner JA: Thyroid-stimulating hormone: Biosynthesis, cell biology, and bioactivity. *Endocr Rev* 1990; 11:354.

71. Manson JM, Wilmore DW: Use of growth hormone in surgery, in Bercu BB (ed): *Basic and Clinical Aspects of Growth Hormone*. New York, Plenum Press, 1988.

72. Marshall JC, Kelch RP: Gonadotropin-releasing hormone: Role of pulsatile secretion in the regulation of reproduction. *N Engl J Med* 1986; 315:1459.

73. Martha PM Jr, et al: Alterations in the pulsatile properties of circulating growth hormone concentrations during puberty in boys. *J Clin Endocrinol Metab* 1989; 69:563.

74. McKusick VA: Mapping the genes for hormones and growth factors and the mutations causing disorders of growth. *Growth Genet Horm* 1989; 5:1.

75. Melmed S: Acromegaly. *N Engl J Med* 1990; 322:966.

76. Moran A, et al: Gigantism due to pituitary mammosomatotroph hyperplasia. *N Engl J Med* 1990; 323:322.

77. Mullis P, et al: Isolated growth hormone deficiency: Analysis of the growth hormone (GH)–releasing hormone gene and the GH gene cluster. *J Clin Endocrinol Metab* 1990; 70:187.

78. Naor Z, et al: Mechanism of action of gonadotropin-releasing hormone on pituitary gonadotropin secretion. *J Reprod Fertil* 1989; 37(suppl):295.

79. Nash JF, Maickel RP: The role of the hypothalamic-pituitary-adrenocortical axis in post-stress induced ethanol consumption by rats. *Prog Neuropsychopharmacol Biol Psychiatry*, 1988; 12:653.

80. Nieman LK, et al: The ovine corticotropin-releasing hormone (CRH) stimulation test is superior to the human CRH stimulation test for the diagnosis of Cushing's disease. *J Clin Endocrinol Metab* 1989; 69:165.

81. Padmanabhan V, Chappel SC, Beitins IZ: An improved *in vitro* bioassay for follicle-stimulating hormone (FSH): Suitable for measurement of FSH in unextracted human serum. *Endocrinology* 1987; 121:1089.

82. Page MD, et al: A clinical update of hypothalamic-pituitary control. *Acta Neurochirurgica [Suppl] (Wien)* 1990; 47:48.

83. Parker LN, Lifrak ET, Odell WD: A 60,000 molecular weight human pituitary glycopeptide stimulates adrenal androgen secretion. *Endocrinology* 1983; 113:2092.

84. Reppert SM, et al: Putative melatonin receptors in a human biological clock. *Science* 1988; 242:78.

85. Richardson DW, Robinson AG: Desmopressin. *Ann Intern Med* 1985; 103:228.

86. Rimoin DL, Graham JM Jr: Syndromes associated with growth deficiency, *Acta Paediatr Scand [Suppl]* 1989; 349:3.

87. Robertson GL, Harris A: Clinical use of vasopressin analogues. *Hosp Pract* 1989; 24:114.

88. Root AW: Neurophysiologic regulation of the secretion of growth hormone. *J Endocrinol Invest* 1989; 12(suppl 3):3.

89. Root AW, Diamond F: The pituitary gland, in Kelly VC (ed): *Practice of Pediatrics*, Philadelphia, Harper & Row, 1982, p 181.

90. Root AW, et al: Subhypothalamic high-intensity signals identified by magnetic reso-

nance imaging in children with idiopathic anterior hypopituitarism. *Am J Dis Child* 1989; 143:366.

91. Rose SR, et al: The advantage of measuring stimulated as compared with spontaneous growth hormone levels in the diagnosis of growth hormone deficiency. *N Engl J Med* 1988; 319:201.

92. Rosenfeld RG, et al: Identification of insulin-like growth factor-binding protein-2 (IGF-BP-2) and a low molecular weight IGF-BP in human seminal plasma. *J Clin Endocrinol Metab* 1990; 70:551.

93. Rudman D, et al: Effects of growth hormone in men over 60 years old. *N Engl J Med* 1990; 323:1.

94. Salomon F, et al: The effects of treatment with recombinant human growth hormone on body composition and metabolism in adults with growth hormone deficiency. *N Engl J Med* 1989; 321:1797.

95. Sano T, Asa SL, Kovacs K: Growth hormone-releasing hormone–producing tumors: Clinical, biochemical, and morphological manifestations. *Endocr Rev* 1988; 9:357.

96. Sapolsky R, et al: Interleukin-1 stimulates the secretion of hypothalamic-corticotropin-releasing factor. *Science* 1987; 238:522.

97. Sasaki A, et al: Multiple forms of immunoreactive growth hormone-releasing hormone in human plasma, hypothalamus, and tumor tissues. *J Clin Endocrinol Metab* 1989; 68:180.

98. Schwartz ID, et al: Diabetes insipidus in children under age 2 years: Experience with intranasal desmopressin (abstract) (DDAVP). *Pediatr Res* 1989; 25:93A.

99. Schwartz ID, et al: Linear growth response to exogenous growth hormone (GH) in children with short stature. *Am J Dis Child* 1990; 144:1092.

100. Shah BR, et al: Familial glucocorticoid deficiency in a girl with familial hypophosphatemic rickets. *Am J Dis Child* 1988; 142:900.

101. Shoemaker J, et al: Induction of first cycles in primary hypothalamic amenorrhea with pulsatile luteinizing hormone–releasing hormone: A mirror of female pubertal development. *Fertil Steril* 1987; 48:204.

102. Shulman DI, et al: Hypothalamic-pituitary dysfunction in primary empty sella syndrome in childhood. *J Pediatr* 1986; 108:540.

103. Silbergeld A, et al: Serum growth hormone binding protein activity in healthy neonates, children, and young adults: Correlation with age, height, and weight. *Clin Endocrinol* 1989; 31:295.

104. Smith IA, Funder JW: Proopiomelanocortin processing in the pituitary, central nervous system, and peripheral tissues. *Endocr Rev* 1988; 9:159.

105. Smith MA, et al: Corticotropin-releasing hormone: From endocrinology to psychobiology. *Horm Res* 1989; 31:66.

106. Spiliotis BE, et al: Growth hormone neurosecretory dysfunction: A treatable cause of short stature. *JAMA* 1984; 251:2223.

107. Stanhope R, Pringle PJ, Brook CGD: The mechanism of the adolescent growth spurt induced by low dose pulsatile GnRH treatment. *Clin Endocri* 1988; 28:83.

108. Stanhope R, et al: Induction of puberty by pulsatile gonadotropin releasing hormone. *Lancet* 1987; 2:552.

109. Sugden D: Melatonin biosynthesis in the mammalian pineal gland. *Experientia* 1989; 45:922.

110. Taylor AL, Fishman LM: Corticotropin-releasing hormone. *N Engl J Med* 1988; 319:213.

111. Thorner MO, et al: Acceleration of growth rate in growth hormone-deficient children

treated with human growth hormone–releasing hormone. *Pediatr Res* 1988; 24:145.

112. Usadel KH: Hormonal and nonhormonal cytoprotective effect by somatostatins. *Horm Res* 1988; 29:83.

113. Van Vliet G, Bergmann P: Glucagon increases the growth hormone response to growth hormone releasing hormone in normal men. Presented at 72nd Annual Meeting of the Endocrine Society 1990, abstract 1092, p 297.

114. Vidaller A, et al: T-cell dysregulation in patients with hyperprolactinemia: Effect of bromocriptine treatment. *Clin Immunol Immunopathol* 1986; 38:337.

115. Vokes TJ, Robertson GL: Disorders of antidiuretic hormone. *Endocrinol Metab Clin North Am* 1988; 17:281.

116. Watanabe S, et al: Leukemia in patients treated with growth hormone. *Lancet* 1988; 1:1159.

117. Weisberg LS: Pseudohyponatremia: A reappraisal. *Am J Med* 1989; 86:315.

118. Williams G, Bloom SR: Regulatory peptides, the hypothalamus and diabetes. *Diabetic Med* 1989; 6:472.

119. Wilson BW, Stevens RG, Anderson LE: Neuroendocrine mediated effects of electro-magnetic-field exposure: Possible role of the pineal gland. *Life Sci* 1989; 45:1319.

120. Wise JE, et al: Phenotypic features of patients with congenital adrenal hypoplasia and glycerol kinase deficiency. *Am J Dis Child* 1987; 141:744.

Chapter 4

Parathyroid Glands, Calcium, Phosphorus, and Vitamin D Metabolism

Allen W. Root

REGULATION OF CALCIUM AND PHOSPHORUS HOMEOSTASIS

Normal Physiology

Calcium, Phosphorus, Alkaline Phosphatase

Calcium is the most abundant cation in the body; 99% of the total body calcium store is present in bone where, together with phosphorus, it forms the skeleton providing the structural support of the body. Although only 1% of body calcium is to be found in the intra- and extracellular fluid spaces, calcium plays an extremely important role as an enzyme cofactor and in interneuronal and neuromuscular transmission, muscular contraction, intracellular communication (see Chapter 1), clotting, protein synthesis and secretion, and cellular proliferation. The extracellular serum concentrations of calcium are maintained within narrow limits by regulation of its intestinal absorption, by metabolites of vitamin D; its resorption from bone, primarily by parathyroid hormone (PTH) and vitamin D metabolites; and its resorption in the renal tubule after glomerular filtration, by PTH and vitamin D metabolites.[60]

More than 80% of the body's store of phosphorus is present in bone. In addition to its structural role, phosphorus is a component of the cell's plasma membrane lipids, high-energy adenosine triphosphate (ATP), DNA, and RNA; it is the key element in cellular function that occurs after protein phosphorylation by many protein kinases.

In serum, calcium circulates in the free, ionized state (Ca^{2+}), which is the biologically significant form; bound to serum proteins, primarily albumin, where it is relatively inert; and in an accessible, complexed, or chelated form. The serum concentration of Ca^{2+} is extremely sensitive to the acid-base balance: when the serum pH rises (alkalosis) more calcium is bound to albumin; when pH falls (acidosis) calcium is released from albumin. In bone, calcium is present in both a rapidly exchangeable compartment in equilibrium with extracellular Ca^{2+} and in a less readily available pool with a slower rate of Ca^{2+} turnover. There is a hypothetical fluid compartment immediately adjacent to the bone surface that is surrounded by a living membrane of osteocyte-like cells. This compartment, which is supersaturated with calcium, has been termed the "bone fluid."[60] The exchange of calcium between bone surface and extracellular fluid may take place through the bone fluid compartment, perhaps under the regulation of PTH. Calcium absorption from the intestine is primarily under the control of 1,25-dihydroxyvitamin D_3 [1,25$(OH)_2D_3$] and is important for the long-term regulation of calcium homeostasis. Changes in the rates of renal glomerular filtration of calcium and of calcium resorption from the distal convoluted renal tubule under the influence of PTH are the most rapid mechanisms for regulation of acute alterations in serum Ca^{2+} levels, but this mechanism has a limited capacity to correct either significant hypocalcemia or hypercalcemia. Resorption of calcium from bone, primarily through PTH stimulation of osteoclast activity, is a relatively rapid mechanism for restoration of calcium levels in hypocalcemia. Even in the complete absence of PTH, the serum Ca^{2+} concentration is maintained at a constant (but low) level, primarily due to resorption of calcium from bone by an undetermined mechanism. Calcitonin inhibits resorption of calcium from bone.

Calcium concentrations are highest in utero and fall rapidly after birth to a nadir at 24 to 48 hours of life, increasing thereafter to a "set point," which is maintained relatively constant. Careful examination reveals that Ca^{2+} concentrations decline slightly over the first 18 months of life and are lower in formula-fed than in human milk-fed infants.[82] There is a diurnal variation in calcium levels with the lowest values in the early morning hours (4 AM). Total, but not ionized, calcium values are lower in summer than in winter. Phosphorus concentrations are highest in the neonatal period and decline slowly through infancy and childhood. Serum concentrations of phosphorus are lower in black than in white infants, in winter than in summer, and in breast-fed as compared with formula-fed infants. It is important to recognize that serum phosphorus concentrations in infants and children (4–7 mg/dL) are considerably higher than levels in adults. The serum concentration of phosphorus also varies diurnally with a pattern reciprocal to that of Ca^{2+}.

There are multiple isomeric forms of alkaline phosphatase. There are separate genes for the intestinal and placental alkaline phosphatases, while one gene located on the short arm of chromosome 1 codes for the liver, bone, and kidney form of this enzyme.[18] The mechanism by which bone alkaline phosphatase synthesized by osteoblasts increases skeletal mineralization is unclear. Alkaline phosphatase had been thought to increase local concentrations of inorganic phosphorus by hydrolyzing phosphomonoesters such as phosphoethanolamine, pyrophosphate, or pyridoxal-5'-phosphate, all natural substrates for alkaline phosphatase, but these compounds are present in such low amounts that they are unlikely to increase greatly the local supply of inorganic phosphorus. It has also been suggested that alkaline phosphatase may act by transporting phosphorus and calcium to the mineralization site, by transphosphorylation, or by removing inhibitors of mineralization such as pyrophosphate from the site of mineralization.[18] However, alkaline phosphatase also regulates the formation of pyrophosphate which is necessary for the initial precipitation of calcium and phosphorus in the formation of hydroxyapatite. None of these proposed modes of action of alkaline phosphatase entirely explains the mechanism(s) by which alkaline phosphatase enhances bone mineralization.

Breast milk, cow milk, and soybean formulas contain sufficient calcium (300, 440, and 600 mg/L, respectively) for normal bone mineralization of the well, full-term infant through the first year of life.[40] However, the amount of phosphorus in human milk (150 mg/L) is less than that in cow milk and soybean formulas (300 and 475 mg/L, respectively), and in vitamin D–deficient, exclusively breast-feeding mothers, phosphorus deficiency may contribute to the development of metabolic bone disease in their infants. Introduction of solid foods in the second half of the first year of life increases phosphorus intake and is generally recommended.[40] Human breast milk contains too little phosphorus for the rapid accretion of bone which takes place in very low-birth-weight infants.

Bone Formation and Resorption

Eighty percent of the skeleton is composed of cortical or compact bone, found primarily in the shafts of the long bones, and 20% is composed of trabecular or spongy bone, located in the vertebrae, flat bones (of the skull and pelvis), and ends of the long bones. The turnover rate of trabecular bone is more rapid than that of compact bone because of its greater surface area, and, therefore, more susceptible to diseases that affect mineralization. Woven bone refers to irregularly distributed, coarsely formed bone seen primarily in areas of rapid bone formation (in the fetus, neonate, and infant, and in healing fracture sites); lamellar bone refers to the organized and ordered pattern seen in mature bone.[6]

Bone may develop either by endochondral or intramembranous bone formation. Intramembranous bone forms in the absence of cartilage by local condensation of mesenchymal cells. These cells are replaced by bone cells that secrete a fibrous matrix which is subsequently ossified.[6,64] Long bones develop from a cartilaginous anlage developed during chondrogenesis.[45] In the embryo the limb buds are composed of a layer of ectoderm covering undifferentiated mesenchymal cells; the latter develop into differentiated chondrocytes, cartilage-specific proteins are synthesized, and the long bone takes shape. The initial cartilage formed is resistant to vascular invasion because of its composition of specific collagens and proteoglycans. Hypertrophic chondrocytes (very large cells with properties different from the differentiated chondrocyte) appear in the middle of the long bone; the hypertrophic chondrocyte secretes proteins that do not inhibit penetration by vascular cells exterior to the cartilage. After invasion by vascular cells, cartilage matrix is destroyed, and the hypertrophic chondrocyte dies and is replaced by an osteoblast which accompanies the vascular cells into the cartilage.

Osteoblasts are derived from the stromal mesenchymal cell system.[60] The osteoblasts secrete bone matrix which is deposited locally on fragmented and incompletely degraded cartilage as the process of osteogenesis begins. This is followed by deposition of calcium and phosphorus, further degradation of residual cartilage, and bone remodeling. The areas of osteogenesis spread from the center of the long bones toward either end where the cartilage growth plate is formed. At the ends of the long bones are the cartilaginous epiphyses which develop a zone of proliferating chondrocytes distal to the hypertrophic chondrocytes. It is the layer of proliferating chondrocytes which permits the long bones to grow linearly. The growth plate then consists of the proliferating chondrocytes, which evolve into the hypertrophic chondrocytes. This zone is invaded by vascular cells and osteoblasts and osteogenesis ensues (Fig 4–1). Secondary ossification centers appear in the epiphyseal cartilage in a relatively reproducible time sequence, permitting estimation of skeletal maturity (bone age). Linear growth ceases when the growth plate has been replaced by bone.

Cartilage growth and bone formation are regulated by a number of extra- and intracartilaginous hormones and growth factors. Growth hormone influences the differentiation of chondrocytes and stimulates local synthesis of insulin-like growth factor I (IGF-I) and perhaps IGF-II, as well as increasing cell membrane receptors for a number of other growth factors.[45] IGF-I and IGF-II, transforming growth factor-β_1 (TGF-β_1), platelet-derived growth factor (PDGF), and basic fibroblast growth factor (bFGF) are present in human bone matrix. IGF-I, IGF-II, TFG-β_1, and PDGF are synthesized by human bone cells in vitro. PTH and estradiol stimulate the release of IGF-I, IGF-II, and TGF-β_1 from bone cells in vitro. These cells also secrete an IGF-binding protein which inhibits binding of IGF-II to its receptor on bone cells. Both IGF-I and IGF-II stimulate the proliferation of human bone cells in vitro; since the concentration of IGF-II in human bone is 10- to 12-fold higher and its in vitro secretion rate is 50-fold greater than those of IGF-I, it is likely that IGF-II is a major growth factor for cartilage. It may also be an important differentiating factor. PDGF and bFGF can also stimulate human bone cell proliferation in vitro while TGF-β_1 appears to be involved in osteoblast and osteoclast differentiation. These factors presumably act in an autocrine or paracrine manner.

Bone formation is coupled to bone resorption; osteoclasts are bone-resorbing cells which develop from bone marrow–derived mononuclear stem cells that also give rise

FIG 4–1.
Cartilage growth plate.

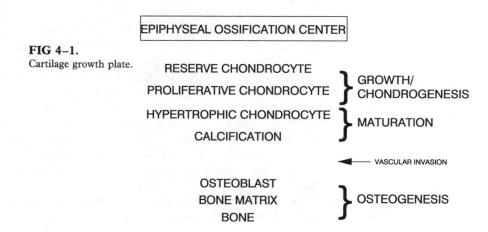

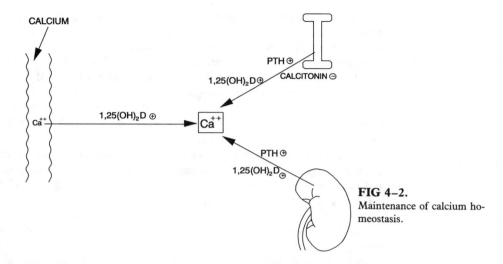

FIG 4–2.
Maintenance of calcium homeostasis.

to monocytes and macrophages. Interleukin-3 is thought to be the cytokine that initiates the differentiation of the stem cell to an osteoclast progenitor cell (stage I); colony-stimulating factor, tumor necrosis factor, TGF-α, and interleukin-1 are important for further differentiation to osteoclast progenitor cell stage II, while PTH, the PTH-related protein, and 1,25(OH)$_2$D$_3$ transform the committed osteoclast progenitor cell to the multinucleated osteoclast.[60] Interleukin-1 is the most potent of the osteotropic cytokines or growth-regulatory factors of immune cell origin.[62] It is effective at concentrations of 10^{-10} to 10^{-12} mol in vitro. Collectively, interleukins-1 and -6, tumor necrosis factor, differentiation-inducing factor, colony-stimulating factor, and TGF-α make up a group of osteoclast activating factors produced by immune cells. Interferon-γ and TGF-β inhibit proliferation and differentiation of osteoclast progenitor cells.[62] Once formed, the osteoclast acts on the endosteal and periosteal bone surfaces, where it adheres to the ruffled border of bone, a series of fingerlike projections which indent the bone. The osteoclast resorbs the mineral phase of bone by secreting acid which dissolves the calcium-phosphorus complex and the organic matrix of bone by secretion of collagenase and lysosomal proteolytic enzymes. After bone resorption is completed, a "reversal phase" ensues in which the resorptive site is "cleansed" by monocytes followed by the appearance of osteoblasts which lay down new bone at the resorptive site. The mechanisms(s) through which bone resorption is coupled to bone formation is unknown. Skeletal coupling factor(s), perhaps secreted by the osteoclasts themselves, have been proposed and include TGF-β$_1$ and TGF-β$_2$, IGF-I and IGF-II, osteoinductive factor, PDGF, and fibroblast growth factor.[60,62]

Sixty-five percent of the skeleton is inorganic mineral and 35% is organic substance, the majority of which is collagen. There are multiple forms of collagen[30]; the collagen molecule consists of three polypeptide chains in the form of a triple helix assembled into fibrils and bundles of fibers. Glycine is present as every third amino acid in the chain, which also contains lysine and proline in abundance.

The peptide chains that form collagen are synthesized (translated) as large peptides on the ribosome, and are processed further by cleavage of the prepropeptide to the propeptide, hydroxylation of lysine and proline, glycosylation of hydroxylysine with galactose and glucose, and inter- and intrachain disulfide bonding leading to association of the three propeptide chains into the triple helix formation characteristic of procollagen.[69,70] The C-terminal region of the propeptide is the site of initiation and direction of triple helix formation leading to assembly of the procollagen molecule.[74] After release of procollagen from the chondrocyte, the N- and C-terminal extensions are removed in the extracellular space and a number of triple helix fragments of collagen aggregate spontaneously and cross-link by oxidative deamination and condensation to form mature collagen.

At least 13 different types of collagen are derived from 25 gene products.[69,71] Type I collagen is found predominantly in bone, tendon, ligament, fascia, and skin, and is composed of two procollagen α_1 and one procollagen α_2 chains whose genes are located on chromosomes 17q21.31–q22.05 (COL1A1) and 7q21.3–q22.1(COL1A2), respectively. It is the most abundant type of collagen. Type II collagen, present in cartilage, vitreous tissue, and nucleus pulposus, is composed of three procollagen α_1 chains (chromosome 12q13.1–q13.3; COL2A1). Type III collagen is present in bone, tendon, arteries, and intestine (chromosome 2q31; COL3A1). Type IV collagen is found in many tissues with basement membranes; it is a dimer composed of one molecule each of procollagen α_1 and α_2 (chromosome 13q34; COL4A1, COL4A2). The mature collagens can be separated into three groups: Group 1 consists of very long α chains with continuous collagen domains which form fibrils, and includes types I, II, III, V, and XI. Type I collagenopathies are characterized by defects which disturb the intracellular assembly of the collagen polypeptide chains and thus its helical structure (osteogenesis imperfecta), or by abnormalities of the processing of procollagen to collagen in extracellular sites (Ehlers-Danlos syndrome, type VII). Defects in type II cartilage formation lead to various chondrodystrophies (chondroepiphyseal dysplasia). Group 2 collagens are composed of long α chains with discontinuous collagen domains, and consist of collagen types IV, VI, VII, and VIII. The group 3 collagens are nonfibrillar, and are composed of short α chains (types IX, X, XII, XIII). Nonfibrillar cartilage molecules are present in bone and cartilage where they stabilize and bridge the fibrillar collagen molecules and link fibrils with other components in the matrix. Procollagen molecules are measurable in serum; their concentrations reflect the synthesis and metabolism of collagen, and secondarily of growth.[74] In normal infants and children the serum concentration of the C-terminal propeptide of type I procollagen is approximately 2,500 μg/L, falling to 50 to 150 μg/L in adults; the serum level of the NH_2-terminal propeptide of type III procollagen in infants is 40 to 50 μg/L; it falls to approximately 7 μg/L by 2 years of age, and to 3 to 4 μg/L in adults.[74]

Several bone matrix noncollagenous proteins have been identified. Osteocalcin (mol wt 6 kDa) is a vitamin K–dependent protein containing three γ-carboxyglutamic acid (Gla) residues synthesized by osteoblasts and is found in bone, dentin, and plasma. Through the Gla residues, osteocalcin binds hydroxyapatite avidly and calcium weakly. Plasma concentrations of osteocalcin reflect osteoblast activity and hence bone formation, although the physiologic role for this peptide is not clear. The active vitamin D metabolite $1,25(OH)_2D_3$ stimulates formation of osteocalcin acting at the level of gene transcription. Osteonectin (mol wt 32 kDa) is a protein that binds collagen and hydroxyapatite and may be important for initiation of matrix calcification. Several of the TGF-β factors (a family of dimeric peptides of mol wt 25 kDa) increase synthesis and secretion of collagen types I through V and numerous other matrix proteins, including osteonectin, by increasing gene transcription and by stabilizing their messenger RNA (mRNA).[76]

Parathyroid Hormone (Fig 4–2)

The parathyroid glands are paired structures derived from the third (inferior pole parathyroids) and fourth (superior pole parathyroids) branchial arches. Occasionally a parathyroid gland may be within the parenchyma of the thyroid or in the mediastinum. There may also be five parathyroid glands on occasion. Parathyroid hormone (mol wt 9.6 kDa) is an 84-amino-acid peptide which raises serum calcium concentrations by increasing calcium resorption in the distal renal tubule, mobilizing calcium from bone by enhancing osteoclast differentiation and activity, and increasing calcium absorption in the intestinal tract through stimulation of renal 25-hydroxyvitamin D (25OHD)–1α-hydroxylase activity and increased production of $1,25(OH)_2D_3$, the biologically active metabolite of vitamin D. However, PTH downregulates the gene for the vitamin D receptor.[73] The gene for human PTH is located on the short arm of chromosome 11 and codes for a 115-amino-acid prepro-PTH molecule that is processed in the endoplasmic reticulum to a 90-amino-acid pro-PTH peptide. The N-terminal 6 amino acids are enzymatically removed leaving the mature 84-residue PTH. The entire biologic activity of PTH resides in the N-terminal 1–34 segment of PTH, while some biologic activity is present in as few as the first 28 amino acids of the N-terminal segment. The N-terminal amino acids arginine and valine are critical for biologic activity. PTH binds to its receptor through residues 25–27 (Arg-Lys-Lys) and through a sequence within the first 15 amino acids as well. In the parathyroid chief cell, the site of PTH synthesis and secretion, PTH is packaged into secretory granules in its mature 84-amino-acid form and secreted intact, primarily in response to a decline in Ca^{2+} concentration.

Adrenergic agonists and prostaglandins (PGE) stimulate, while $1,25(OH)_2D_3$ suppresses, PTH secretion by down-regulating gene activity for this product.[60] Magnesium effects PTH release but not synthesis, as well as the target cell response to PTH. A modest decline in magnesium concentration enhances PTH secretion, but significant hypomagnesemia suppresses PTH release and decreases the osteoclast response to PTH. Parathyroid hormone is co-localized within its secretory granule with secretory protein I or chromogranin A, and the two proteins are released concurrently in response to hypocalcemia. Chromogranin A is a large protein present in many endocrine and neuroendocrine cells, secreted in tandem with the primary cell product. Chromogranin A is a propeptide for a daughter peptide of 49 amino acids which is able to inhibit the secretion of PTH and other protein hormones (including pancreatic insulin, hence its designation as pancreastatin). Chromogranin A and pancreastatin may represent an autocrine mechanism of control of the secretion of PTH and other peptide hormones.[28]

After release, PTH is rapidly degraded to the 1–33 NH_2 and 34–48 COOH terminal fragments; there is relatively little intact bioactive PTH in the circulation. Parathyroid hormone binds to cell membrane receptors, acts through a guanosine

(G)-binding protein to increase adenyl cyclase activity, cyclic adenosine monophosphate (cAMP) production, and phosphoinositide-specific phospholipase and protein kinase activities. In bone the resorptive effects of PTH are enhanced by $1,25(OH)_2D$. The rate of bone formation is also increased by PTH, linked to the increase in bone resorption. However, PTH has a direct inhibitory effect on osteoblast form and function in vitro. The renal tubular reabsorption of amino acids, bicarbonate, and phosphorus is depressed by PTH, leading to systemic acidosis and hypophosphatemia.

A PTH-related protein (PTH-RP) has been identified in patients with humoral hypercalcemia of malignancy, but found to be a normal body product as well.[14,48,65] The gene for PTH-RP is localized to the short arm of chromosome 12 and codes for a 177-amino-acid propeptide. One species of the mature peptide (mol wt 16 kDa) contains 141 amino acids; 8 of the first 13 NH_2 terminal amino acids (70%) of PTH and PTH-RP are identical; the biologic activities of PTH and PTH-RP are similar and they may bind to the same receptor. Thus PTH-RP increases serum calcium concentrations, enhances formation of $1,25(OH)_2D_3$, and modestly increases renal tubular resorption of calcium. PTH-RP increases osteoclast activity and bone resorption, but does not enhance bone formation, in contrast to the effects of PTH. PTH-RP is also synthesized by fetal liver, osteoblasts, adrenal cortex and medulla, keratinocytes, lactating mammary gland, parathyroid glands, and placenta. Messenger RNA transcripts of PTH-RP are present in the gastric mucosa, adrenal, and brain of the rat, but the physiologic role of this agent is unknown in this species. As a consequence of alternative processing of mRNA there are three species of PTH-RP of 139, 141, and 173 amino acids, all of which have the same first 139 residues. In the circulation, PTH-RP is present as NH_2 and COOH terminal fragments, as is PTH.[15] PTH-RP is not the only agent of pathogenetic significance in patients with hypercalcemia of malignancy. Immobilization, bony metastases, a number of cytokines, and production of $1,25(OH)_2D_3$ may result in calcium mobilization in the patient with malignancy. The physiologic role of PTH-RP is not yet clarified, but this protein can enhance differentiation of keratinocytes and stimulate biosynthesis of fibronectin by human skin fibroblasts.[48] The presence of PTH-RP in breast tissue and placenta raises the possibility that it may play a role in fetal and neonatal calcium metabolism.

Calcitonin

Calcitonin is a hypocalcemic peptide with 32 amino acids derived from a large precursor protein (mol wt 17 kDa) encoded on the short arm of chromosome 11. Calcitonin is secreted by the parafollicular (C) cells of the thyroid, but is also synthesized in the anterior pituitary, brain, and intestinal tract. The calcitonin gene also encodes a larger protein—calcitonin gene-related peptide (CGRP)—expressed primarily in the central nervous system. The secretion of calcitonin is increased by a rise in serum Ca^{2+} concentration and by intestinal gastrin, glucagon, secretin, and cholecystokinin, the latter being homeostatic mechanisms by which calcium levels are maintained within narrow limits after ingestion of calcium-containing foods. Calcitonin inhibits PTH and vitamin D–induced osteoclast resorption of bone, acting directly on this cell. Katacalcin, a hypocalcemic peptide derived from the C-terminal region of the procalcitonin molecule, is secreted concomitantly with calcitonin; CGRP can also induce hypocalcemia, but its major effects are on vasodilation.[60]

Vitamin D

The metabolites of vitamin D_3 increase intestinal absorption of calcium, and enhance renal tubular and skeletal reabsorption of calcium.[72] The majority of the body's content of vitamin D is synthesized endogenously. Ultraviolet light (280–305 nM) and heat (37° C) transform cutaneous 7-dehydrocholesterol through an intermediate previtamin D_3 to vitamin D_3 (cholecalciferol) (Fig 4–3). (Vitamin D_2, or ergocalciferol, is derived from plant ergosterol, and differs from vitamin D_3 only by the presence of a double bond on the carbon side chain of the molecule. Vitamins D_2 and D_3 are metabolized and act in a similar manner.) Vitamin D_3 is transported in the blood by a vitamin D–binding protein (DBP) (see Chapter 1) to the liver where the microsomal enzyme, vitamin D–25-hydroxylase, forms $25OHD_3$, or calcidiol. Serum concentrations of $25OHD_3$ generally reflect body stores of vitamin D, are higher in sunny climes, and fluctuate seasonally with highest values in the summer. Serum levels of $25OHD_3$ are higher in white than in black people, as heavily pigmented skin absorbs ultraviolet light. Hepatic formation of $25OHD_3$ may be negatively regulated to a limited extent by $1,25(OH)_2D_3$. After transport to the kidney by DBP, 25OHD is metabolized by cells of the proximal convoluted and straight renal tubules containing the mitochondrial cytochrome P-450 enzyme $25(OH)D$-1α-hydroxylase to the most active metabolite of vitamin D, $1,25(OH)_2D_3$ or calcitriol. Calcidiol and $1,25(OH)_2D_3$ are biologically active, but the activity of $1,25(OH)_2D_3$ is 500- to 1,000-

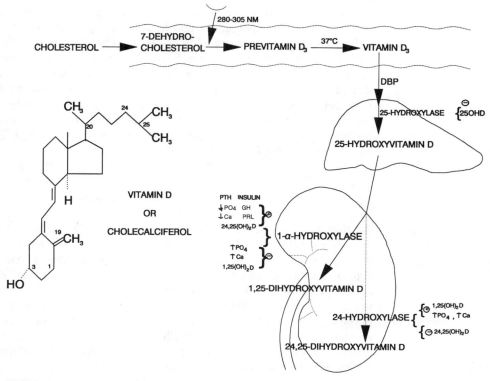

FIG 4–3.
Metabolism of vitamin D. See text.

fold greater than is that of 25OHD$_3$. The substrate 25OHD$_3$ can also be hydroxylated in the kidney to produce 24,25(OH)$_2$D$_3$ and 1,24,25(OH)$_3$D$_3$ as well as a number of other relatively inactive metabolites. The activity of renal vitamin D 24-hydroxylase is stimulated by 1,25(OH)$_2$D$_3$. The activity of renal 25OHD-1α-hydroxylase is stimulated by PTH, low ambient phosphorus and calcium concentrations, 24,25(OH)$_2$D$_3$, and IGF-I[19]; it is inhibited by 1,25(OH)$_2$D$_3$ and high phosphorus levels. Serum concentrations of 1,25(OH)$_2$D$_3$ are increased by thyroid hormone, growth hormone, prolactin, insulin, estrogen (by increasing synthesis of DBP), and calcitonin; activated macrophages, keratinocytes, and the placenta also demonstrate 25OHD-1α-hydroxylase activity.

There are specific nuclear vitamin D receptors (see Chapter 1) which mediate the biologic effects of 1,25(OH)$_2$D$_3$, although the mechanism by which this metabolite acts is incompletely understood. After interaction of 1,25(OH)$_2$D$_3$ and its nuclear receptor, intracellular calcium-binding protein (calbindin) levels and alkaline phosphatase activity increase, either one of which, or both, may be important in intestinal absorption of calcium (and phosphorus whose absorption 1,25(OH)$_2$D$_3$ also regulates). Calcitriol down-regulates genes which control the synthesis of PTH, calcitonin, type I collagen, and a number of cytokines, including interleukin-2, interferon-γ and granulocyte-macrophage colony-stimulating factor (GM-CSF) as well as the proto-oncogene c-*myc*. Calcitriol enhances transcription of genes regulating the nuclear vitamin D receptor, osteocalcin, prolactin, and the oncogenes c-*fos* and c-*fms*.[72]

In bone, 1,25(OH)$_2$D$_3$ increases bone resorption primarily by accelerating maturation of osteoclast precursors and by stimulating osteoblast release of an osteoclast activity factor(s). This metabolite enhances bone formation by increasing local concentrations of calcium and phosphorus and by regulating osteoblast function.[72] In addition to its effects on mineral homeostasis and bone metabolism, 1,25(OH)$_2$D$_3$ also plays an important role in cellular differentiation and growth. Receptors for 1,25(OH)$_2$D$_3$ are found not only in the usual target tissues (intestine, kidney, bone, parathyroid) but also in skin, muscle, placenta, brain, breast, gonads, thyroid, pituitary, pancreas, and thymus as well in circulating B and T lymphocytes and monocytes. In lymphocytes 1,25(OH)$_2$D$_3$ suppresses production of interleukin-2, interferon-γ and GM-CSF, and inhibits proliferation of T and B cells.[56] In monocytes 1,25(OH)$_2$D$_3$ suppresses production of interleukin-1$_\alpha$ and interleukin-1$_\beta$, perhaps the primary mechanism by which 1,25(OH)$_2$D$_3$ suppresses lymphocyte proliferation and function. (In some studies 1,25(OH)$_2$D$_3$ has increased interleukin-1 production.) In the thymus, 1,25(OH)$_2$D$_3$ may play a role in lymphocyte differentiation into helper cells. This metabolite also promotes macrophage differentiation from the monocyte and the expression of surface class II antigen-presenting proteins, enhances phagocytosis, and increases production of hydrogen peroxide, tumor necrosis factor, and heat shock protein. Since, in the absence of vitamin D there is evidence for compromise of immune function, these data suggest an important role for 1,25(OH)$_2$D$_3$ in the regulation or modulation of the immune system. Skin is yet another tissue with receptors for 1,25(OH)$_2$D$_3$, in which this metabolite may be important for terminal differentiation of squamous cells and decreased proliferation of keratinocytes. Indeed, topical 1,25(OH)$_2$D$_3$ has been employed successfully to treat psoriasis, a hyperproliferative disorder,[42] and alopecia occurs in some children with vitamin D resistance and abnormal vitamin D receptors.

Human milk contains less than 100 U/L of vitamin D[40]; it is recommended that infants receive 100 units/kcal of vitamin D ingested up to 400 U/day in older children.[23] Mean serum concentrations of 25OHD$_3$ are similar in black and white infants, but during childhood levels are a bit higher in whites than in blacks. Mean serum values of 1,25(OH)$_2$D$_3$ are slightly higher in black than in white infants and in formula-fed than in human milk-fed infants, and decline to adult levels by 6 months of age.[39,40] During adolescence there is a transient increase in 1,25(OH)$_2$D$_3$ values. Serum concentrations of 25OHD$_3$ are higher in sunny climes and in summer than in winter (reflecting sunlight exposure), while in infants levels of 1,25(OH)$_2$D$_3$ are higher in winter than in summer.[55] Serum concentrations of DBP (370 µg/mL) are independent of race but increase with age during infancy, decrease during the summer, and are lower in human milk-fed than in formula-fed infants.

Other Factors Influencing Bone Metabolism

Thyroid hormone increases osteoclast activity directly and indirectly through activation of cytokines. In thyrotoxic patients or in patients receiving excessive doses of thyroxine, bone mineral density may be decreased and serum and urine calcium levels increased. Estrogens inhibit bone resorption; estrogens and androgens increase bone mineralization in the child and adolescent. Hypogonadism (e.g., Turner syndrome) is accompanied by decreased bone mineral density in midchildhood, while the hypogonadal adolescent may also be osteopenic. Glucocorticoids lead to osteopenia by inhibiting bone formation and bone resorption, impairing the action of 1,25(OH)$_2$D$_3$ on intestinal absorption of calcium and inhibiting osteoblast maturation.[60]

Many cytokines have effects on mineral homeostasis.[60,62] Interleukin-1 is an osteoclast activating factor and increases bone resorption as do tumor necrosis factor and lymphotoxin. On the other hand interferon-γ inhibits the osteoclast activating effect of these cytokines. Prostaglandins (PGE) and TGF-α also enhance osteoclast activity. TGF-β stimulates osteoblast and inhibits osteoclast activity.

DISORDERS OF CALCIUM AND MINERAL HOMEOSTASIS

Hypocalcemia

In utero serum concentrations of calcium are high and increase with gestational age; levels of PTH are low, while serum concentrations of calcitonin are elevated. Immediately after delivery serum calcium levels decline to a nadir by 24 hours of age, remain stable for the next 24 hours, and then increase; serum calcium concentrations fall more rapidly and to lower levels in preterm than in term infants; in infants of less than 32 weeks' gestation serum calcium values recover more slowly than in gestationally more mature neonates.[85] In infants with birth weights less than 1,000 g, serum calcium concentrations may remain low for several weeks after birth.[39] Serum concentrations of phosphorus are also high in utero and increase slightly over the first 2 days of life. During early infancy serum phosphorus concentrations range from 6 to 8 mg/dL. Serum concentrations of magnesium increase in term infants over 48 hours but decline slightly in preterm infants. Cord serum concentrations of calcitonin are highest in infants of less than 32 weeks' gestation, and increase to a peak within 24 hours after birth in both term and preterm neonates, the rise being greater in the more immature infant. Serum levels of PTH also increase within the first 48 hours after birth in full-term infants and in some, but not all, premature infants. Within several days after birth, serum concentrations of calcitonin and PTH fall to stable values.

Concentrations of $25OHD_3$ in cord serum are directly related to those of the mother, which in turn reflect maternal diet, sunlight exposure, and parity. Concentrations of $1,25(OH)_2D_3$ are higher in the cord sera of term infants than in normal adults, and increase over the first several days of life. Concentrations of $1,25(OH)_2D_3$ are often even higher in preterm or low-birth-weight than in full-term infants.

Causes of Hypocalcemia

Table 4–1 lists causes of hypocalcemia in infancy and childhood. Neonatal hypocalcemia (tetany) occurring within the first 48 hours after birth usually reflects a preexisting maternal illness such as toxemia, diabetes mellitus, hyperparathyroidism, or an acquired peripartum illness such as sepsis or respiratory distress. In the infant of the hyperparathyroid mother hypocalcemia usually occurs within the first few days or weeks of life but may not be recognized until the infant is several months of age, particularly if the infant is breast-fed, as human milk has a high ratio of calcium to phosphorus.[35] Hypocalcemia occurring after 48 to 72 hours of life often is due to immaturity of the renal tubular handling of a high phosphorus intake, received either orally or intravenously. Acute hyperphosphatemia may cause profound hypocalcemia in infants and older subjects. Magnesium is essential for PTH secretion and function; hypomagnesemia is a common cause of hypocalcemia in the newborn, with resultant functional hypoparathyroidism. After magnesium administration PTH and calcium values increase rapidly. Neonatal tetany due to prolonged and exaggerated suppression of PTH secretion may persist for up to 21 days after birth before resolving spontaneously. Hypocalcemia of longer duration requires further evaluation. Among the diagnostic considerations is transient congenital hypoparathyroidism, which is characterized by low PTH concentrations in the presence of hypocalcemia which resolves spontaneously after several months of therapy with calcium and analogues of vitamin D. In some instances such patients may be mild examples of the DiGeorge anomaly.[34] In other patients the hypocalcemia and hyperphosphatemia resolve, but the secretion of PTH remains marginal.[9] Persistent congenital hypoparathyroidism may occur sporadically or may be inherited as an autosomal dominant, or autosomal or sex-linked recessive characteristic, due to malformation of the parathyroid glands or to an error in the construction of the gene coding for PTH. When the dysgenetic malformation is mild, hypocalcemia may not be appreciated until mid-childhood or early adolescence.

In older children hypocalcemia may reflect disorders of the parathyroid gland or of the vitamin D system, dietary deficiency of calcium, or critical illness. An abnormal, incompletely processed, and hence hypoactive PTH molecule may be secreted by some patients. Hypoparathyroidism may be part of a larger anomaly of branchial arch formation with malformations of the face, cardiovascular system, and thymus (DiGeorge anomaly). The DiGeorge anomaly is a polytypic developmental field defect

TABLE 4–1.

Causes of Hypocalcemia

Neonatal hypocalcemia	Vitamin D deficiency (see disorders of
Early onset	mineralization)
Maternal illness	Other
Diabetes mellitus	Calcium deficiency
Toxemia	Nutritional deprivation
Hyperparathyroidism	Hypercalciuria
Respiratory distress, sepsis	Hypomagnesemia
Low birth weight	Congenital
Hypomagnesemia	Malabsorption
Late onset	Acquired hypermagnesuria
High phosphorus load	Primary
Hypoparathyroidism	Bartter's syndrome
Transient	Renal tubular acidosis
Permanent	Miscellaneous
Hypoparathyroidism	Acute and chronic renal failure
Congenital	Diuretics
Transient neonatal	Hyperphosphatemia
Familial: autosomal recessive, autosomal dominant,	Hypoproteinemia
sex-linked recessive	Drugs
DiGeorge anomaly	Furosemide
Kenny-Caffey syndrome	Calcitonin
Dyshormonogenesis	Mithramycin
Acquired	Critical illness
Autoimmune	Pancreatitis
Sporadic	Chronic renal failure
Familial (polyglandular syndrome type I)	
Postsurgical, radiation insult	
With excessive iron or copper deposition	
Idiopathic	
Resistance to parathyroid hormone	
Pseudohypoparathyroidism types IA, IB	
Pseudohypoparathyroidism type II	
Pseudohypohyperparathyroidism	
Pseudopseudohypoparathyroidism	

in which an embryologic reactive unit of cephalic neural crest cells fails to enter the third and fourth branchial arches and pouches resulting in cardiac, facial, immunologic, and endocrinologic abnormalities. The spectrum of the DiGeorge anomaly is broad; hypoparathyroidism may be permanent and severe or transient and mild; immunodeficiency may be profound, mild, or absent; when present, the immune defect is often transient with spontaneous remission.[11,34] Characteristic facial features include mandibular hypoplasia, hypertelorism, short philtrum, and malformed or low-set ears. Among the anomalies of the cardiovascular system are interrupted aortic arch type 2, ventricular and atrial septal defects, pulmonic stenosis, right aortic arch, and truncus and pseudotruncus. Deficiency of T lymphocytes (low CD4 cells and low CD4/CD8 ratio) is the most characteristic immune defect. The DiGeorge anomaly may be familial, associated with chromosomal abnormalities (monosony 22q11 or 10p13), other syndromes (Kallmann, Zellweger), or anomalies (velocardiofacial syndrome, holoprosencephaly), or due to teratogens (alcohol, isotretinoin). Because of the wide spectrum of the DiGeorge anomaly, its diagnosis may be difficult, but should be considered in all children with hypoparathyroidism.[34] Another congenital anomaly, the Kenny-Caffey syndrome, is associated with short stature, small, slender long bones with medullary stenosis and thickening of the diaphyseal cortex, and hypoparathyroidism.[53] An abnormality in the processing of PTH may result in the secretion of biologically less active forms of PTH (dyshormonogenesis).

Acquired hypoparathyroidism may be the result of surgical or radiation insult to the parathyroid glands; more commonly it is associated with an autoimmune process. Autoimmune destruction of the parathyroid glands may be an isolated disorder or part of a polyendocrinopathy[7] (Table 4–2). It is difficult to establish the diagnosis of autoimmune hypoparathyroidism in the absence of associated autoimmune diseases or endocrinopathies because specific antibodies against the parathyroid gland are difficult to demonstrate.[78] Antiparathyroid antibodies directed against parathyroid cell surface antigens have been demonstrated in a few patients; these antibodies have stimulated or inhibited PTH release or have had cytotoxic effects. Autoimmune polyglandular disease type I is also termed *autoimmune polyendocrinopathy-candidiasis-ectodermal dysplasia* (APECED). This term highlights the associated disorders of failure of the adrenal cortex, parathyroids, gonads, thyroid, pancreatic beta cells, and gastric parietal cells (leading to pernicious anemia), chronic mucocutaneous candidiasis, and ectodermal dysplasia characterized by alopecia, vitiligo, dystrophic nails and teeth, keratopathy, and chronic active hepatitis.[3] This disorder may be familial. In a study of 68 patients from 54 families in Finland (Table 4–3), Ahonen et al.[3]

TABLE 4–2.

Polyglandular Autoimmune Endocrinopathies*

Type	Endocrinopathies	Associated Disorders
I	Hypoparathyroidism Hypoadrenocortism Hypogonadism Insulin-dependent diabetes mellitus Pernicious anemia	Chronic mucocutaneous candidiasis Vitiligo, enamel hypoplasia, alopecia, keratopathy Malabsorption Chronic active hepatitis
II	Hypoadrenalism Autoimmune thyroid disease Insulin-dependent diabetes mellitus (hypogonadism)	Vitiligo
IIIA	Autoimmune thyroid disease Insulin-dependent diabetes mellitus	
IIIB	Insulin-dependent diabetes mellitus	Pernicious anemia
IIIC	Autoimmune thyroid disease	Alopecia Vitiligo Myasthenia gravis Idiopathic thrombocytopenic purpura

*From Bachrach LK, Foley TP Jr: *Pediatr Rev* 1989; 11:184–191. Used by permission.

TABLE 4–3.

Associated Disorders in Autoimmune Polyglandular Disease Type I (N = 68)*

Endocrinopathy/Disorder	n (%)	Age of Onset (yr)
Hypoparathyroidism	54(79)	1.6–44
Hypoadrenocorticism	49(72)	4.2–4.1
Primary hypogonadism		
Female	15/25(60)	>13
Male	4/28(14)	>16
Insulin-dependent diabe-tes mellitus	8(12)	4.1–37
Pernicious anemia	9(13)	6.1–47
Hypothyroidism	2	
Oral candidiasis	68 (100)	0.1–21
Ungual candidiasis	48(71)	—
Keratopathy	24(35)	1–15
Alopecia	20(29)	0.1–15
Malabsorption	12(18)	0.3–21
Enamel hypoplasia	33/43(77)	<7

*From Ahonen P, Myelarniemi S, Sipila I, et al: *N Engl J Med* 1990; 322:1829–1836. Used by permission.

found 79% of the patients to have hypoparathyroidism, which appeared between 19 months and 44 years; 72% were hypoadrenocortical, presenting between 4 and 41 years; and 60% of the females greater than 13 years of age had primary hypogonadism. Insulin-dependent diabetes mellitus was present in 12% of patients and 13% had pernicious anemia. All 68 patients had or had had oral candidiasis appearing as the first manifestation of this disease between 1 month and 21 years of age. *Candida* infection of the nails was present in 71% of patients. Alopecia was present in 29% (onset 5–30 years), vitiligo in 13% (1 month–15 years), and keratopathy in 35% (1–15 years). The most common association of disorders was hypoparathyroidism, hypoadrenocorticism, and candidiasis (51% of patients). Hypoparathyroidism occurred most commonly between 3 and 5 years and hypoadrenocorticism between 11 and 15 years of age. In 76% of patients, oral candidiasis was the first clinical sign of this disorder. Hypoparathyroidism was the first endocrinopathy, five times more frequent than adrenocortical failure. Further manifestations of the disease continued to appear into the fifth decade of life, but only a few patients succumbed to a component of the disorder itself.

There are several forms of pseudohypoparathyroidism (PHP). Albright's hereditary osteodystrophy or type I PHP is an autosomal or X-linked dominant disorder characterized by a phenotype of short stocky stature, developmental delay, brachymetacarpals and brachymetatarsals, round face, subcutaneous calcifications, hypocalcemia, hyperphosphatemia, increased concentrations of PTH, and neither an increase in urine cAMP nor in phosphorus after PTH administration, denoting end-organ insensitivity to this peptide. The PTH receptor number and binding characteristics have been normal in the limited number of patients studied. The abnormality in this disorder occurs after the interaction of PTH with its receptor. The PTH receptor acts through a Gs-binding protein. In PHP type IA there is a decrease or absence of the activity of this Gs-binding protein which does not transmit the PTH-receptor message to the second-messenger system (adenyl cyclase–cAMP) mediating the action of PTH. Defects in the alpha subunit of the trimeric Gs-binding protein in patients with PHP type IA have been found in many tissues (including platelets and red blood cells) which lead to generalized end-organ resistance to a number of protein hormones including the gonadotropins, thyrotropin, and antidiuretic hormone.

Patten et al.[66] described a single base mutation in the Gs alpha gene of adenine to guanine at position +1, converting the initiator triplet codon from ATG (methionine) to GTG (valine), thus blocking initiation of translation of the normal gene product for the Gs alpha subunit and resulting in the synthesis of an abnormal and inactive subunit. There is molecular heterogeneity in PHP-IA as this particular base defect has not been found in other phenotypic patients with this disorder. In PHP-IB, the clinical phenotype and chemical abnormalities are similar to those of PHP-IA, but Gs-binding protein activity is normal, suggesting a molecular error distal to the G-binding protein. In some subjects the clinical findings of PHP-I are present, but calcium, phosphorus, and PTH concentrations are normal, and after administration of PTH there is a normal increase in the urine excretion of cAMP and phosphorus. This is termed *pseudopseudohypoparathyroidism* (PPHP). Patten et al.[66] found similar gene defects in a son with PHP-1A and his mother with PPHP. They hypothesized that the expression of the abnormal gene in PHP-IA required a second abnormality in the activity of the adenyl cyclase–cAMP generating system. Children with PHP-IA in childhood have evolved into adults with PPHP, suggesting perhaps the appearance of a secondary or alternative pathway for response to PTH in these patients. There is generalized resistance to the action of protein hormones in patients with PHP-I, with variable hypothyroidism, hypogonadism, and mild diabetes insipidus. Neonates with PHP-I may first be identified in infant screening programs for congenital hypothyroidism.

In PHP-II, the phenotype is usually normal, the serum calcium level is low, and the serum concentrations of phosphorus and PTH are high. However, in response to PTH there is an increase in urine cAMP excretion but no phosphaturia. The Gs-binding protein activity is normal. These observations suggest that in PHP-II the molecular defect lies distal to the generation of cAMP, perhaps at the level of protein kinase A or in an alternative pathway important for cellular response to PTH. There may be variable tissue resistance to PTH in some patients. In pseudohypohyperparathyroidism, there is radiologic evidence of hyperparathyroidism indicating skeletal responsiveness to PTH, but of renal resistance to PTH resulting in hypocalcemia, perhaps due to deficiency of $1,25(OH)_2D_3$.

Deficiency of vitamin D (see Disorders of Mineralization below) usually results in compensatory secondary hyperparathyroidism, low-to-normal calcium, and low phosphorus values. Occasionally severe hypocalcemia can be observed in the vitamin D–deficient patient, perhaps because of the dependence of PTH bioactivity on small amounts of $1,25(OH)_2D_3$. In the vitamin D–deficient child with rickets treated with vitamin D, rapid deposition of calcium and phosphorus occurs. If sufficient dietary calcium is not provided to these patients, hypocalcemia may ensue (the "hungry bone" syndrome). Hypocalcemia is observed in patients with absence of renal

25OHD-1α-hydroxylase and in those with abnormal receptors for vitamin D. Since magnesium is required for secretion of PTH and for its metabolic effects, hypomagnesemia can result in hypocalcemia. Magnesium depletion plays a role in the hypocalcemia of the infant of a diabetic woman. A number of drugs can lower serum calcium concentrations, either by inhibition of bone resorption, or by increasing the urinary excretion of calcium (furosemide, citrate, ethylenediaminetetraacetate). Severe hyperphosphatemia due either to chronic or acute renal failure and phosphorus retention, to administration of large quantities of phosphorus intravenously or per rectum, or to massive tissue destruction (i.e., during treatment of leukemia) can lower serum calcium concentrations acutely. In patients with pancreatitis, serum calcium levels fall, in part due to sequestration of calcium in peripancreatic saponified fat. Acute and critical illnesses and sepsis are associated with hypocalcemia. The hypocalcemia of severe illness may be due to administration of large amounts of citrated blood, to the hypocalcemic effects of glucocorticoids and other drugs (cimetidine, anticonvulsants), to functional depression of PTH release (possibly related to an effect of interleukin-1 on increasing intracellular calcium or to associated hypomagnesemia), to decreased renal 25OHD-1α-hydroxylase activity resulting in decreased synthesis of $1,25(OH)_2D_3$, and acquired peripheral resistance to $1,25(OH)_2D_3$.[16,90] Hypocalcemia is also seen in children with hypernatremia and hypokalemia.

Evaluation of Hypocalcemia

Evaluation of the neonate with hypocalcemia begins with the history of maternal health during the pregnancy, the circumstances of the delivery, and the course of the infant after birth. Maternal illnesses (diabetes mellitus, toxemia), preterm or traumatic delivery, or early illness may lead to hypocalcemia in the first 2 days after birth; later onset of hypocalcemia may be the result of high phosphorus intake, intercurrent illness, or other stress. In the hypocalcemic, otherwise well full-term neonate without apparent cause for hypocalcemia, serial measurements of maternal concentrations of calcium, phosphorus, and PTH may reveal occult hyperparathyroidism in the mother. In the infant and young child, hypocalcemia may occur as a consequence of vitamin D deficiency, and therefore information about maternal and infant diet and sunlight exposure may provide diagnostic clues. In the older child and adolescent, the presence of autoimmune disease(s) in the patient or other family members is important information. Hypocalcemia needs to be considered in the differential diagnosis of seizures in the neonate or infant. Generalized seizures may also occur in the older child, although tetany (carpopedal spasm), muscular cramping (particularly with exercise), and paresthesias are more common symptoms of hypocalcemia which may not be recognized initially. Tetany may occur during hyperventilation in patients with hypo- or hyperkalemia, hypomagnesemia or hyper- or hyponatremia. With chronic hypocalcemia increased intestinal motility may lead to steatorrhea and clinical signs of malabsorption. After the newborn period, physical examination of the hypocalcemic subject may not be remarkable, but occasionally signs of increased intracranial pressure (papilledema) or cataract formation (perhaps due to abnormal hydration of the lens) may be seen.[60] The Chvostek sign (facial twitching elicited by tapping the facial nerve) is often present in hypocalcemic children, but is not diagnostic of hypocalcemia as it occurs in patients with other forms of increased neuromuscular irritability and even in normal adolescents with no clinical or biochemical abnormalities. Carpopedal spasm elicited by temporary occlusion of arterial flow to the forearm (Trousseau sign) is a reliable indicator of hypocalcemia and other hyperirritable states.

Recognition of associated ectodermal abnormalities such as mucocutaneous candidiasis, alopecia, vitiligo, and abnormal dentition may focus attention upon evaluation of mineral homeostasis. A characteristic phenotype (see above) suggests the diagnosis of PHP-I, whereas rachitic deformities of the metaphyses of the long bones and costochondral junctions suggest the possibility of hypovitaminosis D. Alopecia associated with hypocalcemia and rickets suggests end-organ insensitivity to $1,25(OH)_2D_3$. In the newborn period evidence of congenital abnormalities of branchial arch development (branchial cleft cysts and sinuses, heart murmur) in association with hypocalcemia raise the possibility of the DiGeorge anomaly.

Laboratory assessment of the child with suspected hypocalcemia should include measurement of total and ionized calcium concentrations (to document that hypocalcemia is not due to hypoproteinemia) and levels of phosphorus, magnesium, creatinine, alkaline phosphatase activity, and PTH. Other studies which may be helpful depending on individual circumstances are measurements of concentrations of $25OHD_3$ (to assess vitamin D stores) and $1,25(OH)_2D_3$. In patients with primary hypoparathyroidism, total and ionized calcium concentrations are low, the level of phosphorus is high, magnesium is usually normal, and alkaline phosphatase activity normal or elevated. The concentration of PTH is inappropriately low for the level of calcium. The choice of assay for measurement of PTH is important. Currently the immunometric method of PTH measurement (in which the PTH molecule is sandwiched between two antibodies which recognize the NH_2 terminal and middle COOH terminal, respectively) adequately separates hypoparathyroid from normal subjects; the middle COOH terminal–specific radioimmunoassay for PTH is also useful for this purpose.[79] Table 4–4 presents data on laboratory studies in different hypocalcemic states. In patients with PHP-I the PTH concentration is high and neither the urinary excretion of cAMP nor that of phosphorus increases following administration of PTH

TABLE 4–4.

Laboratory Data in the Differential Diagnosis of Hypocalcemia*

	Hypopara-thyroidism	Pseudo-hypopara-thyroidism	Hypomag-nesemia	Vitamin D Deficiency	25-Hydroxyvitamin D_3–1α-Hydroxylase Deficiency	Resistance to 1,25-Dihydroxyvitamin D_3	Chronic Renal Disease
Total calcium	↓	↓	↓	↓	↓	↓	↓
Ionized calcium	↓	↓	↓	↓	↓	↓	↓
Phosphorus	↑	↑	↑	↓	↓	↓	↑
Magnesium	N↓	N	↓	N	N	N	N↑
Alkaline phosphatase	N	N	N	↑	↑	↑	↑
Parathyroid hormone	↓	↑	↓	↑	↑	↑	↑
$25OHD_3$	N	N	N	↓	N	N	N
$1,25(OH)_2D_3$	N↓	N↓	N	↓N↑	↓	↑↑↑	↓

*↓ = decreased; ↑ = increased; N = normal.

(now available as the 1–34 NH_2 terminal bioactive fragment). In patients with PHP-II, the phenotype is normal, the serum PTH concentration is increased, and the urinary excretion of cAMP, but *not* that of phosphorus, increases after administration of PTH. Hypomagnesemia and chronic renal disease must also be considered in this evaluation. After establishment of the diagnosis of hypoparathyroidism, definition of its etiology may be difficult unless there is a clearly defined familial inheritance pattern, or it is associated with characteristic congenital anomalies or other (autoimmune) diseases. In patients with "idiopathic" hypoparathyroidism, the disorder may be due to mild dysgenesis of the parathyroid glands with late failure of function or perhaps to an isolated autoimmune disorder.

Treatment of Hypocalcemia

Identification of the cause of hypocalcemia is essential for appropriate therapy. Rapid restoration of plasma calcium concentrations can be accomplished by administration of intravenous (calcium gluconate 10% containing 9 mg/dL elemental calcium, 2 mL/kg over 10 minutes) or oral calcium (calcium glubionate containing 115 mg/5 mL elemental calcium, 75 mg/kg/day). In the hypocalcemic neonate, provision of an intake of calcium and phosphorus in the ratio of 4:1, will usually increase serum calcium values. In hypomagnesemia, administration of Mg^{2+} alone will restore the eucalcemic state. Identification of the cause of hypomagnesemia is important to correct this abnormality. Administration of $1,25(OH)_2D_3$ (0.5–2.0 μg/day) and supplemental calcium (as calcium citrate with 24% elemental calcium) will increase serum calcium and lower phosphorus concentrations in children with persistent primary hypoparathyroidism and PHP. A search for and treatment of associated endocrinopathies and other disorders in children with autoimmune hypoparathyroidism is essential. In patients with PHP, abnormalities of other endocrine systems should be sought as there is frequently generalized resistance to the action of protein hormones, such as thyrotropin, the gonadotropins, and antidiuretic hormone. Exposure to sunlight and provision of adequate dietary vitamin D (2,000–5,000 U/day for several weeks) and calcium is usually sufficient to replete stores in the vitamin D–deficient child. Provision of adequate dietary calcium will result in eucalcemia in those subjects with hypocalcemia due to lack of calcium intake. In all patients with hypocalcemia it is important to determine urine and serum calcium and creatinine levels serially and to avoid hypercalcemia, hypercalciuria, and nephrocalcinosis, adjusting the treatment program and drug regimen to maintain the eucalcemic and eucalciuric states.

Hypercalcemia

Causes of Hypercalcemia

Hypercalcemia may be due to disorders which result in excessive absorption of calcium from the intestine, to increased mobilization of calcium from bone,[36] or to enhanced resorption in the kidney. In neonates, hypercalcemia may result from resorption of calcium from deposits in necrotic subcutaneous fat which have developed because of severe illness and hypotension and by the acquisition of 25OHD-1α-hydroxylase activity by activated macrophages leading to increased production of $1,25(OH)_2D_3$ (Table 4–5). Hypophosphatemic neonates may be hypercalcemic. Hy-

TABLE 4–5.

Causes of Hypercalcemia

Hyperparathyroidism
  Congenital
    Autosomal recessive/dominant
    Multiple endocrine neoplasia types I, IIA, (IIB)
  Acquired (adenoma or hyperplasia)
  Secondary (post–renal transplantation)
Familial hypocalciuric hypercalcemia
Hypervitaminosis D
  Nutritional
  Granulomatous/inflammatory diseases (sarcoidosis, leprosy, tuberculo-
    sis)
Immobilization
Neoplasia
  Parathyroid hormone–like protein
  Osteoclast activating factor(s)
Others
  Hyperproteinemia
  Hypophosphatemia
  Drugs (thiazides, lithium, vitamin A)
  Hyperthyroidism

percalcemia in the neonatal period is rarely due to maternal hypocalcemia or to excessive maternal ingestion of vitamin D.[23] Hypercalcemia in the neonate or infant may be idiopathic, the consequence of increased intake of vitamin D in formula and supplemental vitamins, or a manifestation of familial hypocalciuric hypercalcemia (see below) or of Williams syndrome. The last-named is characterized by elfin facies (dolicocephaly, bitemporal depressions, full cheeks, periorbital fullness, epicanthal folds, prominant nasal tip, wide mouth, long philtrum, and thick lips[59,89]), failure to thrive, developmental delay, supravalvular aortic stenosis, and hypercalcemia in 15% of patients, which usually resolves by 2 to 3 years of age. The pathogenesis of hypercalcemia in Williams syndrome is unknown. It is not associated with excessive maternal ingestion of vitamin D (indeed, mothers who have had excess vitamin D intake during pregnancy have normal children with rare exceptions); serum concentrations of $25OHD_3$ and $1,25(OH)_2D_3$ are usually normal (although occasionally elevated); patients with Williams syndrome seem to have a more responsive hepatic vitamin D–25-hydroxylase system than unaffected subjects and may be "more sensitive" to the effects of vitamin D itself; there is no evidence of excessive PTH secretion in these infants, but calcitonin secretion may be blunted.[23]

In familial (benign) hypocalciuric hypercalcemia (FHH), transmitted as an autosomal dominant trait, the majority of affected persons are asymptomatic despite elevations of total and ionized calcium values. Other features include hypophosphatemia, slightly increased magnesium levels, low urine calcium excretion relative to the elevated serum calcium concentration, and usually normal levels of immunoreactive PTH, which increases or decreases according to alterations in serum calcium values.[37] FHH is distinguished from other forms of hypercalcemia by the absence of hypercalciuria (which usually occurs when the filtered load of calcium exceeds the renal tubular capacity for resorption of this cation), and by mild hypermagnesemia, which is not present in hyperparathyroidism. FHH is benign *except* in the neonate when marked hypercalcemia (>17 mg/dL) may occasionally be life-threatening, requiring emergency parathyroidectomy. In such infants the father is usually the affected parent and the mother is normal; since the affected fetus "requires" a higher than usual in utero calcium level, there is hyperplasia of the fetal parathyroids and excessive PTH secretion which persists postnatally and results in clinical and radiographic findings of hyperparathyroidism (bone demineralization and metaphyseal destructive lesions). The infant that is homozygous for FHH may also develop significant neonatal hypercalcemia. In affected patients serum calcium concentrations are highest in infancy and childhood and then decline to adult values. The pathophysiology of FHH is uncertain, but seems to be associated with an elevated homeostatic set point for calcium necessary for normal cellular function. Parathyroid gland function and histology are usually normal; the cellular calcium response to PTH is normal, although the renal tubular resorptive response to PTH may be slightly exaggerated. Serum levels of $1,25(OH)_2D_3$ are normal, as are bone histology, turnover, and density. In red blood cells the membrane calcium pump mechanism is normal, suggesting that in this tissue calcium channels are normal.

Primary hyperparathyroidism may be sporadic or familial. When familial, it may be transmitted as an autosomal recessive characteristic which is manifest in infancy as failure to thrive and vomiting with severe hypercalcemia (>17 mg/dL), often requiring parathyroidectomy, or which may be a self-limited disorder associated with nephrocalcinosis and renal tubular acidosis.[63] An autosomal dominant form of familial hyperparathyroidism may present in midchildhood with renal calculi, hypercalciuria, and hypercalcemia; familial hyperparathyroidism may also be a component of the dominantly transmitted multiple endocrine neoplasia (MEN) syndromes (see below). Primary hyperparathyroidism is an uncommon disorder in childhood. Mundy[60] found only 7 (4 females) patients less than 19 years of age among 414 patients with this disorder, which is most prevalent between 40 and 60 years of age and most common in females (3:1). Chief cell adenomas occur in 85% and chief cell hyperplasia in 15% of adult patients with primary hyperparathyroidism. Neonatal hyperparathyroidism may occur in the offspring of a hypocalcemic (usually hypoparathyroid) woman, manifested by demineralization and destructive lesions of the bones, occasionally hypercalcemia and hypophosphatemia, and elevated values of PTH; this disorder usually resolves spontaneously.

Although tumors of the pituitary (secreting prolactin, growth hormone, or adrenocorticotropin), thyroid, adrenal cortex, and pancreas (secreting insulin, glucagon, somatostatin, or gastrin) are common in patients with MEN type I (Table 4–6), many subjects with MEN-I have diffuse hyperplasia and not adenomas of the parathyroid glands. In the plasma of patients with MEN-I a factor similar to bFGF has been found which simulates parathyroid mitogenesis; its source and role in the pathophysiology of MEN-I are unknown, but it seems likely that abnormal synthesis, secretion, or function of endocrine gland growth factors are of pathogenetic significance in this disorder.[29] The genetic abnormality resulting in MEN-I lies at chromosome 11q13, where changes in this segment have been found in affected individuals.[84] This region is also the site of a proto-oncogene INT2 which codes for a FGF

TABLE 4–6.

Abnormalities Associated With Multiple Endocrine Neoplasia (MEN) and Hyperparathyroidism

MEN Type	Abnormalities
I	Pituitary tumors (prolactinoma, acromegaly, Cushing syndrome)
	Thyroid
	Pancreatic tumors (gastrinoma, insulinoma, glucagonoma, somatostatinoma)
IIA	Pheochromocytoma
	Medullary thyroid carcinoma
IIB	Medullary thyroid carcinoma
	Pheochromocytoma
	Marfanoid habitus
	Mucosal neuromas

protein that may be involved in the pathogenesis of parathyroid tumors and possibly of MEN-I as well. It has been hypothesized that MEN-I is the result of a two-stage recessive genetic mutation. In the first stage, there is a recessive mutation to a normally dominant, but unexpressed, gene which predisposes the affected subject to tumor formation. After a second mutation of the remaining normal allele, the gene altered by the first mutation is expressed and tumor formation ensues. It is interesting that the gene for PTH also is located on the short arm of chromosome 11.

In patients with MEN-IIA the frequency of hyperparathyroidism is unclear and whether it is a primary disorder or secondary to excessive calcitonin secretion is uncertain. A locus for MEN-IIA has been found on chromosome 10. A marfanoid habitus and mucosal neuromas are characteristic of MEN-IIB. This disorder presents in infancy with feeding disturbances and developmental delay, and the finding of mucosal neuromas on the lips and tongue of an affected infant or child should suggest this entity. It is essential that the disorder be recognized as early as possible so that total thyroidectomy may be carried out during the premalignant phase of parafollicular (C) cell hyperplasia, the precursor lesion of medullary carcinoma of the thyroid. Hyperparathyroidism rarely occurs in MEN-IIB. Secondary hyperparathyroidism is much more common in childhood than is primary hyperparathyroidism. It is associated with chronic renal failure; renal tubular acidosis; abnormalities of vitamin D intake, metabolism, or tissue response; and excessive administration of phosphorus in the treatment of patients with hypophosphatemic rickets. Secondary hyperparathyroidism is seldom associated with hypercalcemia except after successful renal transplantation when the hyperplastic mass of parathyroid tissue may require excision.

Hypercalcemia accompanies excessive intake of vitamin D or one of its metabolites or the excessive production of $1,25(OH)_2D_3$ by macrophages in granulomatous diseases (sarcoid, tuberculosis, leprosy, foreign body). Macrophages in inflammatory tissue may express 25OHD-1α-hydroxylase activity.[2] In contrast to renal tubular cells macrophage 25OHD-1α-hydroxylase activity is insensitive to stimulation by PTH or to inhibition by $1,25(OH)_2D_3$; it is responsive to stimulation by interferon-γ and inhibition by glucocorticoids. Macrophages do not express significant 24-hydroxylase activity, thus permitting accumulation of $1,25(OH)_2D_3$. Granulomatous hypercalcemia is associated with suppressed secretion of PTH, inappropriately increased concentrations of $1,25(OH)_2D_3$, extreme sensitivity to small doses of vitamin D, and suppression with glucocorticoids. In patients with B cell lymphomas or Hodgkin's disease and hypercalcemia, $1,25(OH)_2D_3$ levels are often elevated, suggesting a pathogenetic role for this metabolite. (However, many T and B cell lymphomas are associated with hypercalcemia and low levels of $1,25(OH)_2D_3$ indicating another mechanism(s) for hypercalcemia in these patients.) Excessive oral intake of vitamin A or retinoic acid can lead to hypercalcemia by a direct stimulatory effect on bone resorption. Thiazide diuretics increase renal tubular resorption of calcium and secondarily increase serum calcium concentrations. Lithium carbonate increases serum concentrations of PTH and in turn serum calcium concentrations,[79] but the mechanism by which this agent stimulates PTH secretion is unknown. In excess, theophylline and acetylsalicylic acid also raise serum calcium levels.[68] Excessive ingestion of bicarbonate *and* calcium may result in the milk-alkali syndrome characterized by hypercalcemia, hypercalciuria, systemic alkalosis, but an acid urine (due to excessive renal resorption of bicarbonate owing to suppressed secretion of PTH).

Sudden immobilization leads to "acute disuse osteoporosis," hypercalciuria, and hypercalcemia. This occurs most frequently in rapidly growing adolescents who are immobilized because of a severe injury, but is also seen in younger children placed at bed rest and in adults with spinal cord injuries. Continued osteoclast activity that is uncoupled from osteoblast function leads to resorption of bone without compensatory increase in bone formation, suggesting that the primary abnormality in immobilization hypercalcemia lies in one (or more) of the skeletal growth factors, or with an agent such as the PTH-RP.[48] Malignancy-related hypercalcemia may be due to bone destruction by metastases acting locally, or to production of $1,25(OH)_2D_3$ as in B cell lymphomas and related neoplasms, but in the majority (75%) of adults without osseous metastases it is due to the tumor production of PTH-RP which shares a common amino acid structure with PTH at the NH_2 terminal, occupies the PTH receptor, and has many of the biologic effects of PTH.[15] These include increase in bone and renal tubular resorption of calcium, and increase in urinary excretion of nephrogenous cAMP and phosphorus.[48] In contrast to native PTH, in bone PTH-RP uncouples resorption from formation, whereas in hyperparathyroidism the two processes are linked. Tumors may suppress $1,25(OH)_2D_3$ synthesis, but these may not be due to an effect of intact PTH-RP on renal 25OHD-1α-hydroxylase activity, but perhaps to a fragment of this protein or yet another peptide, as intact PTH-RP administered to rats in vivo increases $1,25(OH)_2D_3$ values, and in vitro it stimulates renal 25OHD-1α-hydroxylase activity.[48]

In addition to PTH-RP and $1,25(OH)_2D_3$, tumors produce many other hypercalcemic agents.[61] These include TGF-α, which enhances osteoclastic activity by increasing the number of osteoclasts and suppressing osteoblast function; TGF-β, which increases bone resorption through an effect on osteoclast activity mediated by prostaglandins, but which also inhibits osteoclast activity in some systems; and prostaglandins (particularly PGE_2), interleukin-$1_α$, interleukin-$1_β$, tumor necrosis factor, and lymphotoxin, which enhance osteoclast bone resorption by increasing osteoclast differentiation, stimulating osteoclast activity, and inhibiting osteoblast activity.

Thyrotoxicosis causes hypercalcemia by a direct effect of thyroid hormone on bone resorption, perhaps through stimulation of bone-resorbing factors. In thyrotoxic patients and those on large doses of thyroxine, hypercalciuria, osteopenia, and hypercalcemia may be observed.[68] Hypercalcemia has also been reported in hypothyroid infants. In patients with adrenocortical insufficiency, serum calcium concentrations may be high, although the pathophysiologic mechanism is unclear. Glucocorticoids enhance vitamin D catabolism and depress intestinal calcium absorption and bone calcium resorption; therefore, absence of the effects of this hormone may cause calcium levels to rise. Hypercalcemia also occurs, for reasons that are not clear, during the recovery phase of acute renal failure and in patients with chronic renal and liver disease, in those receiving parenteral nutrition (with too little phosphorus intake), and in adults with Paget's disease, particularly if they are immobilized or receiving thiazide diuretics.[68]

Evaluation of Hypercalcemia

Infants with hypercalcemia fail to thrive (Fig 4–4). Subjects with Williams syndrome have a characteristic facies, later onset of supravalvular aortic stenosis, and statural and developmental delay. In a child with hyperparathyroidism, a renal calculus or pathologic fracture through an area of osteitis fibrosa cystica may be the presenting symptom. Except in the neonate in whom severe hypercalcemia may cause lethargy and hypotonia, children with FHH are asymptomatic and usually are first identified by a chemical screen, which reveals an elevated serum calcium concentration, or in a family survey. Hypercalcemia may be associated with neurologic symp-

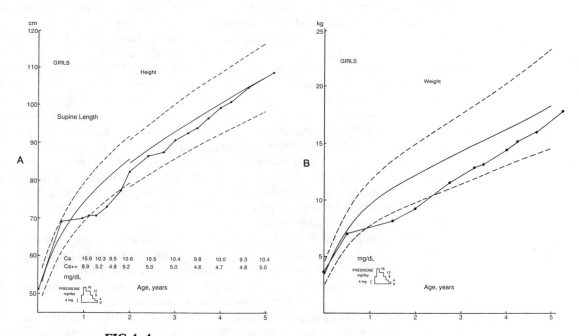

FIG 4–4.
Effects of hypercalcemia on linear growth (**A**) and weight (**B**) in an infant girl with idiopathic hypercalcemia. Note the arrest of growth and weight gain between 0.5 and 1.1 years when the infant was hypercalcemic, and the improvement with treatment.

toms ranging from drowsiness and confusion to depression or irritability, to stupor and coma; anorexia, vomiting, and constipation (rarely diarrhea) are common gastrointestinal symptoms, while polydipsia and polyuria reflect the increased osmotic load of the hypercalcemic state leading to hypercalciuria and nephrocalcinosis which impair urinary concentrating ability. A comprehensive family history is essential to identify patients who may be members of a kindred with inherited hyperparathyroidism, MEN, or FHH. The pattern of the hypercalcemic child's growth and development should be recorded. His or her vitamin and drug exposure should be sought, as should a history of diseases known to be associated with hypercalcemia such as peptic ulcers and pancreatitis. Physical examination may reveal subcutaneous masses in a hypercalcemic neonate, stigmata of the Williams syndrome, thyrotoxicosis, hypoadrenalism, or associated abnormalities (galactorrhea). Blood pressure may be elevated as calcium increases myocardial contractility, shortens the ventricular systolic phase, and decreases the QT interval on the electrocardiogram.

Laboratory data that are helpful include measurement of serum (plasma) total and ionized calcium concentrations and urine calcium levels, and serum phosphorus, creatinine, PTH, $25OHD_3$, and $1,25(OH)_2D_3$ concentrations. In patients with hypervitaminosis D, $25OHD_3$ levels are high. There is mild hypokalemia due to hypercalciuria-induced polyuria. Classically, patients with hyperparathyroidism have hypercalcemia, hypercalciuria, hypophosphatemia, and elevated concentrations of PTH and $1,25(OH)_2D_3$, in association with radiographic evidence of subperiosteal resorption. Currently, the immunoradiometric measurement (IRMA) of the intact PTH molecule seems to be most useful in identifying the patient with hyperparathyroidism and, in the absence of causes of secondary hyperparathyroidism, establishes the diagnosis of primary hyperparathyroidism.[79] Ancillary studies of parathyroid function, such as measurement of PTH secretory responses to hypocalcemia and hypercalcemia and of nephrogenous cAMP excretion, are usually unnecessary. Localization of hyperfunctioning parathyroid tissue may be difficult, but in my opinion should be undertaken in children prior to surgical exploration of the neck. The noninvasive methods for localization of parathyroid adenomas include high-resolution ultrasonography with 10- or 7.5-MHz transducers in which parathyroid tumors appear hypoechoic or anechoic; thallium-technetium subtraction scanning in which ^{201}Tl is taken up by both thyroid and parathyroid tissues owing to their high blood flow, and technetium accumulates only in the thyroid (and salivary glands), subtraction of the technetium image from the thallium uptake leaves the parathyroid visible; computed tomography (CT) with high-resolution features for soft tissues aided by the use of contrast agents which accumulate in thyroid and parathyroid tissue; magnetic resonance imaging (MRI) with equipment specifically designed for imaging of the neck and chest. Other noninvasive localizing techniques include intravenous digital subtraction angiography and cine-CT. (For a discussion of these techniques, see Eisenberg et al.[26])

The localizing technique of choice is at this time unclear. Individually, each of the methods discussed above localizes the adenoma in 55% to 80% of patients. The use of CT and thallium-technetium or ultrasound identifies the adenoma in 88% of patients.[26] These data apply to adults as there is little experience in children. Invasive procedures to identify hyperfunctioning parathyroid tissue are usually reserved for patients in whom the initial exploratory surgery has been unsuccessful. These techniques include arteriography and venous sampling of PTH concentrations. When considering the possibility of MEN in association with hyperparathyroidism, a search for other hyperfunctioning endocrine tumors is important.

The diagnosis of FHH is established by the absence of clinical symptoms, a positive family history (after survey of the parents and siblings), and low urine calcium excretion relative to serum calcium levels.[37] In patients with inflammatory or granulomatous diseases, renal insufficiency, leukemia, lymphoma, or other diseases, the primary disease is usually apparent. In subjects with hypercalcemia due to production of PTH-RP by malignant tumors, the serum concentration of this protein is increased.[15]

Treatment of Hypercalcemia

The management of the child with hypercalcemia requires accurate identification of the cause of the disorder. Acutely, serum calcium concentrations can be decreased by hydration (with twice maintenance volumes of 0.5–1.0 normal saline), which increases renal filtration of calcium and impairs its proximal renal tubular reabsorption, and by use of loop duretics (furosemide and ethacrynic acid), which depress calcium resorption in the loop of Henle. These agents require prior hydration of the patient and continuous replacement of ongoing losses of water and electrolytes.[5] Acute decline in calcium concentrations can also be achieved by the administration of calcitonin and the antibiotic mithramycin. Derivatives of pyrophosphate (bisphosphonates), which inhibit bone resorption, and phosphates, which bind calcium in the gut, have also been used to lower serum calcium concentrations. Glucocorticoids decrease calcium concentrations, particularly in patients with excessive vitamin D intake or generation; they are relatively ineffective in patients with hyperparathyroidism. In such patients removal of the parathyroid adenoma or resection of the hyperplastic parathyroid glands (with autotransplantation of part of one gland into a forearm or abdominal wall pocket) is appropriate therapy. Associated endocrinopathies must be addressed in such patients. Patients with FHH require follow-up but little intervention, unless a neonate with severe hypercalcemia should be delivered and parathyroidectomy is required; clearly newborns in such families should have serial measurements of calcium levels prospectively. Disease-specific treatment is indicated in disorders associated with hypercalcemia.

Disorders of Mineralization

Decreased bone mass (osteopenia) may be due to a paucity of bone matrix upon which to deposit bone mineral because of its inadequate formation or rapid destruction, or to subnormal amounts of calcium and phosphorus in matrix which is due either to abnormalities of mineral availability or deposition or excessive resorption of deposited minerals. Bone accretion is most rapid in utero as calcification of the fetal skeleton begins at 8 weeks' gestation. Between 25 and 36 weeks' gestation the fetus accumulates 114 to 130 mg/kg/day of calcium and 65 to 80 mg/kg/day of phosphorus.[39] By term the fetal skeleton has accumulated 30 g of calcium and 17 g of phosphorus. Postnatally the rate of bone deposition remains high. The bone mineral content measured by single photon absorptiometry of the left radius increases from 0.02 to 0.10 g/cm^2 between 24 and 40 weeks' gestation; bone mineral density increases progressively in human mild-fed and formula-fed infants in the first year of life[40]; by 12 to 35 months of age the bone mineral content (left radius) is 0.2 g/cm^2 in white infant males, increasing further to 0.27 g/cm^2 between 3 and 6 years and to 0.33 g/cm^2 by 7 years.[40,54] Bone mineral content is lower in white female infants but reaches white male values by 5 years. In black children bone mineral content is higher than in white children; it is higher in black males than in black females between 1 and 7 years of age.[54] Bone mineral content increases with age, height, and weight. Human milk-fed and formula-fed infants have similar bone densities after 1 year of age, although at 3 to 6 months of age bone mineral density is slightly lower in breast-fed than in formula-fed babies. In adolescents and adults, bone mineral content is higher in males than in females and in blacks than in whites. Maximum bone mass accumulation occurs in the second and third decades of life, indicating the critical period of adolescence in this process.[33]

Normal bone formation requires adequate intakes of protein, calcium, and phosphorus in age-appropriate amounts; although vitamin D is synthesized endogenously, supplemental vitamin D is necessary for very low-birth-weight infants and is generally recommended for infants and children although its necessity in breast-fed infants of well-nourished, sun-exposed mothers is unclear.[44] However, to insure adequate vitamin D intake, it is generally recommended that all full-term infants receive 100 units/day (2.5 µg) of vitamin D per 100 kcal of formula up to 400 units/day (10µg), that children and adolescents ingest 400 units/day of vitamin D, and that pregnant and lactating women receive 600 units/day (15 µg) of vitamin D.[23,39] The daily administration of more than 400 units of vitamin D to very low-birth-weight infants (1,000–1,500 g) does *not* seem to improve bone mineralization in this population which is significantly at risk for osteopenia and rickets.[25,27] Provision of adequate calcium (approximately 200 mg/kg/day) and phosphorus (100 mg/kg/day) is essential for adequate bone mineralization in this group of infants.[25,42] During the first year of life infants retain between 140 and 200 mg of calcium and 70 to 85 mg of phosphorus daily.[40] During the first 20 years of life females accumulate approximately 140 mg of calcium daily while males retain 164 mg/day. During adolescence calcium retention rates increase two- to threefold indicating the necessity for intakes of calcium of 1,000 mg/day at this critical period.[57] It has been estimated that approximately one-half of bone mass is accreted during childhood, 45% during puberty, and 5% late in the second and early in the third decades of life.[77] Thereafter, bone mass is stable until resorption exceeds formation; gradual reduction in bone mass occurs in midadulthood accelerating transiently after menopause in the female. Both cortical bone and trabecular bone are lost with aging.

Causes of Disordered Bone Mineralization

Table 4–7 lists causes of disordered mineralization of bone. Dietary deficiency of vitamin D is unusual in the United States provided milk fortified with this vitamin is ingested and there is adequate exposure to sunlight. In the low-birth-weight preterm infant, vitamin D stores are low as the bulk of maternal 25OHD$_3$ is transferred to the fetus in the third trimester. Although the low-birth-weight infant is at risk for os-

TABLE 4–7.

Disorders of Mineralization

Abnormalities of vitamin D
  Nutritional deprivation
    Low-birth-weight infants
    Socioeconomic factors
    Malabsorption/hepatobiliary dysfunction
    Anticonvulsant drugs
  Metabolic errors
    Deficiency of 25-hydroxyvitamin D_3–1α-hydroxylase
    Abnormal receptor for 1,25-dihydroxyvitamin D_3 ($\pm$ alopecia)
  Chronic renal disease
Deficiency of calcium
  Nutritional deprivation
  Hypercalciuria
Deficiency of phosphorus
  Nutritional deprivation (low-birth-weight infant)
  Hyperphosphaturia
    Familial hypophosphatemia
    Renal tubular acidosis
      Fanconi's syndrome
      Primary
    Oncogenic
Hypophosphatasia
  Perinatal, infantile, childhood, adult
  Pseudohypophosphatasia
Inhibitors of mineralization (aluminum, diphosphonates)
Idiopathic juvenile osteoporosis/osteopenia
  Hypogonadism
    Gonadal dysgenesis
    Hypogonadotropism
  Malnutrition
    Cystic fibrosis
    Anorexia nervosa
  Cranial radiation
  Diabetes mellitus
  Drugs (glucocorticoids, aluminum)
  Hyperparathyroidism
Osteogenesis imperfecta types I, II, III, IV
Osteopetrosis
  Autosomal recessive/dominant/intermediate
  With associated disorders (deficiency of carbonic anhydrase II)
  Other forms of osteosclerosis
    Pyknodysostosis
    Progressive diaphyseal dysplasia

---

teopenia, fractures, and rickets, provision of more than 400 U/day of vitamin D does not lower the incidence of osteopenia below 20% in this population.[27] Of greater pathogenetic significance in the metabolic bone disease of prematurity are deficiencies of calcium and particularly of phosphorus.[42,50] Adequate intake of calcium and phosphorus by supplementation of human milk or commercial formula or by parenteral alimentation ameliorates or prevents this disorder. However, low-birth-weight infants remain osteopenic relative to full-term infants, whether breast-fed or formula-fed, at 1 year of age and perhaps even at older ages.[1] Characteristically, vitamin D deficiency rickets occurs in the exclusively breast-fed term infant born to a multigravida, vegetarian, black woman whose exposure to sunlight is limited owing to a mode of dress that covers most of her body.[39] The disorder occurs late in the first year of life, often in the winter. Deficiency of vitamin D is usually associated with low normal concentrations of calcium (although severe hypocalcemia may occur also), low serum phosphorus levels, increased alkaline phosphatase activity, low urine calcium and phosphorus values, and increased concentrations of PTH and aminoaciduria resulting from secondary hyperparathyroidism. Serum concentrations of $25OHD_3$ are low and plasma levels of $1,25(OH)_2D_3$ variable (low, normal, or high) in these patients.

Vitamin D deficiency may occur in patients with disorders of fat absorption, but rarely in patients with chronic liver disease or biliary obstruction is an abnormality of vitamin D–25-hydroxylase present. Vitamin D deficiency in these patients is secondary to its malabsorption due to deficiency of bile acids.[38] Gastrectomy, small intestinal bypass or resection (for the management of morbid obesity), and pancreatic insufficiency may lead to vitamin D deficiency, although in children with cystic fibrosis vitamin D deficiency is mild or absent. Several anticonvulsant drugs (phenytoin, barbiturate, glutethimide) lead to increased hydroxylation and subsequent urinary loss of inactive (water-soluble) metabolites of vitamin D. Rickets does occur in children treated with these drugs, especially if they are bedridden and not exposed to sunlight. Autosomal recessive abnormalities in the synthesis or response to $1,25(OH)_2D_3$ have been described. In patients with congenital deficiency of $25OHD$-1α-hydroxylase (vitamin D–dependent rickets type I), the clinical and biochemical stigmata of rickets are present, but concentrations of $25OHD_3$ are normal or high and those of $1,25(OH)_2D_3$ low. End-organ insensitivity to $1,25(OH)_2D_3$ (inappropriately termed vitamin D-"dependent" rickets type II) is characterized by hypocalcemia, severe rachitic deformities, and in some subjects alopecia. Plasma concentrations of $1,25(OH)_2D_3$ are extremely high (>300 pg/mL) and secondary hyperparathyroidism develops.

Several point mutations in the gene for the vitamin D receptor have been described which probably account for the lack of response to $1,25(OH)_2D_3$. An abnormal gene structure has been localized to the ligand-binding portion of the vitamin D receptor in four children from three related families in whom there was no nuclear binding of $1,25(OH)_2D_3$. In these children there was a single base mutation in exon 7 (cytosine to adenine) which led to an ochre termination codon (thymidine-adenine-adenine, TAA) instead of the codon for tyrosine (thymidine-adenine-cytosine, TAC) normally found at this point (amino acid 292, nucleotide 970) in the mRNA for the vitamin D receptor.[75] Thus a large portion of the $1,25(OH)_2D_3$ binding region was deleted from the vitamin D receptor of these subjects. In two other families, each with two children with end-organ insensitivity to $1,25(OH)_2D_3$, the base abnormalities leading to defects in response to this metabolite were present in the zinc finger DNA binding domain of the vitamin D receptor. In one family the substitution of adenine for guanine led to insertion of aspartic acid (GAC) instead of glycine (GGC) at amino acid 30 of the vitamin D receptor at a position near the tip of the first zinc finger; in another family, substitution also of adenine for guanine led to insertion of glutamine

(CAA) in place of arginine (CGA) at position 70 of the vitamin D receptor located near the tip of the second zinc finger.[44] Although the phenotype of patients with insensitivity to vitamin D is similar, there is marked genetic heterogeneity in this disorder.

Chronic renal disease leads to renal osteodystrophy and osteopenia by two interrelated mechanisms: decrease in renal 250HD-1α-hydroxylase activity due to decrease in renal mass, increased phosphorus levels, and acidosis results in decreased synthesis of $1,25(OH)_2D_3$ and functional vitamin D deficiency with decreased calcium absorption from the intestine; depressed intestinal calcium absorption and increased phosphorus retention due to impaired renal function lead to lowering of calcium levels and secondary hyperparathyroidism which increases bone resorption. In patients dialyzed with solutions of high aluminum content or in those receiving aluminum-containing phosphate-binding agents orally, there may be accumulation of this cation in bone where it interferes with osteoclast and osteoblast function and inhibits matrix formation and calcium-phosphorus deposition.[58] Thus, in patients with renal insufficiency there is increased bone resorption and decreased deposition of calcium with resultant severe clinical symptoms (pain on weight-bearing, increased fracture rate, growth retardation, and deformities) unless proper medical management prevents these complications.

Decreased calcium intake, most often in preterm infants but in older children as well, leads to decreased mineralization, as does chronic hypercalciuria. Dietary deprivation of phosphorus is perhaps the most significant pathogenetic factor in the osteopenia of prematurity. Phosphorus depletion also occurs in patients with various forms of renal tubular acidosis and in the occasional patient with a mesenchymal tumor (oncogenous rickets) which secretes a hyperphosphaturic agent which has not yet been identified. Hyperphosphaturic hypophosphatemic rickets has also been recorded in children with the linear sebaceous nevus syndrome, due to a phosphaturic substance produced by the nevus that also seems to depress synthesis of $1,25(OH)_2D_3$.[81] Hypophosphatemia, hyperphosphaturia, hypercalciuria, and rickets have been described in several children.[22] These children have appropriately increased concentrations of $1,25(OH)_2D_3$ and increased gastrointestinal absorption of calcium and phosphorus; these features, in addition to the hypercalciuria, distinguish this syndrome from the more common form of hypophosphatemic rickets (see below). Children with hypercalciuric hypophosphatemic rickets respond well to phosphorus supplementation alone; additional vitamin D is not necessary and may result in hypercalcemia. The basic defect in renal handling of phosphorus in these subjects has yet to be identified.

Familial hypophosphatemic rickets is an X-linked dominant disorder (occasionally inherited as an autosomal recessive or dominant trait) with variable expressivity and more prominent clinical manifestations in the hemizygous male than in the heterozygous female. However, the disorder is often severe in the affected female. Familial hypophosphatemic rickets is the most common form of rickets in the United States. It is characterized by rachitic bone deformities, short stature, hypophosphatemia, and hyperphosphaturia. There may be decreased intestinal absorption of phosphorus in some children, but the primary abnormality is increased urinary excretion of this element as its renal tubular resorption is decreased. In addition, plasma concentrations of $1,25(OH)_2D_3$ are inappropriately low for the serum concentration of phosphate, and decline when serum phosphate levels are raised.[21] The set-point for 250HD-1α-hydroxylase activity in response to low phosphate concentrations appears to be lower in patients with familial hypophosphatemic rickets than in normal subjects. The secretory response of $1,25(OH)_2D_3$ to PTH is blunted in these patients also; these children do not have secondary hyperparathyroidism (unless treated with excessive amounts of phosphorus). Although the primary metabolic defect has not been identified, abnormalities in the transport of phosphorus across (renal and muscle) cell membranes and in the response of the renal proximal convoluted tubule to a low phosphorus environment seem likely. The latter may be a manifestation of the inability of the cells of the renal proximal convoluted tubule to transport phosphorus intracellularly. Intramyocellular concentrations of inorganic phosphate are lower in patients with familial hypophosphatemic rickets than in controls and increase after administration of $1,25(OH)_2D_3$.[24] There may also be an element of resistance to the effects of $1,25(OH)_2D_3$ in the intestine, as large doses of this agent are required to increase calcium absorption.

Hypophosphatasia is a congenital defect in the production of the (bone/kidney/liver) alkaline phosphatase isoenzyme (also termed tissue-nonspecific alkaline phosphatase), but not in the synthesis of intestinal and placental isoenzymes of alkaline phosphatase.[18] This disorder may occur sporadically or it may be inherited as an autosomal recessive characteristic (occasionally as an autosomal dominant trait). The gene for (bone/kidney/liver) alkaline phosphatase is present on the short arm of chromosome 1. In one neonate with lethal hypophosphatasia, a missense mutation in the gene for this alkaline phosphatase has been identified.[87] In this infant substitution of adenine for guanine led to an exchange of threonine for alanine resulting in the production of inactive protein. In some patients synthesis of an abnormal form of alkaline phosphatase has been characterized, while in others defective regulation of the gene for alkaline phosphatase has been suggested. It is likely that considerable molecular heterogeneity is present in patients with similar clinical pictures.

There are several clinical forms of hypophosphatasia.[18] *Perinatal hypophosphatasia* is a lethal form of the disorder occurring in utero; the fetus has short, bowed, and fractured long bones, soft skull, narrowed chest, a rachitic rosary, and flaring of metaphyses. Death usually results from respiratory insufficiency due to the abnormal thoracic rib cage. *Infantile hypophosphatasia* appears within the first 6 months of life and is characterized by signs of decreased mineralization including short stature, varus or valgus deformities of the long bones, rachitic rosary, and metaphyseal widening, accompanied by hypotonia, failure to thrive, and constipation. Approximately 50% of affected infants will die, often of respiratory infections. *Childhood hypophosphatasia* is characterized by symptoms which vary from premature loss of primary dentition to the more classic physical and radiologic signs of rickets. *Adult hypophosphatasia* may be subclinical and identified only when an offspring manifests the childhood form, or there may be a history of premature loss of dentition or of rickets in childhood or of an increased rate of fractures. The biochemical hallmarks of hypophosphatasia are low or absent serum alkaline phosphatase activity and increased urinary excretion or plasma concentrations of the natural substrates for alkaline phosphatase—phosphoethanolamine, pyrophosphate, or pyridoxal-5'-phosphate. In patients with *pseudohypophosphatasia,* a clinical and biochemical picture similar to that of hypophosphatasia is present, but the serum alkaline phosphatase activity is normal when assessed by the synthetic substrates ordinarily utilized in the clinical chemistry laboratory.

Less common forms of rickets have been reported including its occurrence in the neonates of mothers who had received infusions of magnesium sulfate to stop premature labor during the second and third trimesters,[52] and in a child with deficiency of 11β-hydroxysteroid dehydrogenase and mineralocortcoid excess.[12]

Osteoporosis is a decrease in the amount of bone,[77] often associated with decrease in the quantity of the organic, structural component of bone, and secondarily with a decrease in the amount of mineral in bone. Osteoporosis is observed in children and teenagers with primary and secondary hypogonadism. Sixty percent to 80% of girls with Turner's syndrome have decreased bone mineralization beginning in the prepubertal years, where it is seen primarily in the shaft of the long bones; during puberty vertebral density is decreased in girls with Turner syndrome relative to the increased vertebral density noted during normal puberty.[77] Histologic examination of bone biopsies from subjects with Turner syndrome suggests an increase in bone resorption, somewhat similar to that seen in patients with postmenopausal osteoporosis. On the other hand, histologic evidence of decreased bone formation has also been reported in these patients.[77] Since osteopenia begins in midchildhood in girls with Turner syndrome, it is unclear if the abnormality is due to lack of sex hormones at this age or to a defect in bone formation contingent on the abnormal chromosome. Both growth hormone and estrogens appear to increase bone density in girls with Turner syndrome.[49,77]

In contrast to the osteopenia of Turner syndrome, patients with juvenile osteoporosis experience significant generalized and vertebral demineralization and fractures of the vertebrae and long bones. There are probably many causes of this disorder, the majority of which have not been identified. Patients with cystic fibrosis have osteopenia, usually not due to deficiency of vitamin D, but to suboptimal nutrition (and probably protein deprivation).[31] Adolescent girls with anorexia nervosa have decreased vertebral bone density, related both to nutritional deprivation and estrogen deficiency.[8] In addition, stress-related hypercortisolism may contribute to the osteoporosis of these patients.[51] Osteoporosis of the spine has been reported in survivors of childhood acute lymphoblastic leukemia who had received chemotherapy and cranial (but not spinal) irradiation, but not in patients who had received chemotherapy (antimetabolites and glucocorticoids) alone.[32] The mechanism by which cranial irradiation leads to osteoporosis is unknown; it has been suggested that hyposomatotropism and decreased production of IGF-I may be involved. Osteoporosis occurs in children with diabetes mellitus (possibly due to insulin deficiency) and those who have received spinal irradiation. I have seen boys with Marfan syndrome and osteoporosis. Homocystinuria and lysinuric protein intolerance have been reported as causes of osteopenia in childhood,[17] perhaps due to deprivation of amino acids necessary for collagen formation or to generalized protein malnutrition.

Chronic glucocorticoid excess leads to osteopenia by inhibiting protein and collagen synthesis, by increasing the rate of bone resorption through enhancement of PTH secretion, by inhibiting calcium absorption from the intestine through a direct effect on the intestinal cell, and by increasing the urinary excretion of calcium.[41] In hyperparathyroid patients bone density is decreased due to increased osteoclast resorption of calcium and destruction of matrix. Prolonged parenteral hyperalimentation may result in osteopenia by any of several mechanisms, including provision of too little protein, vitamin D, calcium, or phosphorus necessary for bone matrix formation and mineralization; by induction of acidosis and hypercalciuria; and by increasing the body's load of aluminum contained in casein hydrolysate and calcium gluconate, which inhibits mineralization of matrix by inhibiting the differentiation and functioning of osteoblasts.[47] Bisphosphonates and other compounds may also inhibit bone formation.

Osteogenesis imperfecta (OI) is a heterogeneous cluster of disorders of type I (skeletal) collagen formation[20] characterized by osseous fragility and increased fracture rate which varies in severity from lethal to subclinical forms. *Osteogenous imperfecta type I* is an autosomal dominant disorder with increased bone fragility and osteoporosis, blue scleras, and presenile conductive hearing loss in the patient or family.[80] It occurs in 1 in 30,000 births. Type IA is associated with normal dentition and type IB with abnormal dentition (dentinogenesis imperfecta). Patients with OI type IB have an increased frequency of fractures at very early ages (some at birth) and shorter stature than do patients with type IA. *Osteogenesis imperfecta type II*, an autosomal recessive form, is a lethal disease; the infant may be stillborn or die within hours to weeks after birth. There are three subtypes (A, B,C) characterized by subtle roentgenographic findings in the ribs (beaded or dysplastic) and long bones. Patients with OI type IIB survive longer than do infants with OI types IIA and IIC. *Osteogenesis imperfecta type III* is an autosomal recessive form of nonlethal OI. These patients have blue scleras at birth and pale blue or white scleras when older. Distinction from other types of OI requires a positive family history and prolonged observation of the clinical course. This is a severe form of OI resulting in fractures and deformities of the long bones, kyphoscoliosis, and frontal and temporal bossing and other features of facial dysplasia.

Osteogenesis imperfecta type IV is an autosomal dominant type of variable severity and is capable of survival into adulthood. The frequency of fractures decreases after puberty. These patients have light blue or white scleras and the frequency of hearing loss is less than OI type I. Two subtypes of OI type IV have been identified, those without (type IVA) and with (type IVB) dentinogenesis imperfecta. In addition, there are patients with OI who cannot be precisely characterized by present criteria. Many genetic abnormalities have been identified in patients with OI; these range from deletions or insertions within the gene coding for type I collagen to single base substitutions leading to abnormal amino acid constituents (often cysteine for glycine) in collagen within the pro-alpha$_1$ or -alpha$_2$ subunit, all of which lead to abnormal formation of the basic triple helix collagen unit and consequent structural fragility of bone.

Osteopetrosis is marked by a generalized increase in bone density (osteosclerosis), abnormalities of bone modeling, and an increase in the frequency of fractures. Histologic examination of osteopetrotic bone reveals areas of unresorbed calcified cartilage throughout the skeleton. There are three clinical types of osteopetrosis: an infantile, lethal, autosomal recessive form; a more mild autosomal dominant form; and an intermediate form.[4,88] The infantile type is characterized by failure to thrive, anemia, recurrent fractures, and hepatosplenomegaly noted within the first several months of life. The volume of bone marrow is decreased, requiring extramedullary hematopoiesis; the infant is susceptible to infections; the bony canals through which the cranial nerves pass are narrowed, resulting in loss of vision, hearing, and other cranial nerve function. Intermediate, less severe forms of autosomal recessive or dominant osteopetrosis have been observed in older children and adults. In some children osteopetrosis may be but one of a number of congenital anomalies. The autosomal dominant form is recognized in late childhood or in adults and is subdivided into two types on the basis of radiologic characteristics. In addition to diffuse osteosclerosis common to all subjects with osteopetrosis, type I patients have a sclerotic, enlarged cranial vault and sclerotic vertebrae without thickening of the end plate; in type II, sclerosis is most marked at the base of the skull; there is thickening of the vertebral end plates, and subcristal sclerosing bands of bone are present in the pelvis. Patients with autosomal dominant osteopetrosis may be asymptomatic or have a history of osteomyelitis or osteoarthritis, backaches, headaches, bone pain, facial nerve paresis, amblyopia, or deafness.[13,88] Osteopetrosis is caused by defective bone resorption, presumably due to a primary abnormality in osteoclast function or in the microenvironment necessary for such activity.

Osteopetrosis has also been associated with neuronal storage disease, an abnormal form of PTH, and deficiency of interleukin-2 or carbonic anhydrase II.[88] Patients with deficiency of carbonic anhydrase II have renal tubular acidosis, diffuse osteosclerosis which ameliorates over time, and cerebral calcifications. In osteoclasts carbonic anhydrase II is necessary for generation of the acid required for dissolution of bone mineral. This enzyme is also present in erythrocytes, kidney, and brain. Another form of osteosclerotic bone dysplasia is pyknodystosis, an autosomal recessive disorder characterized by growth retardation and disproportionate short stature with short limbs, macrocephaly, frontal prominence, beaked nose and other facial findings, and an increased fracture rate.[88]

Progressive diaphyseal dysplasia is an autosomal dominant osteosclerotic disease associated with new bone formation at the ends of the long bones resulting in widening of the diaphyses and later the metaphyses, with irregular bone surfaces. There may be macrocephaly, prominent forehead, decreased muscle mass, and some pain in affected children.[88]

Evaluation of Disorders of Mineralization

The history and physical examination are critically important in the evaluation of an infant or child with a disorder of mineralization. The family history of a heritable disorder (familial hypophosphatemic rickets, insensitivity to vitamin D, renal tubular acidosis, osteogenesis imperfecta, osteopetrosis, or other osteosclerotic disorder) will direct attention to this disorder in the patient. Maternal history during gestation, feeding practices, associated illnesses, fracture rate, and other details, or physical findings typical of rickets or other stigmata characteristic of metabolic bone disease guide further evaluation. Measurement of serum and urine calcium and phosphorus levels, serum electrolytes, blood pH, creatinine, PTH, metabolites of vitamin D, and alkaline phosphatase activity will identify patients with nutritional deprivation of vitamin D, insensitivity to $1,25(OH)_2D_3$, inadequate intake or excessive loss of calcium or phosphorus, abnormalities of alkaline phosphatase activity, hyperparathyroidism, and so forth. Radiologic examination will identify patients with rickets, osteopenia (which may be further quantified by measurement of bone mineral density, the most useful procedure being dual photon absorptiometric study of trabecular bone in the lumbar spine), osteogenesis imperfecta, osteopetrosis, or osteosclerotic bone disorders. Bone biopsy may be necessary on occasion for histologic examination and to quantify the dynamics of bone formation, resorption, and turnover. Specific identification of genetic defects in the vitamin D receptor, collagen, the osteoblast and osteoclast, and of other familial diseases will become increasingly available as the technology of molecular biology expands. The entire spectrum of clinical, laboratory, and radiologic data must be correlated to reach a diagnosis.

Management of Disorders of Mineralization

In the low-birth-weight infant adequate amounts of calcium (200 mg/kg/day orally), phosphorus (100 mg/kg/day orally), and vitamin D (400 units/day) should be administered as soon after birth as possible to prevent the osteopenia and rickets of prematurity. If parenteral alimentation is required, provision of adequate calcium, phosphorus, and vitamin D must also be considered.[67] Administration of 400 U/day of vitamin D will maintain adequate vitamin D stores in breast-fed and formula-fed infants and in children; slightly larger amounts are required initially in vitamin D–deprived subjects (2,000–5,000 U/day for several weeks). Children receiving anticonvulsant drugs who live in northern climes require approximately 2,000 U/day of vitamin D; children maintained indoors require supplemental vitamin D. Patients with deficiency of 250HD-1α-hydroxylase respond nicely to physiologic doses of $1,25(OH)_2D_3$ alone. In children with abnormalities of the vitamin D receptor, high doses of $1,25(OH)_2D_3$ (10 μg/day or more) may ameliorate the disorder; some of these patients may respond to $24,25(OH)_2D_3$; in other patients long-term intracaval infusion of calcium through a jugular venous catheter may be feasible.[86] In patients with chronic renal disease (or those receiving parenteral nutrition), aluminum exposure should be minimized and adequate $1,25(OH)_2D_3$ provided to maintain normal serum calcium levels and prevent secondary hyperparathyroidism.

Children with familial hypophosphatemic rickets require supplemental phosphorus (1–3 g of elemental phosphorus) and $1,25(OH)_2D_3$ (65–75 ng/kg/day initially, decreasing to 30 ng/kg/day after radiologic healing) to promote healing of the rickets. Whether aggressive therapy is warranted in such children is uncertain, as there are conflicting data concerning the effect of treatment on final height, and there is a significant risk of hypercalcemia, hypercalciuria, nephrocalcinosis, and renal failure.[10,21,83]

Treatment of osteoporosis requires specific identification of the pathophysiology of the osteopenia. Hypogonadal children can receive sex hormones. Those with protein malnutrition respond to an adequate diet. A variety of agents have been employed in the treatment of osteoporosis in the adult, including calcium supplementation, sodium fluoride (which does increase bone formation), calcitonin, vitamin D, and phosphonates, with variable success.

Some children with osteopetrosis have been treated with high doses of

1,25$(OH)_2D_3$ with variable response. Others have responded to bone marrow transplantation with repopulation of normal osteoclasts.[4,88] Patients with osteogenesis imperfecta are managed symptomatically and require careful orthopedic supervision.[20] Children with hypophosphatasia are very sensitive to vitamin D and easily become hypercalcemic and hypercalciuric. Temporary improvement has been reported in infants with the lethal form of hypophosphatasia after infusion of plasma rich in alkaline phosphatase activity taken from adults with Paget disease.[18,88] Appropriate dental and orthopedic care is required.

REFERENCES

1. Abrams SA, Schanler RJ, Tsang RC, et al: Bone mineralization in former very low birth weight infants fed either human milk or commercial formula: One year follow-up observation. *J Pediatr* 1988; 114:1041–1044.
2. Adams JS: Vitamin D metabolite-mediated hypercalcemia. *Endocrinol Metab Clin North Am* 1989;18:765–778.
3. Ahonen P, Myelarniemi S, Sipila I, et al: Clinical variation of autoimmune polyendocrinopathy-candidiasis-ectodermal dysplasia (APECED) in a series of 68 patients. *N Engl J Med* 1990; 322:1829–1836.
4. Anast CS: Neonatal mineral metabolism and congenital osteopetrosis, in Martin TJ, Raisz LG (eds): *Clinical Endocrinology of Calcium Metabolism*, New York, Marcel Dekker, Inc, 1987, pp 287–316.
5. Attie MF: Treatment of hypercalcemia. *Endocrinol Metab Clin North Am* 1989; 18:807–828.
6. Aurbach GD, Marx SJ, Spiegel AM: Metabolic bone disease, in Wilson JD, Foster DW (eds): *Textbook of Endocrinology*, ed 7. Philadelphia, WB Saunders Co, 1985, pp 1218–1255.
7. Bachrach LK, Foley TP Jr: Thyroiditis in children. *Pediatr Rev* 1989; 11:184–191.
8. Bachrach LK, Guido D, Katzman D, et al: Decreased bone density in adolescent girls with anorexia nervosa. *Pediatrics* 1990; 86:440–447.
9. Bainbridge R, Mughal Z, Mimouni F, et al: Transient congenital hypoparathyroidism: How transient is it? *J Pediatr* 1987; 111:866–868.
10. Balsan S, Tieder M: Linear growth pattern in patients with hypophosphatemic vitamin D–resistant rickets: Influence of treatment regimen and parental height. *J Pediatr* 1990; 116:365–371.
11. Bastian J, Law S, Vogler L, et al: Prediction of persistent immunodeficiency in the DiGeorge anomaly. *J Pediatr* 1989; 115:391–396.
12. Batista MC, Mendon BB, Kater CE, et al: Spironolactone-reversible rickets associated with 11β-hydroxysteroid dehydrogenase deficiency syndrome. *J Pediatr* 1986; 109:989–993.
13. Bollerslev J: Autosomal dominant osteopetrosis: Bone metabolism and epidemiological, clinical and hormonal aspects. *Endoc Rev* 1989; 10:45–67.
14. Broadus AE, Mangin M, Ikeda K, et al: Humoral hypercalcemia of cancer. Identification of a novel parathyroid hormone-like peptide. *N Engl J Med* 1988; 319:556–563.
15. Burtis WJ, Brady TG, Orloff JJ, et al: Immunochemical characterization of circulating parathyroid hormone–related protein in patients with humoral hypercalcemia of cancer. *N Engl J Med* 1990; 322:1106–1112.

16. Cardenas-Rivero N, Chernow B, Stolko MA, et al: Hypocalcemia in critically ill children, *J Pediatr* 1989; 114:946–951.
17. Carpenter TO, Levy HL, Hottrop ME, et al: Lysinuric protein intolerance presenting as childhood osteoporosis. Clinical and skeletal response to citrulline therapy. *N Engl J Med* 1985; 312:290–294.
18. Caswell AM, Russell RGG, Whyte MP: Hypophosphatasia: Pediatric forms. *J Pediatr Endocrinol* 1989; 3:73–92.
19. Caverzasio J, Montessuit C, Bonjour JP: Stimulatory effect of insulin-like growth factor-I on renal Pi transport and plasma 1,25-dihydroxyvitamin D_3. *Endocrinology* 1990; 127:453–459.
20. Cetta G, Ramirez F, Tsipooras P (eds): Third International Conference on Osteogenesis Imperfecta. *Ann NY Acad Sci* 1988; 543:1–187.
21. Chan JCM, Alon U, Hirschmann GM: Renal hypophosphatemic rickets. *J Pediatr* 1985; 106:533–544.
22. Chen C, Carpenter T, Steg N, et al: Hypercalciuric hypophosphatemic rickets, mineral balance, bone histomorphometry, and therapeutic implications of hypercalciuria. *Pediatrics* 1989; 84:276–280.
23. Chesney RW: Requirements and upper limits of vitamin D intake in the term neonate, infant and older child. *J Pediatr* 1990; 116:159–166.
24. Clarke GD, Kainer G, Conway WF, et al: Intramyocellular phosphate metabolism in X-linked hypophosphatemic rickets. *J Pediatr* 1990: 116:288–292.
25. Cooke R, Hollis B, Conner C, et al: Vitamin D and mineral homeostasis in the very low birth weight infant receiving 400 IU of vitamin D. *J Pediatr* 1990; 116:423–428.
26. Eisenberg H, Pallotta J, Sacks B, et al: Parathyroid localization, three-dimensional modeling and percutaneous ablation techniques. *Endocrinol Metab Clin North Am* 1989; 18:659–700.
27. Evans JR, Allen AC, Stinson DA, et al: Effect of high dose vitamin D supplementation on radiographically detectable bone disease of very low birth weight infants. *J Pediatr* 1989; 115:779–786.
28. Fasciotto BH, Gore SU, Bourdeau AM, et al: Autocrine regulation of parathyroid secretion by chromogranin A (secretory protein-I) and potentiation of secretion by chomomografin A and pancreastatin antibodies. *Endocrinology* 1990; 127:1329–1335.
29. Fitzpatrick LA: Hypercalcemia in the multiple endocrine neoplasia syndromes. *Endocrinol Metab Clin North Am* 1989: 18:741–752.
30. Fleischmajer R, Olsen BR, Kuhn K (eds): Structure, molecular biology, and pathology of cartilage. *Ann NY Acad Sci* 1990; 580:1–592.
31. Gibbens DT, Gilsanz V, Boechat MI, et al: Osteoporosis in cystic fibrosis. *J Pediatr* 1988; 113:295–300.
32. Gilsanz V, Carlson ME, Roe TF, et al: Osteoporosis after cranial irradiation for acute lymphoblastic leukemia. *J Pediatr* 1990; 117:238–244.
33. Gilsanz V, Gibbens DT, Roe TF, et al: Vertebral bone density in children: Effect of puberty. *Radiology* 1988; 166:847–850.
34. Greenberg F: What defines DiGeorge anomaly? *J Pediatr* 1989; 115:412–413.
35. Hanukoglu A, Chalew S, Kowarski AA: Late onset hypocalcemia, rickets and hypoparathyroidism in an infant of a mother with hyperparathyroidism. *J Pediatr* 1988; 112:751–754.
36. Harrison HE, Harrison HC: *Disorders of Calcium and Phosphate Metabolism in Childhood and Adolescence.* Philadelphia, WB Saunders Co, 1979, pp 1–314.
37. Heath H III: Familial benign (hypocalciuric) hypercalcemia. A troublesome mimic of mild primary hyperparathyroidism. *Endocrinol Metab Clin North Am* 1989; 18:723–739.

38. Heubi JE, Hollis BW, Tsang RC: Bone disease in chronic childhood cholestasis. II. Better absorption of 25-OH vitamin D than vitamin D in extra hepatic biliary atresia. *Pediatr Res* 1990; 27:26–31.

39. Hillman LS. Nutritional factors affecting mineral homeostosis and mineralization in the term and preterm infant, in Simmons DJ (ed): *Nutrition and Bone Development*, New York, Oxford University Press, 1990, pp 55–92.

40. Hillman LS. Mineral and vitamin D adequacy in infants fed human milk or formula between 6 and 12 months of age. *J Pediatr* 1990; 117:S134–S142.

41. Hodgson SF. Corticosteroid-induced osteopenia. *Endocrinol Metab Clin North Am* 1990; 19:95–111.

42. Holick MF: 1,25-Dihydroxyvitamin D_3 and the skin: A unique application for the treatment of psoriasis. *Proc Soc Exp Biol Med* 1989; 191:246–257.

43. Holland PC, Wilkinson AR, Diez J, et al: Prenatal deficiency of phosphate, phosphate supplementation and rickets in very-low-birthweight infants. *Lancet* 1990; 335:697–701.

44. Hoogenboezem T, Degenhart HJ, DeMuinck Keizer-Schrama SMPF, et al: Vitamin D metabolism in breast-fed infants and their mothers. *Pediatr Res* 1989; 25:623–628.

45. Horton WA: The biology of bone growth. *Growth Genet Horm* 1990; 6:1–4.

46. Hughes MR, Malloy PJ, Kieback DG, et al: Point mutations in the human vitamin D receptor gene associated with hypocalcemic rickets. *Science* 1988; 242:1702–1705.

47. Hurley DL, McMahon MM: Long-term parenteral nutrition and metabolic bone disease. *Endocrinol Metab Clin North Am* 1990; 19:113–131.

48. Insogna KL: Humoral hypercalcemia of malignancy. The role of parathyroid hormone-related protein. *Endocrinol Metab Clin North Am* 1989; 18:779–794.

49. Kirkland RT, Lin T-H, LeBlanc AD, et al: Effects of hormonal therapy on bone mineral density in Turner syndrome, in Rosenfeld RG, Grumbach MM (eds): *Turner Syndrome*, New York, Marcel Dekker, Inc, 1990, pp 319–325.

50. Koo WWK, Sherman R, Succop P, et al: Serum vitamin D metabolites in very low birth weight infants with and without rickets and fractures. *J Pediatr* 1989; 114:1017–1022.

51. Kreipe RE, Forbes GD: Osteoporosis: A "new morbidity" for dieting female adolescents? *Pediatrics* 1990; 86:478–480.

52. Lamm CI, Norton KI, Murphy RJC, et al: Congenital rickets associated with magnesium sulfate infusion for tocolysis. *J Pediatr* 1988; 113:1078–1082.

53. Lee WK, Vargas A, Barnes J, et al: The Kenny-Caffey syndrome: Growth retardation and hypocalemia in a young boy. *Am J Med Genet* 1983; 14:773–782.

54. Li J-Y, Specker BL, Ho ML, et al: Bone mineral content in black and white children 1 to 6 years of age. Early appearance of race and sex differences. *Am J Dis Child* 1989; 143:1346–1349.

55. Lichtenstein P, Specker BL, Tsang RC, et al: Calcium-regulating hormones and minerals from birth to 18 months of age: A cross-sectional study. I. Effects of sex, race, age, season and diet on vitamin D status. *Pediatrics* 1986; 77:883–890.

56. Manolagas SC, Hustmyer FG, Yu X-P: 1,25-Dihydroxyvitamin D_3 and the immune system. *Proc Soc Exp Biol Med* 1989; 191:238–245.

57. Matkovic V, DeKanic D, Kostial K: Calcium, teenagers and osteoporosis, in *Osteoporosis: Current Concepts. Seventh Ross Conference on Medical Research*, 1987, pp 64–66.

58. McCarthy JT, Kumar R: Renal osteodystrophy. *Endocrinol Metab Clin North Am* 1990; 19:65–93.

59. Morris CA, Demsey SA, Leonard CO, et al: Natural history of Williams syndrome. *J Pediatr* 1988; 113:318–326.

60. Mundy GR: *Calcium Homeostasis: Hypercalcemia and Hypocalcemia.* London, Martin Dunitz Ltd, 1989, pp 1–248.
61. Mundy GR: Hypercalcemia factors other than parathyroid hormone-related protein. *Endocrinol Metab Clin North Am* 1989; 18:795–806.
62. Mundy GR: Immune system and bone remodeling. *Trends Endocrinol Metab* 1990; 1:307–311.
63. Nishiyama S, Tomoeda S, Inoue F, et al: Self-limited familial hyperparathyroidism associated with hypercalciuria and renal tubular acidosis in three siblings. *Pediatrics* 1990; 86:421–427.
64. Ogden JA: Histogenesis of the musculoskeletal system, in Simmons DJ (ed), *Nutrition and Bone Development,* New York, Oxford University Press, 1990, pp 3–36.
65. Orloff JJ, Wu TL, Stewart AF: Parathyroid hormone-like proteins: Biochemical responses and receptor interactions. *Endoc Rev* 1989; 10:476–495.
66. Patten JL, Johns DR, Valle D, et al: Mutation in the gene encoding the stimulatory G protein of adenylate cyclase in Albright's hereditary osteodystrophy. *N Engl J Med* 1990; 322:1412–1419.
67. Pelegano JF, Rowe JC, Carey DE, et al: Simultaneous infusion of calcium and phosphorus in parenteral nutrition for premature infants: Use of physiologic calcium/phosphorus ratio. *J Pediatr* 1989; 114:115–119.
68. Pont A: Unusual causes of hypercalcemia. *Endocrinol Metab Clin North Am* 1989; 18:753–764.
69. Pyeritz RE: Heritable defects in connective tissue. *Hosp Pract* 1987; 22:153–168.
70. Ramirez F, Boast S, D'Alessia M, et al: Fibrillar collagen genes. Structure and expression in normal and diseased states. *Ann NY Acad Sci* 1990; 580:74–80.
71. Ramirez F, DeWet W: Molecular biology of the human fibrillar collagen genes. *Ann NY Acad Sci* 1988; 543:109–116.
72. Reichel H, Koeffler HP, Norman AW: The role of the vitamin D endocrine system in health and disease. *N Engl J Med* 1989; 320:980–991.
73. Reinhardt TA, Horst RL: Parathyroid hormone down-regulates 1,25-dihydroxyvitamin D receptors (VDR) and VDR messenger ribonucleic acid in vitro and blocks homologous up-regulation of VDR in vivo. *Endocrinology* 1990; 127:942–948.
74. Ristelli J, Ristelli L: Growth and collagen. *Growth Growth Factors* 1989; 4:159–164.
75. Ritchie HH, Hughes MR, Thompson ET, et al: An ochre mutation in the vitamin D receptor gene causes hereditary 1,25-dihydroxyvitamin D_3 resistant rickets in three families. *Proc Natl Acad Sci USA* 1989; 86:9783–9787.
76. Roberts AB, Heine UI, Flandersk C, et al: Transforming growth factor-β. Major role in regulation of extracellular matrix. *Ann NY Acad Sci* 1990; 580:225–232.
77. Rubin KR: Osteoporosis in Turner syndrome, in Rosenfeld RG, Grumbach MM (eds): *Turner Syndrome,* New York, Marcel Dekker, Inc, 1990, pp 301–317.
78. Salvi M, Fukazawa H, Bernard N, et al: Role of autoantibodies in the pathogenesis and association of endocrine autoimmune disorders. *Endoc Rev* 1988; 9:450–466.
79. Segre GV: Advances in techniques for measurement of parathyroid hormone. Current applications in clinical medicine and directions for future research. *Trends Endocrinol Metab* 1990; 1:243–247.
80. Sillence DO: Osteogenesis imperfecta nosology and genetics. *Ann NY Acad Sci* 1988; 543:1–15.
81. Skovby F, Svejgaard E, Moller J: Hypophosphatemic rickets in linear sebaceous nevus sequence. *J Pediatr* 1987; 111:855–857.
82. Specker BL, Lichtenstein P, Mimouni F, et al: Calcium regulating hormones from

birth to 18 months of age: A cross-sectional study II. Effects of sex, race, age, season and diet on serum minerals, parathyroid hormone and calcitonin. *Pediatrics* 1986; 77:891–896.

83. Stickler GB, Morgenstern BZ: Hypophosphatemic rickets: Final height and clinical symptoms in adults. *Lancet* 1989; 2:902–905.

84. Thakker RV, Bouloux P, Wooding C, et al: Association of parathyroid tumors in multiple endocrine neoplasia type 1 with loss of alleles on chromosome 11. *N Engl J Med* 1989; 321:218–224.

85. Venkataraman PS, Tsang RC, Chen I-W, et al: Pathogenesis of early neonatal hypocalcemia: Studies of serum calcitonin, gastrin and plasma glucagon. *J Pediatr* 1987; 110:599–603.

86. Weisman Y, Bab I, Gazit D, et al: Long-term intracaval calcium infusion therapy in end-organ resistance to 1,25-dihydroxyvitamin D. *Am J Med* 1987; 83:984–990.

87. Weiss MJ, Cole DEC, Ray K, et al: A missence mutation in the human liver/bone/ kidney alkaline phosphatase gene in lethal hypophosphatasia. *Proc Natl Acad Sci USA* 1988; 85:7666–7669.

88. Whyte MP: Heritable metabolic and dysplastic bone disease. *Endocrinol Metab Clin North Am* 1990; 19:133–173.

89. Williams syndrome—The enigma continues (editorial). *Lancet* 1988; 2:488–489.

90. Zaloga GP, Chernow B: The multifactorial basis for hypocalcemia during sepsis. Studies of the parathyroid hormone–vitamin D axis. *Ann Intern Med* 1987; 107:36–41.

Chapter *5*

Thyroid Gland

Wellington Hung

The thyroid gland produces the thyroid hormones thyroxine (T_4), and 3,5,3′-triiodo-thyronine (T_3) whose classic action is the regulation of the rate of cellular oxidation in virtually all tissues.

The median part of the thyroid gland originates in the embryo during the 3- to 4-mm stage by proliferation and invagination of the medial endoderm of the foregut at the level of the first and second pharyngeal pouches. The lateral thyroid anlage arises from the fourth pouch and becomes elongated and enlarges laterally to become bilobed with the pharyngeal region contracting to become a narrow stalk, the thyroglossal duct. This duct normally atrophies and the thyroid continues to grow and simultaneously migrates caudad. When it fails to atrophy, it may retain as a cystic mass in the midline of the neck, somewhere between the base of the tongue and the hyoid bone. A thyroglossal cyst should be considered in any patient presenting with an enlarging cystic mass in the midline of the neck. A thyroglossal duct cyst should be removed surgically. A pyramidal lobe of the thyroid can result from retention and growth of the lower end of the thyroglossal duct. The pyramidal lobe usually undergoes gradual atrophy.

The parathyroid glands are derived from the third and fourth pharyngeal pouches. The ultimobranchial body is derived from a portion of the fourth pharyngeal pouch and migrates to the thyroid where it gives rise to the C cells of the thyroid gland. Evidence indicates that these C cells are the source of calcitonin. Variations involving the development of the thyroid are of two types:

1. Failure of thyroid gland to develop, which results in congenital hypothyroidism.

2. Differentiation in abnormal locations, including persistence of a thyroglossal duct or tract. This represents an arrest in the usually descent of part or all of the thyroid to the usual location.

NORMAL ANATOMY

The thyroid gland is bilobed and the lobes are connected by an isthmus. The isthmus usually overlies the region of the second to fourth tracheal cartilages. The right lobe of the thyroid is often the larger of the two lobes in children. The right lobe tends to enlarge more than the left lobe in disorders associated with diffuse increase in size.

The weight of the "normal" thyroid gland in children varies from one region of the world to another and appears to be greater in areas of relative iodine deficiency. Within the United States, regional variations are encountered.[35] Since weight is an important criterion in the pathologic diagnosis of goiter, these regional variations, as well as the variations associated with age, must be recognized.

HYPOTHALAMIC-PITUITARY-THYROID INTERRELATIONSHIPS

Thyroid-stimulating hormone (TSH) secretion is stimulated by thyrotropin-releasing hormone (TRH) (Fig. 5–1). The structure of TRH has been shown to be pyroglutamyl-histidyl-prolinamide, and this tripeptide has been synthesized. TRH is produced by several hypothalamic nuclei and is secreted into the hypophyseal portal system and carried to the anterior pituitary gland. Here TRH interacts with cell membrane receptors on the thyrotroph, resulting sequentially in activation of adenyl cyclase, increased production of cyclic adenosine monophosphate (cAMP), and increased secretion of TSH, which results in stimulation of T_4 and T_3 formation in the thyroglobulin molecule.

The secretion of TSH is pulsatile. In children and adolescents serum TSH concentrations exhibit a circadian rhythm. The serum TSH levels reach a nadir in the late afternoon, rise to a peak around midnight, remain on a plateau for several hours, and then decrease. The nocturnal rise is sleep-independent.

Feedback control of TSH secretion occurs at both the pituitary and hypothalamic levels. At the pituitary, low levels of circulating thyroid hormones result in increased TSH secretion, while elevated levels of thyroid hormones suppress TSH secretion. Feedback inhibition by thyroid hormones on the thyroid gland itself has been described.

The cytologic differentiation of the pituitary gland begins at approximately 8 weeks of gestation and periodic acid–Schiff (PAS)–positive basophils are first detected at approximately 9 weeks of gestation. TSH is produced and stored in the basophilic cells of the anterior pituitary gland. TSH has been identified in fetal pituitaries at 12 to 14 weeks of gestation.

Excellent reviews of normal development of the thyroid gland in the fetus have

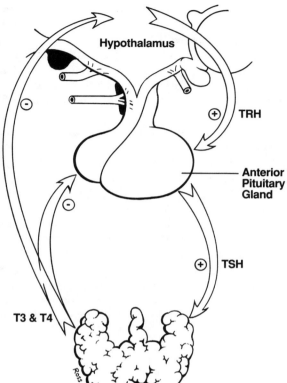

FIG 5–1.
Schematic diagram of hypothalamic-
pituitary-thyroid axis. See text.

been published.[3,21] The fetal hypothalamic-pituitary-thyroid axis begins to develop at the end of the first trimester and maturation continues in the second trimester. The concentration of TSH in the fetal pituitary gland and serum is very low before 18 weeks and increases between 18 and 24 weeks. Activation of the fetal pituitary-thyroid axis at this time is presumably mediated by TRH since hypothalamic TRH is detectable in the fetus by the tenth week of gestation and increases thereafter.

The thyroid gland will develop and store colloid as well as synthesize small amounts of hormones in the absence of the pituitary gland. The fetal thyroid is capable of binding iodine and concentrating radioactive iodine by 10 weeks of gestation. This is of importance since maternal administration of therapeutic amounts of radioactive iodine after the tenth week of gestation can result in fetal radiothyroidectomy and sever congenital hypothryoidism.

Fetal serum T_4 is measurable in low concentrations by the 11th to 12th week of gestation, which suggests that it appears in the circulation about a week after initiation of intrathyroidal hormone synthesis. After the 18th to 20th week of gestation, serum T_4 increases progressively until term, at which time the mean T_4 level is 11.2 ± 0.43 μg/dL. Fetal serum free thyroxine (FT_4) increases with increasing gestational age until term; the mean FT_4 is 2.9 ± 0.1 ng/dL.

Serum T_3 levels in the fetus less than 30 weeks of age are below the detectable limits of radioimmunoassay (RIA) but gradually increase to term levels of 40 ng/dL. This constitutes a state of relative T_3 deficiency. 3,3',5'-triiodothyronine (reverse T_3, RT_3) is a normal component of human serum and extrathyroidal metabolism of T_4 is an important source of RT_3 in humans. The fetal thyroid gland contains only small amounts of RT_3 and it seems that most of RT_3 is derived from monodeiodination of T_4 in peripheral tissues. RT_3 has minimal metabolic activity compared with T_4 and T_3. Fetal T_4 metabolism differs markedly from that during extrauterine life in that T_4 is metabolized predominantly to RT_3 rather than to T_3 as in postnatal life. Serum RT_3 levels exceed 250 ng/dL early in the last trimester and decrease steadily to term. The high rate of RT_3 production seems to be reflected in high RT_3 levels in amniotic fluid. Amniotic fluid T_4, T_3, and TSH concentrations do not correlate well with the fetal thyroid state. By contrast, amniotic fluid RT_3 levels are relatively high by 15 weeks of gestation and appear to be of fetal origin.

TSH exerts its effect by binding to a specific receptor on the thyroid cell membrane. Binding of TSH activates adenylyl cyclase in the thyroid cell which converts intracellular adenosine triphosphate (ATP) to AMP. Cyclic AMP then initiates a series of biochemical events.

Data derived from studies during pregnancy suggest that the placenta is relatively impermeable to the thyroid hormones and TSH. Concentrations of TSH, T_4, T_3, and FT_3 in fetal blood do not correlate with paired maternal hormone values at any time during pregnancy.

THYROID HORMONE SYNTHESIS

Iodine and amino acids are essential substrates for the formation of the thyroid hormones T_4 and T_3. After iodide is absorbed from the gastrointestinal tract, it enters the iodine pool of the body. From this pool iodide is removed by trapping in the follicular cells of the thyroid gland or is excreted in the urine. Immediately after entrance of iodide into the thyroid, iodination of organic compounds occurs. This is dependent upon oxidation of iodide to iodine. Thyroid hormones are first synthesized as a prohormone, thyroglobulin (Tg), the substrate of the iodination reaction. Thyroglobulin is a glycoprotein (mol wt approximately 660 kDa) consisting of amino acids connected in peptide linkage.

Thyroglobulin is a normal secretory product of the thyroid gland in man and can be measured by RIA in the serum, but interlaboratory variations exist because an international standard has not been developed. Term newborn infants have cord Tg levels significantly less than those of premature infants, but greater than those of adults.[51] The mean cord serum Tg level of term female infants (31.1 ± 8.9 ng/mL) has been found to be significantly greater than that of term male infants (26.1 ± 7.7 ng/mL). It was concluded that the sex difference in cord serum Tg levels related principally to changes in body composition accompanying increasing birth weight rather than to sexually determined phenomena. Serum Tg levels decrease progressively with age in children and adolescents to adult values. In normal adults a mean

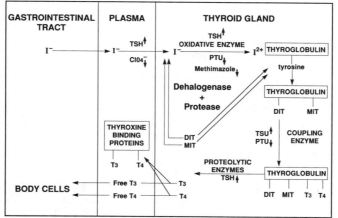

FIG 5–2.
Diagram of synthesis of thyroid hormones. See text.

serum value of 5.1 ng/mL with a range of less than 1.6 to 20.7 ng/mL has been reported. Stimulation of the thyroid gland with TSH produces an increase in serum Tg levels while suppression of TSH release decreases serum Tg levels.

In neonates with congenital hypothyroidism there is a good correlation between the presence of thyroid tissue and the presence of Tg in the serum. Infants with athyreosis have undetected Tg, whereas in those with thyroid tissue demonstrated by thyroid scanning, serum Tg is present.

Organic iodine is incorporated into tyrosine residues within Tg, a large glycoprotein. Sequential iodination, first at the 3 and then at the 5 position, occur to form monoiodotyrosine (MIT) and diiodotyrosine (DIT). MIT and DIT are coupled through an ether linkage to form T_4 and T_3. Both coupling and iodination require oxidative conditions, both may involve the same perioxidase, and both are inhibited by thiourea derivatives.

Within Tg, the usual ratio of DIT/MIT is approximately 2:1, that of T_4/T_3 is approximately 3:1. Proteases and peptidases digest Tg releasing iodotyrosines and iodothyronines. A diagram of the pathway of thyroid hormone synthesis is presented in Figure 5–2; each step is enzymatically dependent.

TRANSPORT OF THYROID HORMONES

Transport of T_4 and T_3 is largely in plasma bound to proteins. Approximately 75% of serum T_4 is bound to an interalpha globulin (T_4-binding globulin or TBG); 20% is bound to albumin and 5% to a prealbumin, throxine-binding prealbumin (TBPA). T_4 binds with approximately ten times the affinity of T_3 to these carrier proteins and this accounts for the much greater concentration of T_4 than T_3 found in normal plasma. In addition, a small amount of T_4 is loosely attached to red blood cells. It is estimated that although free and bound T_4 are in equilibrium, at any given time only 0.016% to 0.064% of the total circulating T_4 is not bound. This tiny fraction is referred to as *free thyroxine* (FT$_4$). Although quantitatively insignificant, the free hormone concentration indicates more accurately the metabolic status of the individual, since only in this form can it traverse the cellular membranes and exert its function.

ACTION OF THYROID HORMONES

The thyroid hormones have profound effects on both growth and development and stimulate the metabolic rates of many processes. The mechanism of stimulation is not clear but the hormones seem to act on the energy-producing electron-transfer process in the respiratory enzyme systems of the mitochondria. Thyroid hormones are also involved in increasing transcription of messenger RNA (mRNA), probably via cAMP.[14] There is no single site of action which explains the variety of physiologic changes caused by thyroid hormones. In pediatric patients important actions on body growth and maturation result from the direct effect of the thyroid hormones on tissue growth and its permissive effect on growth hormone secretion.

At one time it was thought that T_4 was the major biologically active thyroid hormone and T_3 was only of minor importance. However, it has been shown that T_3 may be the only functional thyroid hormone and that the biologic activity of T_4 may depend entirely on its peripheral conversion to T_3. It may be that T_4 serves as a prohormone but is also capable of hormone activity.

PHYSIOLOGIC CHANGES IN THYROID FUNCTION DURING THE PEDIATRIC AGE RANGE

Laboratory Tests

Thyroid-Stimulating Hormone

Serum TSH can be measured by RIA and the conventional RIA can easily detect patients with primary hypothyroidism, but the ability of RIA to differentiate low normal from abnormally low values is limited because of assay insensitivity. A new assay has been developed which has a high specificity, lower limit of detection, wider range, and quicker speed of analysis than RIA.[44] These new assays have been termed *ultrasensitive* or *high-sensitive TSH assays* and are based on immunoradiometric assay (IRMA). In these assays, the antibody rather than the antigen is labeled, and usually two separate monoclonal or polyclonal antibodies of different specificity are used to react with separate sites on the TSH molecule and sandwich the molecule between two relatively large antibody molecules.

Suppression of the TSH level measured by sensitive assays has been shown to be highly predictive of a suppressed response to TRH, thus obviating the need in most situations for the TRH stimulation test (see below). In hypothyroid patients these assays help differentiate primary from secondary and tertiary causes. Additionally, these assays should increase the ability to establish the adequacy of thyroid hormone replacement therapy in primary hypothyroidism.

In the newborn infant, there is a great increase in serum TSH concentration at the time of birth. The increase is probably already occurring at the time of delivery because TSH levels in umbilical cord blood are higher than those in maternal blood.

TSH levels (not measured by ultrasensitive assay) in cord sera range between 1 and 20 μU/mL. An acute increase in levels occurs within the first minutes of life, and peak values are observed approximately 30 minutes following delivery. Levels decrease rapidly thereafter, falling to 50% of the peak values by 2 hours of life. TSH concentrations decrease further, so that by 48 hours of age, they are only slightly higher than cord blood values.

The complete explanation for this striking increase in TSH concentrations is not known. The stress of vaginal delivery is not the stimulus, since babies born by cesarean section manifest the same phenomenon. There is evidence that the increase in levels, at least in part, may be due to the drop in body temperature experienced by the newborn during the first hours of life. It has recently been demonstrated that TRH-degrading activity is initially absent in human cord blood, appears after 3 days of life, and reaches adult euthyroid plasma levels after 5 days of life. This finding may be involved in the control of TRH activity and, therefore, in TSH regulation.

Beyond the newborn period, serum TSH levels do not change much with age. However, a recent report suggests that serum TSH levels decline progressively with age in children and adolescents.[51] The reason for the discrepancy in findings is not known. Normally, serum TSH concentrations measured by IRMA range between 0.5 and 3.8 μU/mL.

Thyrotropin-Releasing Hormone

Synthetic TRH causes release of TSH from the anterior pituitary glands of normal children. Serum TSH levels increase in normal children and adolescents within 10 minutes after the intravenous (IV) administration of TRH, peak at 20 to 45 minutes, and then decline to baseline levels by 2 hours. The TRH test allows us to (1) distinguish hypothalamic TRH deficiency from pituitary TSH deficiency as the cause of hypothyroidism; (2) evaluate pituitary TSH reserve; and (3) offer a confirmatory test for hyperthyroidism. As mentioned above, the availability of ultrasensitive assays for TSH may obviate the need to perform a TRH test in many instances. Adverse reactions to synthetic TRH have been reported.[45]

Thyroxine-Binding Proteins

After secretion from the thyroid gland, more than 99% of T_4 and T_3 are bound to three plasma thyroid-binding proteins: T_4-binding globulin (TBG), the principal protein; T_4-binding prealbumin (TBPA); and albumin. Only a very small fraction of plasma T_4 and T_3 is free and therefore bioactive. Serum TBG concentration can be measured by RIA. The serum concentration of the three thyroid hormone-binding proteins vary with pathologic and physiologic states.

Alterations in TBG concentration or binding usually do not affect the FT_4, and therefore it is useful to measure this if one suspects an abnormality in the serum level of T_4-binding proteins. There are two methods to measure FT_4: resin T_3 uptake (T_3RU), which is an indirect measurement, and by direct measurement. T_3RU, or one of its modifications, is more widely used than the direct measurement method.

A single TBG gene has been located on the long arm of the X chromosome.[69] TBG variants have been identified and typed.[55] The significance of these variants is not clear at the present time.

The binding capacity range of TBG in the newborn (15–23 μg/dL) is approximately 1.5 times the normal adult level, whereas that in the mother is about 2.5 times the normal adult level. The TBG concentration is high (5.2 ng/dL) in cord blood and decreases to adult levels (2.1–5.2 mg/dL) by 13 to 14 years of age. Serum concentrations of TBG at term are higher in healthy full-term newborns than in the small-for-gestational age (SGA) newborn. Serum concentrations of TBG in the SGA newborns are higher than those found in premature newborns. A positive correlation is present between serum TBG and thyroid hormone concentrations.

Serum concentrations of TBPA are higher in the full-term newborn than in the SGA newborn. However, the serum concentration of TBPA is lower in the SGA newborn than in the premature newborn. The T_4-binding capacity of albumin in cord blood is higher than that of the mother at the time of delivery. Serum concentrations are significantly higher in the full-term newborn than in low-birth-weight newborns. Pronounced changes in serum concentrations of thyroid hormone–binding proteins occur in early infancy and these changes are related to the postnatal age as well as to the maturity of the infants.

Protein-Bound Iodine (PBI)

The PBI is a measure of the amount of iodine bound to circulating proteins. The PBI is normally 1.0 to 1.5 µg/dL higher than the T_4 iodine. Its clinical usefulness is nullified by the administration of organic or inorganic compounds. The PBI should *not* be used as a thyroid function test.

Thyroxine

Peak serum concentrations of T_4 in the newborn are reached 24 hours after birth (Table 5–1) and then decrease slowly over the first weeks of life. Healthy premature and SGA newborns have qualitiatively similar but quantitatively decreased changes in T_4 when compared with full-term newborns. During the first 7 weeks of life serum

TABLE 5–1.

Age-Related Levels for Serum Thyroxine (T4), Triiodothyronine (T3), Reverse T_3, T_4-Binding Globulin (TBG), T_3 Resin Uptake (T_3 RU), and Thyroid Weight*†

Age	T_4 (µg/dL)	T_3 (ng/dL)	Reverse T_3 (ng/dL)	TBG (mg/dL)	T_3 RU (%)	Thyroid Weight (gm mean ± SD)
Cord						
30 wk	9.4 (5.7–15.6)					
35 wk	10.1 (6.1–16.8)					
40 wk	10.9 (6.6–18.1)					
45 wk	11.7 (7.1–19.4)					
Term	10.8 (6.6–17.5)	50 (14–86)	224 (100–501)	5.4 (1.4–9.4)	0.90 (0.75–1.05)	
1–3 days	16.5 (11.0–21.5)	420 (100–740)			1.15 (0.90–1.40)	1.5 ± 0.7
1–4 wk	12.9 (8.2–16.6)		90 (26–290)	5.0 (1.0–9.0)	1.00 (0.80–1.15)	1.4 ± 0.6
1–12 mo	11.2 (7.2–15.6)	175 (105–245)	40 (11–129)	4.8 (2.0–7.6)	0.98 (0.88–1.12)	2.0 ± 0.9
1–5 yr	10.5 (7.3–15.0)	168 (105–269)	33 (15–71)	4.2 (2.9–5.4)	0.99 (0.88–1.12)	3.9 ± 2.0
6–10 yr	9.3 (6.4–13.3)	150 (94–241)	36 (17–79)	3.8 (2.5–5.0)	1.00 (0.88–1.12)	5.3 ± 2.1
11–15 yr	8.1 (5.6–11.7)	133 (83–213)	41 (19–88)	3.3 (2.1–4.6)	1.02 (0.88–1.12)	9.6 ± 5.1
16–20 yr	8.0 (4.2–11.8)	130 (80–210)	41 (25–80)	3.4 (2.2–4.6)	1.01 (0.85–1.14)	

*Data from references 18, 20, 35.
†Unless otherwise noted, values are mean ±2 SD.

T_4 levels are significantly lower in SGA than in full-term infants and even lower values are present in premature infants. After approximately 50 days of age, comparable serum T_4 levels are present in all three maturity groups of infants. Between 1 and 15 years of age there is a gradual decrease in concentration of T_4 with increasing age.

Free Thyroxine

The level of FT_4 is less than 0.1% of the total circulating T_4 concentration. The mean cord level of FT_4 is higher than the mean maternal level, but the difference is not statistically significant.[75] Serum FT_4 levels peak at 24 hours of life and then decrease slowly over the first weeks of life. Similarly to T_4, serum FT_4 levels correlate positively with increasing gestational age and birth weight.[60] FT_4 levels decrease progressively with age during childhood.

Triiodothyronine and Free Triiodothyronine

The FT_3 is approximately 0.3% of the total T_3 concentration. Serum T_3 and FT_3 levels in the full-term infant increase three to six times within 4 hours of birth. Changes in serum concentrations of T_3 in infancy are related to postnatal age as well as to the maturity of the infant. Serum T_3 levels decrease with age during childhood and adolescence (see Table 5–1) as do FT_3 levels.[20]

Reverse Triiodothyronine

Concentrations of RT_3 are high in cord blood of the human newborn and slowly decrease after birth. Serum RT_3 concentrations increase slightly with age during childhood.[20]

Thyroidal Uptake of Radioactive Iodine

Studies of radioactive iodine uptake by the neonatal thyroid gland have shown an early increase in uptake as a result of increased TSH stimulation. The mean 24-hour uptake during the first 2 days of life in full-term infants has been found to be 62%, and 72% in premature infants within the first 3 days of life. The initially elevated 24-hour uptake values return to normal values of 10% to 40% by 5 days of age. After the first month of life, the 24-hour uptake of radioactive iodine by the thyroid is quantitatively similar throughout infancy, childhood, adolescence, and adulthood. The mean thyroidal uptake has been found to be slightly but significantly higher in females than in males from childhood through adolescence.

Normal values for 24-hour thyroidal ^{123}I uptake vary geographically because of regional variations in dietary iodine content and must therefore be determined locally for each part of the country.

This test is currently being used less frequently in pediatric patients than in the past because of several factors: (1) the increased intake of stable iodides through food preservatives, antiseptics, and drugs has lowered the normal range of uptake so that it may not discriminate between normal subjects and patients with hypothyroidism; (2) although ^{123}I reduces the dose of radiation to the thyroid gland as compared with ^{125}I or ^{131}I, some tissue radiation is still present; and (3) the test is time-consuming and moderately expensive.

Radiologic Studies

An anatomic image of the thyroid gland can be obtained by scintiscanning. Thyroid scanning may be performed with either ^{123}I or with technetium 99m pertechnetate. Computed tomography (CT) and magnetic resonance imaging (MRI) of the thyroid gland can produce excellent images but at great expense. To date no significant advantages have been shown over high-resolution sonography in evaluating thyroid masses.[43] It should be remembered that iodinated contrast used in CT can interfere with thyroid function tests for weeks.

Ultrasonography is useful for determining thyroid size in pediatric patients and in determining the cause of diffuse goiters. Thyroid volume in normal controls aged 5 to 16 years and living in a non–iodine-deficient area have been published.[31] There was no significant difference in thyroid volume between boys and girls in this study. There was a gradual increase in volume with age. The volume in 5- to 6-year-olds ranged from 1.0 to 1.7 mL (mean 1.3 mL), and in 15- to 16-year-olds from 4.1 to 10.1 mL (mean 7.0 mL).

Uptake of Radioactive L-Triiodothyronine (Thyroid Hormone Binding Ratio [THBR] or T_3 Uptake Test)

Uptake tests of T_3 provide information about the available binding sites of TBG. They measure the partition of added radioactive T_3 between serum TBG and a second binder such as a resin under conditions of controlled temperature and time. Labeled T_3 distributes itself between the free or available binding sites of the TBG and the secondary binder. The results are reported either as the percentage of labeled T_3 taken up by the resin or as the percentage uptake of labeled T_3 relative to a standard or a normal control serum pool. Normal values vary with the test procedure and the individual laboratory. T_3 resin uptake varies shortly after birth, but does not change significantly between 1 and 15 years of age.

Free Thyroxine Index

A free T_4 index (FTI), calculated by multiplying the serum T_4 concentration by the T_3 RU value, provides a guide for interpreting abnormal T_4 values caused by elevation or depression of the TBG level. If the T_4 level is high because of an elevated TBG level, the T_3 RU will be low. In this situation, the FTI will be within the normal range, reflecting a normal FT_4 level. Conversely, a low TBG level causing a low T_4 level will lead to a increased T_3 RU and will result in a normal FTI.

Human Breast Milk

The precise concentrations of T_3 and T_4 present in human milk are not agreed upon. Levels of T_3 and T_4 in various reports differ widely probably because sampling methods were different and in some studies extracted milk was analyzed while in other studies nonextracted milk was used. It has been suggested that sufficient thyroid hormone is present in human milk to mitigate the effect of congenital hypothyroidism.[7] However, other studies have shown that breast-feeding does not impair the detection of congenital hypothyroidism in neonatal screening programs.[25] RT_3 levels are low in human milk and apparently do not change with the duration of lactation.

Defects in Thyroxine-Binding Globulin

Alterations in TBG concentration lead to changes in results of thyroid function tests that complicate their interpretation. Congenital TBG deficiency may occur. The frequency of detection of TBG deficiency in female newborns is approximately 1:25,000 compared with 1:2,800 in male newborns, for an overall frequency of 1:5,000.[55] Familial TBG deficiency occurs in a X-linked dominant inheritance pattern.[33] Affected males show essentially absent TBG levels and most of the females show levels that are lower than normal. The importance of recognizing this deficiency is stressed in order to avoid treating these patients for hypothyroidism. The diagnosis will be apparent by obtaining a serum TBG level, T_3 RU, TSH, or FT_4. Serum TSH, FT_4, TBPA, and albumin concentrations are normal. Elevated serum Tg levels have been found but the mechanism causing the increase is not known.

Congenital familial elevation of TBG also occurs. This condition is inherited as a X-linked dominant trait.[9] The patients are euthyroid and have increased serum T_4 and TBG levels, variably increased T_3 levels, decreased T_3 RU, and normal TSH and FT_4 levels. The estimated incidence of congenital elevation of TBG is 1:40,000 births.[71]

Changes in TBG capacity can result from administration of hormones, or drugs, and in physiologic and disease states (Table 5–2). In addition, there are drugs and

TABLE 5–2.

Causes of Abnormal Binding of Thyroxine Binding Proteins*

	TBG	TBPA
Hypothyroidism	↑	
Genetic	↑ or ↓	N
Estrogens	↑	↓
Pregnancy	↑	↓
Hepatic disease	↑ or ↓ or N	↓
Acute intermittent porphyria	↑	N
Prolonged perphenazine therapy	↑	
Uncompensated acidosis	↓	
Androgens	↓	↓
Anabolic steroids	↓	
Nephrosis	↓	
Severe hypoproteinemia	↓	
Phenytoin (Dilantin)	↓	
Glucocorticoids (high dosage)	↓	↓
Aspirin	N	↓
Acute stress		↓
Chronic illness		↓
Thyrotoxicosis		↓

*TBG = thyroxine-binding globulin; TBPA = thyroxine-binding prealbumin; ↑ = increased; ↓ = decreased; N = normal.

TABLE 5–3.

Agents That Alter Extrathyroidal Metabolism of Thyroid Hormones

Accelerate thyroid hormone peripheral metabolism	Inhibit conversion of T_4 to T_3
Phenytoin (Dilantin)	Propylthiouracil
Carbamazepine (Tegretol)	Glucocorticoids
Phenobarbital	Propranolol
	Iodinated contrast agents
	Amiodarone (Cordarone)

substances which alter the extrathyroidal metabolism of thyroid hormones and thereby affect their serum concentration. Some of the agents used in pediatric patients are listed in Table 5–3.

Laboratory Tests in Thyroid Disorders

A excellent review of the use of laboratory tests in diagnosing thyroid dysfunction has recently been published and the reader is referred to it.[67]

HYPOTHYROIDISM

Etiology

Causes of hypothyroidism in pediatrics are listed in Table 5–4. Since most of the congenital and acquired causes are similar, they are discussed together. The terms *cretinism* or *congenital hypothyroidism* are used when thyroid deficiency is present before or at birth. The terms *acquired hypothyroidism* or *juvenile hypothyroidism* are used when a previously normal infant, child, or adolescent subsequently develops thyroid deficiency.

Circulating antithyroid antibodies are found in a higher percentage of sera from mothers of nongoitrous cretins than in normal control mothers. These antibodies can cross the placenta. They are probably not destructive to the fetal thyroid. The possible role, if any, of circulating or cellular antithyroid antibodies in the causation of congenital athyreosis is not clear. Thyroid dysgenesis is the most common cause of congenital hypothyroidism in nonendemic areas and is approximately two times more common among females than males.[21] Thyroid dysgenesis includes aplasia, ectopy, and hypoplasia of the thyroid gland. In North America the relative incidence of each group is 40%, 25%, and 25%, respectively, of the total patients with thyroid dysgenesis.[22] Ectopy of the thyroid gland is an important cause of hypothyroidism. This cause of hypothyroidism is frequently not detected and is thought to be idiopathic unless a scintiscan is made over the lingual or thyroid area following administration of a radioisotope. Approximately 75% of patients with lingual thyroid glands do not have any functional tissue. Ectopic thyroid glands must be included in the differential diagnosis of midline lingual and sublingual masses. The amount of ectopic thyroid tissue present is usually insufficient to prevent hypothyroidism. Such tissue can respond to TSH stimulation by increasing in size. All children with lingual or sublingual thyroid glands should have a trial of full-replacement thyroid hormone therapy before surgical excision is contemplated. Thyroid therapy will prevent further hypertrophy and hyperplasia. Surgical intervention should be reserved only for those children in whom there is dysphagia, dysphonia, ulceration, or hemorrhage due to a lingual thyroid gland, or if the ectopic thyroid gland fails to decrease in size following an adequate course of treatment with thyroid hormones. There is no evidence in the literature that lingual or sublingual thyroid glands are malignant in children or adolescents.

In infants the combination of elevated plasma TSH and normal or low-normal T_4 levels suggests the presence of thyroid ectopy. Infants with aplasia or hypoplasia of the thyroid gland have high serum TSH and low T_4 levels.

Hypothyroidism may occur because of a hereditary enzymatic deficiency which prevents the normal synthesis of T_4 and T_3[37] (see Table 5–5). Patients with enzymatic defects may present with a goiter and hypothyroidism, with a goiter but with euthyroidism, or with hypothyroidism which occurred prior to development of a goiter; most of these diseases are familial. Since the thyroid gland is not always palpable, infants with congenital goitrous cretinism cannot always be differentiated *clinically* from those with athyreotic cretinism. Diagnosis depends on very specific tests of the various steps in thyroid hormone synthesis and release. Hereditary enzymatic defects are the second most common cause of congenital hypothyroidism.[21] Pendred's syndrome consists of a goiter due to a peroxidase defect with euthyroidism or mild hypothyroidism, and nerve deafness.

Congenital hypothyroidism may be due to TRH deficiency or insensitivity or both; TSH deficiency; or thyroid gland unresponsiveness to TSH. Sporadic and

TABLE 5–4.

Causes of Hypothyroidism*

Congenital
    Thyroid dysgenesis (partial or complete athyreosis)
    Ectopic thyroid gland
    Inborn errors of synthesis
    Hypothalamic-pituitary-thyroid axis abnormalities
        TRH deficiency, insensitivity
        TSH deficiency
        Thyroid gland unresponsiveness to TSH
    Iodine deficiency (endemic cretinism)
    Transplacental passage of antithyroid drugs, chemicals, agents
    Peripheral resistance to thyroid hormone
Acquired
    TRH/TSH deficiency
    Postthyroidectomy
    Post-^{131}I therapy
    Goitrogenic induced (PTU, methimazole, iodide excess, cobalt)
    Postsuppurative or nonsuppurative thyroiditis
    Chronic lymphocytic thyroiditis
    Infiltrative disease of the thyroid (cystinosis, histocytosis X)
    Post–craniospinal irradiation therapy

*TRH = thyroid-releasing hormone; TSH = thyroid-stimulating hormone; PTU = propylthiouracil.

TABLE 5–5.

Hereditary Defects in Thyroid Hormone Synthesis or Action Causing Hypothyroidism*†

	Inheritance	Goiter	Plasma	
			T_4	TSH
Iodide concentration defect in thyroid, salivary, and gastric gland	Autosomal recessive	+	↓	N or ↑‡
Peroxidase defect (unable to convert inorganic iodide into organic form)	Autosomal recessive	+	N or ↓	N or ↓‡
Absence of iodotyrosine deiodinase	Autosomal recessive	+	N or ↓	N or ↑‡
Defect in coupling of iodotyrosines to form iodothyronines	Autosomal recessive	+	N or ↓	N or ↑‡
Defect in thyroglobulin synthesis	Autosomal recessive	+	N or ↓	N or ↑‡
Failure of thyroid to respond to TSH	Autosomal recessive?	–	↓	↑
Syndromes of thyroid hormone resistance	Autosomal recessive or autosomal dominant	±	↑	N or ↑

*Adapted from Lever EG, Madeiros-Neto GA, DeGroot LJ: *Endocr Rev* 1983; 4:213.
†T_4 = thyroxine; TSH = thyroid-stimulating hormone; + = present; – = absent; ± = present or absent; ↓ = decreased; ↑ = increased; N = normal.
‡Depends on age of patient and degree of defect.

familial isolated TSH deficiency has been reported. A TRH test will usually delineate whether a patient has a hypothalamic or pituitary deficiency as the cause of hypothyroidism. If serum TSH levels increase or the TSH response is prolonged, the defect is in the hypothalamus; absence of TSH response to TRH indicates a defect in pituitary TSH production. Thyroid gland unresponsiveness to TSH has been reported. The suggested defect in this disorder is a coupling abnormality between the TSH receptor and the TSH receptor–adenyl cyclase system.

Iodine deficiency is the cause of endemic cretinism in certain parts of the world. The infants usually, but not always, have goiters at birth.

The administration of antithyroid drugs such as propylthiouracil (PTU) or methimazole during pregnancy can cause congenital goiter and hypothyroidism. Iodides taken during pregnancy can cause goiters and hypothyroidism. After birth, the goiter usually disappears with or without thyroid therapy. Temporary thyroid therapy may be necessary in the newborn with a large goiter in order to prevent asphyxiation, or in the newborn with overt signs of hypothyroidism.

Cretinism can occur following maternal radioactive iodine therapy given for treatment of Graves' disease. The human fetal thyroid gland can accumulate maternally administered ^{131}I by the 12th week of gestation.

Chronic lymphocytic thyroiditis (CLT) is the most common cause of acquired hypothyroidism in pediatrics and is discussed below. Hypothyroidism may occur as a consequence of direct irradiation to the thyroid gland as a result of craniospinal irradiation for therapy of malignant disease. Clinical hypothyroidism can occur in cystinosis or histiocytosis owing to infiltrative lesions of the primary disease within the thyroid gland.

Clinical Manifestations

Pediatric patients with hypothyroidism differ considerably in appearance, depending on the age when the deficiency occurs and its duration and severity before therapy is instituted. In complete athyreotic cretinism, symptoms may be present at birth but more commonly occur during the first 2 months of life. Smith et al.[66] have emphasized that athyreotic newborns have variable signs and symptoms of hypothyroidism which should suggest to the physician the need for prompt evaluation. These features include prolonged gestation with large size at birth; large posterior fontanel; respiratory distress; hypothermia; peripheral cyanosis; hypoactivity; feeding difficulties; constipation; abdominal distention with vomiting; prolonged jaundice; and edema.

Respiratory distress may be associated with nasal "congestion," hoarse cry, and cyanosis, and is caused by myxedema of the tongue, epiglottis, pharynx, and larynx. Myxedema is edema in skin, other tissues, and serous cavities secondary to hypothyroidism. It is due to increased extravasation of plasma proteins and lack of a compensatory increase in lymph flow and protein return rate. Hyperbilirubinemia may be the only obvious symptom in the neonate and may persist for as long as 7 weeks. The skin can be pale, dry, cool, and circulatory mottling may be present. Heart murmurs are frequently present and if cyanosis is also present, congenital heart disease may be suspected. One study found normal myocardial function in the immediate newborn period in infants with congenital hypothyroidism and concluded that early thyroid hormone therapy may prevent abnormal cardiac function.

The facial features become coarse and puffy (Fig 5–3). The tongue becomes broad and thick as the neonate gets older. The base of the nose becomes broad and flattened. Linear growth can slow down in the first month of life. Mental retardation occurs if the diagnosis is not made. Diminished physical activity is a prominent finding. Any infant that must be awakened for feedings and rarely cries must be suspected of having hypothyroidism. A protuberant abdomen with an umbilical hernia can occur but is a nonspecific finding. Galactorrhea has been reported in congenital hypothyroidism.

If the infant remains untreated, macroglossia and lethargy increase. The skin is dry, thickened, and cool. Puffy edema may appear about the eyes and in the supraclavicular area. The hair may become dry and brittle. Early diagnosis is mandatory because mental and developmental retardation increases and neurologic sequelae may appear.

Patients developing hypothyroidism in early childhood differ from cretins in their clinical manifestations. Symptoms may appear gradually over several years. Linear growth and eruption of teeth become retarded. Mental sluggishness may develop but mental retardation does not occur if the hypothyroidism develops after the second year of life.

If hypothyroidism has been present since infancy, infantile body proportions persist. Cold intolerance, dry skin, constipation, and muscle weakness are common findings.

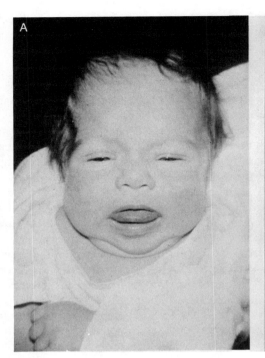 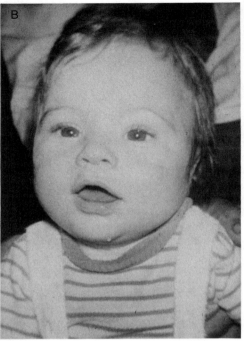

FIG 5–3.
A, hypothyroid infant with typical cretinoid facies, dull appearance, and myxedema of face, eyelids, lips, and tongue. (From Becker KL: *Principles and Practice of Endocrinology and Metabolism.* Philadelphia JB Lippincott Co, 1990, p 381. Used by permission.)
B, same patient after therapy. Note disappearance of myxedema.

Although unusual, musculoskeletal syndromes can be the presenting complaint in children with hypothyroidism. Slipped capital femoral epiphysis may occur. Neurologic dysfunction can occur. Sensorineural hearing loss may occur in sporadic congenital hypothyroidism and the physician should test for hearing loss in any patient with congenital hypothyroidism.

An infrequently recognized syndrome in hypothyroid children is the Kocher-Debré-Semélaign syndrome. This syndrome consists of muscular hypertrophy in children with hypothyroidism. The muscular hypertrophy is generalized and involves particularly the muscles of the extremities, giving the child a "herculean" appearance. The muscular hypertrophy disappears with thyroid therapy. The pathogenesis of the muscle hypertrophy has not been elucidated but seems to be related to the severity and duration of the hypothyroidism.

Myocardial dysfunction, pericardial effusion, and asymmetric septal hypertrophy have been recognized in children with hypothyroidism.[16] However, it has been suggested that the commonly observed enlarged cardiac silhouette seen in hypothyroid children is due to pericardial effusion in the presence of normal cardiac contractility and chamber size and not to a myxedematous myocardium.

In the older child and adolescent, growth retardation is a common finding (Fig

5–4). Hypothyroid effects on the neuromuscular and circulatory systems occur as they do in younger patients. Significant delay in sexual maturation is characteristic. Multicystic ovaries occur frequently in girls with hypothyroidism.

A rare syndrome consisting of severe hypothyroidism and isosexual precocity occurs.[10] The underlying pathophysiology is not clear. It has been suggested that TRH stimulates release of FSH but not LH in both normal and hypothyroid children.[10] Plasma LH, FSH, and prolactin have been elevated in some of these children and return to normal after thyroid hormone therapy.[10] The serum prolactin level may be elevated owing to increased TRH secretion. In girls, breast development and estrogenization of the vagina are present but axillary and pubic hair are not present. In boys, testicular enlargement is inappropriate for the degree of virilization present. Histologic examination of the testes reveals predominantly tubular development without increase in Leydig cell number. After treatment with thyroid hormone, the signs of hypothyroidism and sexual precocity regress. Complete sexual maturation then occurs at the normal age.

Laboratory Studies

Thyroid scanning or ultrasound studies may provide the etiology of the hypothyroidism.[47] In primary hypothyroidism serum TSH levels are high while in secondary and tertiary hypothyroidism serum TSH levels are low or undetectable. Serum T_4, T_3, and T_3 RU are low as is the alkaline phosphatase level. Increased serum myoglobin and creatine kinase levels occur in the presence of hypothyroid myopathy. Plasma somatomedin C concentrations are low in congenital and acquired hypothyroidism. Plasma Tg levels are undetectable or very low in patients with athyreosis. However,

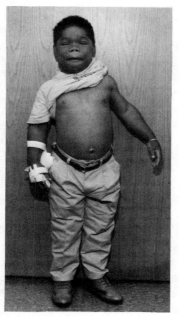

FIG 5–4.
Fifteen-year-old hypothyroid youth with height age of a 6-year-old and bone age of a 4-year-old.

it is possible that such levels may be present in a patient with a defect in Tg synthesis or secretion.

In children and adolescents with hypothyroidism, up to 65% of them may be anemic. However, infants with congenital hypothyroidism may have polycythemia and be at risk to develop potential complications (hyperviscosity syndrome).[73] The pathogenesis is unclear. Infants with congenital hypothyroidism may have hypercalcemia. They have an intolerance to an acute calcium load and a deficient calcitonin response to calcium infusion. Therefore, vitamin D supplementation should be recommended with caution. Hypoglycemia with clinical symptoms has been rarely reported in hypothyroidism and the etiology is most likely multifactorial. Elevation in sweat chloride may occur in hypothyroidism and normalizes with thyroid hormone therapy. The etiology is not known.

Electroencephalographic (EEG) changes occur in hypothyroidism. These consist of low amplitude waves in infants and an excessive amount of slow activity in children. With thyroid therapy the EEG usually reverts to normal patterns. Infants with congenital hypothyroidism have a high incidence of selective caudal brainstem dysfunction demonstrable by brainstem auditory evoked potentials that can be corrected with therapy.[49] Changes in brain maturation associated with hypothyroidism have been detected by MRI.[2]

The bone age is retarded and in primary hypothyroidism the retardation in skeletal maturation is usually greater than that in linear growth. Epiphyseal dysgenesis or stippling of the epiphyses can be present. With thyroid therapy the epiphyseal dysgenesis regresses and the radiographic appearance reverts to normal as does the bone age. Enlargement of the sella turcica can be seen in primary hypothyroidism owing to pituitary hypertrophy.[29] These changes can return to normal with thyroid therapy.

Therapy

The objective of treatment is to establish euthyroidism as rapidly as is safe for the patient. Thyroid hormone preparations available fall into two general categories: crude animal thyroid gland preparations and synthetic hormones. The former includes dessicated thyroid and purified porcine thyroglobulin and these preparations should no longer be prescribed.

Synthetic hormone preparations are available as the sodium salt of levothyroxine L-T_4, liothyronine L-T_3 or a 4:1 mixture of both (liotrix). The major differences between the two synthetic hormones are in their relative potency, rapidity of onset of action, and biologic half-life. On the basis of weight, L-T_3 is approximately three times as potent as L-T_4. When given orally, L-T_3 is more completely absorbed than L-T_4. L-T_3 also produces metabolic changes more rapidly than biologically equipotent amounts of L-T_4. The effects of L-T_3 dissipate faster because of more rapid peripheral metabolism and excretion. The L-T_4-L-T_3 mixture, liotrix, has been synthesized as a physiologic replacement. It has been shown that L-T_4 products are not all equivalent. The mean tablet T_4 content and tablet-to-tablet variability of T_4 content may vary significantly from one brand to another. It is therefore important that patients consistently receive one product, whether it be proprietary or generic (see Table 5–6). We believe that L-T_4 is the preparation of choice.

TABLE 5–6.

Synthetic Thyroid Hormone Preparations

Preparation	Generic Name	Brand Name	Available Strengths	T_4/T_3 Ratio
L-Thyroxine (T_4) sodium salt	Levothyroxine	Synthroid	Tablets: 0.025, 0.05, 0.075, 0.1, 0.112, 0.125, 0.15, 0.175, 0.2, 0.3 mg Injectable: 200 and 500 μg in 10 mL vials	1:0
		Levothroid	Tablets: 0.025, 0.05, 0.075, 0.1, 0.125, 0.15, 0.175, 0.2, 0.3 mg Injectable: 200 and 500 μg in 6 mL vials	
L-Triiodothyronine (T_3) sodium salt	Liothyronine	Cytomel	Tablets: 2, 25, 50 μg	0:1
L-Thyroxine–L-triiodothyronine mixture	Liotrix	Thyrolar ¼, ½, 1, 2, 3	Tablets: levothyroxine and liothyronine: 12.5/3.1 μg, 25/6.25 μg, 50/12.5 μg, 100/25 μg, 150/37.5 μg	4:1
		Euthroid ½, 1, 2, 3	Tablets: levothyroxine and liothyronine: 30/7.5 μg, 60/15 μg, 120/30 μg, 180/45 μg	

Patients treated with L-T_4 have levels of serum T_4 that are slightly higher than normal and those treated with L-T_3 have a lower than normal serum T_4 level when a euthyroid state is reached. Therapy with liotrix can result in an elevated serum T_3 level and normal or low serum T_4 levels.

In very young infants it is important to establish a euthyroid state as promptly as possible in order to protect the brain from damage. However, caution is recommended in the therapy of markedly hypothyroid neonates and infants because of the possible presence of a myxedematous myocardium. Vigorous therapy may cause cardiac failure or serious arrhythmias. Liothyronine has been used in the treatment of cretins without complication as long as the patients were properly monitored.

The initial single daily oral dose of L-T_3 in full-term newborns with congenital hypothyroidism is 0.025 to 0.05 mg. In premature infants the starting dose is 0.025 mg/day and the dose can usually be increased to 0.05 mg/day in 4 to 6 weeks. In infants and children with hypothyroidism, the initial dose of L-T_4 is approximately 100 μg/m²/day.[1]

Suppression of serum TSH to normal levels has been used as the best index of adequate therapy in primary hypothyroidism. Infants with congenital hypothyroidism may have an abnormal "threshold" for inhibition of TSH secretion in that the feedback set-point seems to be increased so that excessive levels of T_4 may be necessary to suppress the TSH levels.[54] Therefore, normal serum TSH levels must *not* be used as the only criterion of adequacy of therapy. Serum TSH values may remain above the accepted normal range for as long as 24 months, despite normal concentrations of serum total T_4 and T_3 produced by replacement therapy.[54] Simultaneous measurement of TSH, T_4, and T_3 provides the most comprehensive assessment of replacement therapy. Measurement of TSH levels is of no value in secondary or tertiary hypothyroidism and measurement of FT_4 and free T_3 (FT_3) is of value.

Other indicators of adequate replacement therapy include normal growth and development and normal skeletal maturation. Studies in patients with congenital hypothyroidism treated in the first weeks of life and followed up to 9 years of age have shown their linear growth to be within the normal ranges. However, patients with prolonged acquired hypothyroidism may not achieve normal adult height.[57] The deficit in adult height is related to the duration of hypothyroidism before therapy.

Indications of excessive therapy may be nervousness, excitability, tremors, tachycardia, and hypertension. One must remember that the previously placid infant or child can be expected to become more active when returned to a euthyroid state. Pseudotumor cerebri has been reported following initiation of T_4 therapy. Excessive thyroid therapy may cause delayed neurologic development or behavioral dysfunction. Premature craniosynostosis and slipped capital femoral epiphysis have also been reported as complications of thyroid therapy.

Transient Disorders of Thyroid Function in the Newborn

Hypothyroidism is transient in approximately 10% of newborns diagnosed as having congenital hypothyroidism.[22] Transient disorders of thyroid function that may occur in the newborn include hypothyroxinemia, hyperthyrotropinemia, primary hypothyroidism, and the euthyroid sick syndrome (Table 5–7).

Transient Hypothyroxinemia

All preterm infants have some degree of hypothyroxinemia. This has been discussed previously and is presumed to be related to immaturity of the hypothalamic-pituitary axis. Transient hypothyroxinemia is defined as transient low serum T_4 and normal serum TSH concentrations with subsequent normal values without therapy or after a month or more after cessation of treatment.[37] Low serum FT_4 and normal TSH responses to TRH are present. Preterm low-birth-weight infants will usually have normal serum T_4 levels by 4 to 6 weeks of age. Transient hypothyroxinemia may also occur in term newborns but the incidence is much lower.

There is controversy related to the advisability of treatment at the time of detection of the hypothyroxinemia since it is difficult to predict whether the thyroid insufficiency will be transient or permanent. Delange et al.[15] recommend treatment because of the

TABLE 5–7.

Transient Disorders of Thyroid Function in the Newborn

Disorder	Serum*			
	T_3	FT_4	T_4	TSH
Hypothyroxinemia	Low	Low	Low	Normal
Hyperthyrotropinemia	Normal	Normal	Normal	High
Primary hypothyroidism	Low	Low	Low	High
Euthyroid sick syndrome				
Low T_3 syndrome	Low	Normal	Normal	Normal
Low T_4 syndrome	Low	Low	Low	Normal
High T_4 syndrome	Low	High	High	Normal

*T_3 = triiodothyronine; FT_4 = free thyroxine; T_4 = thyroxine; TSH = thyroid-stimulating hormone.

possibility of brain damage secondary to thyroid hormone insufficiency. They suggest treatment with T_3 which is suitable for distinguishing between transient and permanent hypothyroidism without interruption of therapy. The recommended daily dose of T_3 is 5 μg/kg body weight and is divided into three doses given every 8 hours. A progressive increase of serum T_4 during therapy occurs in transient but *not* in permanent hypothyroidism. The increase of serum T_4 in the presence of normal serum TSH levels suggests an increasing responsiveness of the thyroid gland to TSH.

In the New England Congenital Hypothyroidism Collaborative program the incidence of transient hypothyroxinemia was 1:19,000.[37] Sixty-five percent of patients with *transient* hypothyroxinemia were *males*, while 75% of patients with *permanent* hypothyroidism were *females*.

Transient Hyperthyrotropinemia

Transient hyperthyrotropinemia is manifested by elevated serum TSH and normal T_4 levels. Immaturity of the hypothalamic-pituitary-thyroid axis may be an etiologic factor. This disorder may last as long as 9 months.[46] It is known that prenatal and perinatal exposure to iodine-containing antiseptic agents or iodine-containing contrast agents can cause transient hyperthyrotropinemia. It is not clear whether thyroid therapy should be given even though the recommendation has been made to do so.[46]

Transient Primary Hypothyroidism

Transient primary hypothyroidism may occur as the result of transplacental passage of antithyroid drugs, thyrotropin-binding inhibitory immunoglobulins or thyroid growth-blocking immunoglobulins associated with maternal thyroid disorders,[23] or topical or oral iodides received by the mother. Perinatal exposure to iodine-containing antiseptic agents can also cause transient primary hypothyroidism as well as transient hyperthyrotropinemia.

Euthyroid Sick Syndrome (Nonthyroidal Illnesses)

Profound alterations in peripheral thyroid hormone metabolism may occur in patients with severe nonthyroidal illnesses of either acute or chronic nature. Despite low serum T_3 or T_4 levels these patients are euthyroid as evidenced by normal basal TSH concentrations and a normal TSH response to TRH administration. This syndrome is called the *euthyroid sick syndrome* (ESS). A low serum T_3 level is usually present associated with normal or increased RT_3 levels and normal FT_4 and TSH levels.

Preterm infants with respiratory distress syndrome (RDS) have been the most frequently reported pediatric patients with ESS. In children a variety of illnesses have been associated with ESS including severe gastroenteritis, acute leukemia, renal failure, severe burns, and untreated insulin-dependent diabetes mellitus. The abnormal thyroid function studies gradually return to normal as the sick neonate or child improves from the primary illness.

There are difficulties in the interpretation of thyroid function tests when patients are initially seen who have severe nonthyroidal illness. It has been suggested that measurement of serum TSH provides the most reliable differentiation between patients with primary hypothyroidism and those with ESS. Serum RT_3 levels are elevated or normal in ESS and *low* in hypothyroid patients. Patients with ESS do not require thyroid hormone therapy.

In newborn infants the site of blood sampling must be considered for proper interpretation of serum levels of thyroid hormones and their binding proteins. Simultaneous levels of thyroid hormones and their binding proteins in peripheral veins and in the aorta and central veins have been compared. It was found that newborns in good clinical condition had serum levels of T_4 and thyroid hormone binding proteins which were significantly higher in peripheral veins than in the aorta and central veins. The median increases were 6% to 8%. In newborns with RDS, serum T_4 and TBG were lower in peripheral than in central veins.

Congenital Hypothyroidism

Neonatal Screening

The clinical diagnosis of congenital hypothyroidism during the neonatal period can be difficult and is frequently missed. For this reason, systemic neonatal screening programs for congenital hypothyroidism have been established.[22] Most regional screening programs employ measurements of T_4 in blood collected on filter paper at the same time that blood is collected for detecting phenylketonuria before the newborn is discharged from the hospital.[36] Alternative methods of screening include measurement of cord blood or dried blood samples on filter paper, TSH testing, and T_4 assay. TSH testing of patients with low T_4 results obtained from filter paper spots provides the most comprehensive screening, identifying infants with primary hypothyroidism and those at risk for secondary hypothyroidism and TBG deficiency. Screening by T_4 assay alone results in lower detection rates and a higher incidence of borderline and false-positive results. Most current mass screening programs in North America use filter paper spot T_4 testing with follow-up filter paper spot TSH testing of samples with the lowest 3% to 5% of T_4 results.[22] In suspicious or positive patients, the diagnosis must be confirmed by *serum* determination. There is a large overlap in the range of RT_3 levels in cord blood of hypothyroid and normal newborns which makes measurement of RT_3 as a screening test impractical.

The results of neonatal thyroid screening programs for congenital hypothyroidism support the conclusion that newborn screening is effective in early detection of congenital hypothyroidism. In North America, 1,046,362 infants had been screened by August 1978.[22] In this series, 277 infants with congenital hypothyroidism were detected and 7 infants were missed, resulting in an overall incidence of 1 in 3,684 births. Only 8 of the 277 detected infants were suspected clinically before the results of testing were known. Approximately 95% of the infants had primary hypothyroidism (an incidence of 1 in 4,254 births) and 5% had secondary or tertiary hypothyroidism (an incidence of 1 in 68,200 births). TBG deficiency was estimated to occur in 1 in 8,913 births.

There appears to be a racial difference in the incidence of congenital hypothyroidism diagnosed during neonatal screening. In the state of Georgia, the incidence in white infants was 1:5,526 while in black infants the incidence was 1:32,377.[8]

Prognosis for Intellectual and Neurologic Development

In congenital hypothyroidism, studies show that the earlier the diagnosis is made and therapy started, the better the prognosis for intelligence. In the era before neonatal screening for hypothyroidism, Smith and associates[65] reported that 10 of 22 patients treated within 6 months of birth had an intelligence quotient (IQ) of 90 or greater, but 18 of the 22 had neurologic sequelae. Recent results of 9- to 10-year follow-up psychometric studies of newborns detected by screening programs are very encouraging.[48] It has been suggested that progressive loss of intelligence potential starts from birth but if treatment is begun before 1 month of age, intelligence remains within the normal range. The prognosis also appears to be related to the etiology of the congenital hypothyroidism. In infants with athyreosis, only 41% had an IQ above 85; in infants with inborn errors of synthesis, only 4% had an IQ above 85; while in infants with an ectopic thyroid gland, 78% had an IQ above 85.[42] In congenital hypothyroidism the extent of retardation in skeletal maturation may predict the infant's developmental potential.

It remains to be proved if the majority of children treated early will escape significant neurologic deficits in later life. It appears that neurologic damage may begin prenatally but serious sequelae occur if treatment is delayed beyond 3 months of age.[65] There is evidence that some hypothyroid children treated before 6 weeks of age have signs of minimal brain dysfunction when evaluated later. The potential for intellectual and neurologic development appears to be related to the exact etiology, age of onset, duration, and age at diagnosis and treatment. There does not seem to be a risk of permanent intellectual impairment if hypothyroidism is acquired after 2 years of age.

Acute Ingestion of Excessive Amounts of Thyroxine

The consequences of accidental acute excessive ingestion of thyroid hormone in infants and children have been documented.[39] The outcome depends on the age of the patient and duration of exposure to the hormones. The initial serum levels of T_4 and T_3 do not correlate with the development of symptoms or signs of toxicity. The patients are generally asymptomatic for the first 24 hours after ingestion. Symptoms occur as T_4 is converted to T_3, which may require up to 72 hours. It has been concluded that the majority of patients with acute excessive ingestion of thyroid hormone do not have severe effects and may be managed conservatively as outpatients.[39] However, controversy exists regarding therapy.

Confirming the Diagnosis in the Patient Receiving Therapy

One problem in pediatrics is the patient receiving thyroid hormone replacement in whom the indications for therapy have not been well documented. There are several methods of evaluating such patients. One approach is to discontinue therapy for 6 to 8 weeks and follow objective clinical changes, supplemented by serial serum T_4 and TSH determinations. In normal persons it takes 6 to 8 weeks for the hypothalamic-pituitary-thyroid axis to recover from prolonged suppression. If the serum T_4 and TSH are normal at 6 to 8 weeks, the parents and patient can be reassured that thyroid therapy is not indicated. Patients who receive large doses of thyroid hormone for prolonged periods of time may develop a temporary defect in endogenous TRH secretion or reserve which requires as long as 28 months before returning to normal.[62] If there is reluctance to stop therapy, the patient can be given an equivalent dose of

L-T$_3$ for 1 month. Liothyronine is then discontinued and 10 days later thyroid function can be determined by measurement of serum T$_4$ and TSH. The 10-day period of thyroid hormone deprivation makes it unlikely that severe symptoms of hypothyroidism will appear if the patient indeed has hypothyroidism.

THYROID AUTOANTIBODIES

A variety of circulating antibodies have been described in patients with thyroid disease. Tests to detect these antibodies are not routinely available nor is their use indicated in all patients. Autoimmune antibodies against thyroglobulin (antithyroglobulin antibody, ATG) and thyroid (antimicrosomal antibody, AMA) are the principal autoantibodies. ATGs are not cytoxic whereas AMAs fix complement and are cytotoxic to thyroid follicular cells. It has been shown recently that AMA is directed predominately against membrane thyroid peroxidase enzyme–antithyroid peroxidase antibodies (anti-TPO). ATG and anti-TPO are hallmarkers of autoimmune thyroid disease, particularly Hashimoto's thyroiditis. In practice, one usually orders both tests, but AMAs are more often positive in Hashimoto's thyroiditis and Graves' disease. These tests are particularly helpful in the diagnosis of Hashimoto's thyroiditis or goiter of unknown etiology in a euthyroid patient.

Graves' disease is accepted as an autoimmune disorder, in which an antibody stimulates the thyroid gland. The antibody is referred to as *thyroid-stimulating antibody* (TSAb), and by some as *thyroid-stimulating immunoglobulin* (TSI). Other antibodies to the TSH receptor, the TSH receptor antibodies (TRAb), do not stimulate the thyroid gland. The nonstimulating TSH receptor antibodies can be detected by their ability to prevent binding of TSH to its receptor, and are termed *TSH binding-inhibiting immunoglobulin* (TBII) or *thyrotropin-displacing immunoglobulin* (TDI).

Thyroid growth-stimulating antibodies (TGI) have been described in patients with Graves' disease or simple goiters and may contribute to development of large goiters.[6]

Serum antithyroid hormone autoantibodies (anti-T$_3$ antibody and anti-T$_4$ antibody) may be present in patients with thyroid and nonthyroid disorders. The autoantibodies produce a discrepancy between physical findings and laboratory data of thyroid function. These discrepancies are caused by interference of the autoantibodies in the RIA for T$_3$ or T$_4$ and cause unexpectedly high or low total and free hormone values. The clinician should remember that when the concentrations of serum thyroid hormones measured by RIA are not compatible with clinical findings, the presence of abnormal binding by serum autoantibodies should be considered and the serum tested. Modified RIAs for free thyroid hormone which are not interfered with by antithyroid hormone autoantibodies are available.

HYPERTHYROIDISM

Graves' disease in children is hyperthyroidism associated with diffuse hyperplasia of the thyroid gland. The various types of hyperthyroidism seen in pediatric patients

TABLE 5–8.

Types of Hyperthyroidism

Diffuse toxic goiter (Graves' disease)
Toxic nodular goiter (Plummer's disease)
Chronic lymphocytic thyroiditis (hashitoxicosis)
Thyroid carcinoma
Exogenous iodine-induced (Jod-Basedow phenomenon)
Thyroid-stimulating hormone (TSH)–producing pituitary tumor
Inappropriate secretion of TSH
Factitious hyperthyroidism

are listed in Table 5–8. *Hyperthyroidism* can be defined as a hypermetabolic state resulting from excess production of T_4 or T_3 or both.

Etiology

Investigations in recent years have shown significant progress in delineating the pathogenesis of Graves' disease. There is increasing evidence that this form of hyperthyroidism has an autoimmune pathogenesis[13] (see above section, Thyroid Autoantibodies). Graves' disease occurs in higher frequency in patients with certain HLA types. It is associated in whites with HLA-DR3 and in Japanese with HLA-B35. The defect that predisposes to Graves' disease is not known. Possible mechanisms include (1) genetically programmed presentation of a thyroid-specific antigen; (2) a tissue-specific defect in suppressor T cell activity; and (3) an idiotype–anti-idiotype reaction.

Histopathologically the thyroid follicles are small with marked hypertrophy and hyperplasia of acinar cells. The follicles contain scant amounts of colloid. Lymphocytic infiltration is present in varying degrees.

Graves' disease in pediatric patients is five times more frequent in girls than in boys.[28] It may appear at any age with a peak incidence being reached during adolescence.

A wide variety of disorders occur in association with Graves' disease. It is not surprising that other autoimmune endocrine diseases such as Addison's disease, diabetes mellitus, idiopathic hypoparathyroidism, and CLT are among them. Nonendocrine autoimmune disorders such as pernicious anemia, idiopathic thrombocytopenia purpura, rheumatoid arthritis, vitiligo, lupus erythematosus, and myasthenia gravis also occur in association with Graves' disease. There is an increased incidence of Graves' disease in patients with Down and rubella syndromes.

Ophthalmopathy may be an invariable component of Graves' disease. The pathogenesis is unclear. However, patients with Graves' ophthalmopathy have serum antibodies that bind to both extraocular muscle and orbital fibroblasts, stimulate synthesis of glycosaminoglycans by orbital fibroblasts, and have cytotoxic effects on eye muscle cells.[32]

Clinical Manifestations

The onset of symptoms and signs is usually gradual. Common complaints include emotional lability, nervousness, irritability, increased sweating, increased appetite with or without weight loss or gain, heat intolerance, weakness, tremors, and an increased number of bowel movements. A tender, painful goiter is a rare complaint. Less recognized gastrointestinal symptoms include nausea, vomiting, and abdominal pain. Deterioration in school performance is not an uncommon complaint.

Physical findings include a goiter, usually tachycardia, increased systolic blood pressure with a widened pulse pressure, warm and moist skin, mild exophthalmos, lid retraction, and stare. The goiter is diffuse and firm and in the majority of patients a bruit is heard. However, it should be remembered that Graves' disease can occur without a goiter. Increased height age may be present. Cardiac findings may include mitral

Graves' ophthalmopathy in children and adolescents has been viewed as a relatively benign entity. An incidence of approximately 50% of ophthalmopathy has been found by ophthalmologists in unselected populations of children and adolescents with Graves' disease. Most cases of Graves' ophthalmopathy, especially those occurring in younger children, are mild. Asymmetric proptosis occurred in 13% of patients in one series and seemed to be correlated with greater severity of the Graves' disease and increasing age of onset of the disease. A tendency toward more severe ophthalmopathy with increasing age at onset of the disease (middle to late teens) was noted.

Laboratory Findings

Serum T_4, FT_4, T_3, FT_3, and T_3RU are elevated in almost all patients. The TSH level is abnormally low when measured by an ultrasensitive assay. TSH receptor antibodies are present in most pediatric patients. Antithyroid antibodies may be detected in low titers unless the patient also has CLT in which instance the titers may be moderately to markedly elevated. Elevated serum Tg levels are present. Serum Tg cannot be determined in all patients because of the presence of ATGs in many patients. Endogenous ATGs interfere with the RIA for Tg. Serum Tg levels are low in factitious hyperthyroidism.

The bone age is frequently advanced. A radiographic indication of advanced bone maturation in adolescence is early costochondral calcification. It has been suggested that premature craniosynostosis is a common feature of juvenile Graves' disease.

Reversible compensated functional cardiomyopathy may occur as manifested by diminished left ventricular reserve demonstrated by radionuclide angiocardiography.

The 24-hour ^{131}I thyroidal uptake is almost always elevated. Rarely a patient is so hyperthyroid that an early uptake (2–4 hours) is markedly elevated and the 24-hour uptake returns to normal. It is therefore important to obtain a 2- or 4-hour uptake determination as well as a 24-hour uptake in hyperthyroid patients. CLT presenting with hyperthyroidism has been reported and the diagnosis confirmed histologically.[17] These patients have clinical and laboratory evidence of hyperthyroidism with a normal or elevated ^{131}I thyroidal uptake. Patients with CLT and hyperthyroidism have been reported with *low* ^{131}I thyroidal uptake. It is important to differentiate this disorder from that with elevated ^{131}I thyroidal uptake because the hyperthyroid state is transient and specific antithyroid therapy is contraindicated.

The T_3 suppression test is of diagnostic help in mild hyperthyroidism. Normal patients will show a suppression of a second ^{131}I thyroid uptake to below 50% of the initial uptake value on the seventh and eighth day after taking T_3. Patients with hyperthyroidism will fail to show this suppression. Another study which has been used to document the presence of Graves' disease in questionable cases is the TRH test. Patients with Graves' disease fail to respond normally to TRH. However, both the T_3 suppression and TRH stimulation tests are probably unnecessary with the availability of ultrasensitive TSH assays.

Differential Diagnosis

Hyperthyroidism associated with goiter, exophthalmos, tachycardia, widened pulse pressure, nervousness, and weight loss presents no diagnostic difficulty. Very rarely, a differential diagnosis includes:

1. Simple goiter in an emotionally labile or nervous patient.
2. Hypermetabolic states such as pheochromocytoma or organic heart disease may be considered but it would be unusual to also have an accompanying goiter (unless Sipple's syndrome is present; see discussion of medullary thyroid carcinoma below).

Treatment

Controversy exists among endocrinologists concerning the therapy of hyperthyroidism in children and adolescents because no available therapy is ideal; each has distinct advantages and disadvantages. All of the conventional methods of treatment, namely antithyroid drugs, surgery, and radioactive iodine, have strong advocates. The selection of treatment depends on many factors, including the age and sex of the patient, severity and duration of the disease, size of the thyroid gland, presence of other complicating conditions, availability of experienced surgeons, ability of the patient and family to cooperate, and fear of the effects of ionizing irradiation on the thyroid and its potential genetic effects.

The parents and the patient (if old enough to understand) should be told from the outset that control does not mean cure and that lifelong surveillance is essential regardless of the method of treatment. Medical management consists of (1) symptomatic and (2) specific treatment.

Symptomatic Therapy

In the extremely toxic patient bed rest and sedation may be of help. β-adrenergic blocking agents such as propranolol are useful in rapid control of tremors, agitation, and severe tachycardia or cardiac arrhythmia. Propranolol is contraindicated if the patient has asthma or complete heart block.

The dosage ranges from 2.5 to 10.5 mg/kg/day orally with a maximal dose of 120 mg/day. Doses must be given every 6 to 8 hours if constant effectiveness is to be achieved. Side effects include mainly bradycardia and hypoglycemia.

Specific Therapy

Antithyroid drugs are probably the most widely used form of therapy for hyperthyroidism in the pediatric population. Their use is based on the assumption that control of hyperthyroidism for a period of time will reverse the disease process or that the disease will undergo spontaneous remission.

The thioamide derivatives impede thyroid hormone synthesis by blocking organification of tyrosine and the coupling of MIT and DIT to form T_4 and T_3. Propylthiouracil also inhibits peripheral deiodination of T_4.

PTU and methimazole (Tapazole) are the drugs used in the United States. It has been suggested that antithyroid drugs have a immunosuppressive effect on thyroid activity in Graves' disease.[18] In the United States, PTU is prescribed approximately 10 times more often than methimazole. There are important differences between the drugs. PTU has a serum half-life of 1 hour while methimazole has a serum half-life of 6 to 8 hours. Methimazole is considered to be 10 times more potent than PTU but some studies suggest it may be 100 times more potent. PTU has less ability than methimazole to cross the placenta and into breast milk.

The usual initial daily dose of PTU is 300 mg in divided doses; that of methimazole is 30 mg divided into three equal doses given approximately every 8 hours. Other daily dosage schedules for PTU include 150 mg/m^2 or 5 to 6 mg/kg body weight. The initial dose is given for 4 to 6 weeks depending on the rapidity of response. Measurement of simultaneous serum T_4, T_3, and TSH is extremely helpful in adjusting the proper dose. The serum T_4 level may be low and the T_3 level high in an occasional patient during the course of therapy. The serum T_3 level does not correlate well with clinical status and does not indicate the presence of hyperthyroidism, nor does the low T_4 level indicate hypothyroidism. When discordance of serum T_4 and T_3 levels is present; the TSH concentration may clarify the thyroid status.

The daily maintenance dose of PTU is 100 to 150 mg and for methimazole, 10 to 15 mg. One study suggests that a single daily dose of methimazole is adequate in children and adolescents. The recommended duration of therapy ranges from 12 to 36 months. Some physicians add thyroid hormone to the thioamide regimen because they believe combined therapy allows for more precise and consistent long-term control. One study concluded that the median time for children to remission on medical therapy is 4.5 years and approximately 25% of a cohort of patients receiving medical therapy will have a remission in 2 years.[40] Unresponsiveness to PTU owing to "resistance" is very rare and a recent study found that most patients thought to be "resistant" were actually not taking the medication.

Another agent used to treat Graves' disease is ipodate sodium (Oragrafin). Ipodate sodium is an iodinated radiocontrast agent which inhibits the conversion of T_4 to T_3. The oral dose is 3 g/day.

Adverse effects of PTU and methimazole include nausea, headaches, rash, urticaria, arthralgia, and arthritis and these effects appear more frequently with high drug doses. The most common drug reaction is probably transient leukopenia (white blood cell count below 4,000/mm^3). Antithyroid drug–induced leukopenia is benign and transient. Mild leukopenia occurs commonly in *untreated* Graves' disease. More serious reactions include agranulocytosis, thrombocytopenia, collagen-vascular–like syndromes, toxic hepatitis, and diffuse interstitial pneumonitis. Agranulocytosis is a syndrome characterized by fever, bacterial infection, and a granulocyte count below 250/mm^3. Both PTU and methimazole can cause agranulocytosis. The onset of agranulocytosis is sudden and cannot be predicted by routine blood counts.[11] There is evidence that the cause of agranulocytosis is autoimmune in nature. All patients receiving antithyroid drugs should be told to stop the medication immediately if fever and an oral or upper respiratory infection occurs, and their physician should be notified.

Thrombocytopenia may occur in association with *untreated* Graves' disease. Etiologic mechanisms for this association include autoimmunity and hypersplensim induced by hyperthyroidism. It is important to obtain a complete blood and platelet count before starting antithyroid therapy in order to be sure that severe leukopenia or thrombocytopenia are not already present. The reported incidence of major complications in children has ranged from 3% to 40%.[4]

The contraindications to medical therapy are drug toxicity and patient noncompliance. The main disadvantages of medical therapy are the relatively long period of therapy required and the necessity of patient compliance.

Remission figures among different series of medically treated patients range from 30% to 61%. If a patient relapses after an adequate course of medical therapy, a choice of continuation of medical therapy or other methods of therapy can be given. Patient noncompliance is a major reason for the failure of medical therapy. Patients who undergo permanent remission after drug therapy require lifelong observation since hypothyroidism can occur as a late sequela.

At the present time there is no single reliable method available for predicting clinical remission or relapse of hyperthyroidism following a course of treatment with antithyroid drugs. A reduction in goiter size to normal correlates fairly well with remission. Thyroid hormone suppression testing, measurement of serum Tg, and measurement of the T_3/T_4 ratio have not proved to be reliable indicators. The possible relationship between HLA type and relapse has been investigated. The results are conflicting, some workers showing a significant association between the presence of HLA-B8 or HLA-DW3/DR3 and relapse while others do not. Measurement of TRAb titers may in time prove to be the best predictor of remission or relapse. In general, studies have shown that TRAb titers tend to decline in most patients after medical therapy, and that a remission is more likely if TRAb titers become normal after therapy; in contrast, if they remain elevated, relapse is highly probable. The choice of treatment of Graves' disease probably does not significantly affect the clinical course of Graves' ophthalmopathy.

Surgery

Surgical treatment offers the advantage of rapid control of hyperthyroidism. Surgery must be performed by experienced surgeons. The patient must be treated with antithyroid drugs until euthyroidism is achieved. Iodide in the form of Lugol's solution, three to five drops in water once or twice daily given 1 to 2 weeks prior to surgery involutes the thyroid and makes it less vascular and friable, thus simplifying surgery. Potential disadvantages of surgery include mortality, hypothyroidism, hypoparathyroidism, injury to the recurrent laryngeal nerve, and laryngotracheal edema sometimes requiring tracheotomy.

The reported surgical series of hyperthyroidism do not allow precise comparison of results. The reasons are obvious: (1) surgical skills, experience, and technique differ from surgeon to surgeon; (2) no precise method is available for determining the amount of thyroid tissue left in the neck; and (3) follow-up periods vary from study to study. These variables must be remembered in reviewing the reported data. The reported incidence of recurrent hyperthyroidism ranges from 0% to 9%; for hypothyroidism, 12.5% to 66%; and for permanent hypoparathyroidism, 0% to 6%. Postoperative hypothyroidism can be immediate and permanent, occurring within the first 2 postoperative months; immediate and transient; or delayed and permanent. Patients that have undergone subtotal thyroidectomy require lifelong observation for detection of hypothyroidism.

Indications for surgery in juvenile hyperthyroid patients include (1) toxicity to antithyroid drugs; (2) failure to cure after an adequate course of medical therapy; (3) lack of patient or parent compliance; and (4) failure of medical therapy to decrease the size of a large conspicuous goiter.

Radioactive Iodine

The use of ^{131}I in the treatment of hyperthyroidism in pediatric patients is controversial, and opinions about its use remain divided. The advantages of ^{131}I are that its administration is simple and it is effective therapy. The disadvantages include the high incidence of hypothyroidism; complete control requires weeks or months; and the long-term effect on induction of neoplasia and the potential genetic effects are unknown.

Studies of the long-term results of ^{131}I treatment of hyperthyroid pediatric patients are few.[26,38,59] The prevalence of hypothyroidism in post ^{131}I–treated patients has been as high as 92% in one series of 51 children and adolescents.[26] It has been recommended that replacement doses of thyroid hormones be prescribed to every ^{131}I treated patient and be continued for life.[59] A review of 273 pediatric patients treated with ^{131}I revealed no increased incidence of leukemia, birth defects, or infertility.[59] Nodules of the thyroid developed following therapy in 16 patients. Chromosomal studies performed in children born to parents previously treated with ^{131}I have revealed no abnormalities. There are reports of two children who received ^{131}I therapy before 13 years of age and developed surgically proven hyperparathyroidism,[38] suggesting a causal relationship between ^{131}I therapy and hyperparathyroidism.

Neonatal Graves' Disease

This is a rare condition in which approximately 1% of mothers with active or previously active Graves' disease are born with neonatal Graves' disease.[79] It is caused by transplacental passage of TRAb. The onset of hyperthyroidism occurs within the first few days of life; the symptoms are usually transient, lasting 1 to 3 months. The TRAb has a half-life of approximately 1 month (similar to other IgG) and disappears from the neonate's circulation, at which time spontaneous remission occurs. In a small number of neonates the hyperthyroidism is more prolonged than would be expected from the rate of catabolism of the TRAb. These neonates may represent cases of early-onset Graves' disease superimposed on neonatal Graves' disease due to transplacental passage of TRAb.[27] In these patients the Graves' disease may not be self-limited or benign. The mortality rate ranges from 15% and 20% and sequelae include craniosynostosis and intellectual impairment. Infants of mothers receiving antithyroid drugs may be protected from the effects of TRAb for up to 10 days after delivery. After that time, the protective effects of the drugs disappear, and the persisting maternal TRAb may cause neonatal hyperthyroidism. Because this delayed response may be overlooked, the clinician should follow the neonates closely.

TRAb measurements may be of specific importance in predicting the likelihood of neonatal hyperthyroidism occurring in the offspring of a woman who has either active Graves' disease, or a history of the disorder. It appears that with a certain minimal level of TRAb in the maternal blood at term, the expectation of neonatal hyperthyroidism is very high.[79]

The clinical features include prematurity, goiter, exophthalmos, tachycardia, hypertension, hyperirritability, congestive heart failure, jaundice, hepatosplenomegaly, and thrombocytopenia.[27] Laboratory diagnosis can be made on the basis of elevated serum T_4 and T_3 levels. Cord TSH levels measured by ultrasensitive assays are below the normal range.

Therapy depends on the severity of the symptoms. Mildly affected newborns require close observation and no therapy. In moderately affected newborns, iodides orally, one drop every 8 hours, may be given together with either PTU or methimazole. The daily dose of PTU or methimazole is 5 to 10 mg/kg or 0.5 to 1.0 mg/kg, respectively in divided doses given every 8 hours. In the neonate in whom oral administration of PTU is difficult, rectal administration of PTU is possible and is effective.[72] In life-threatening situations, propranolol in a dosage of 2 mg/kg/day may be used in conjunction with PTU or methimazole and iodide. Propranolol should not be used alone because of known associated complications and hazards in the neonate. Ipodate sodium at a dose of 100 mg/day has been used in place of PTU or methimazole in the neonate. Supportive measures include the use of oxygen, digitalis, and antibiotics when indicated. Precautions should be taken to prevent tracheal obstruction if the goiter is large. Surgery is rarely necessary to relieve the obstruction.

Thyroid Storm

Thyroid storm is a potentially life-threatening complication of Graves' disease but is rare in the pediatric patient. Characteristically, fever, marked tachycardia, apathy, stupor or coma, cardiac failure, and circulatory collapse are present.

Large doses of PTU, 300 to 600 mg/day in divided doses every 2 hours, may have to be given. Iodine given orally or sodium iodide IV in a dose of 1 to 2 g is given. Iodides potentiate PTU inhibition of thyroid hormone synthesis and, in addition, block thyroid hormone release. Hypothermia is of help in treating hyperpyrexia. Since excessive catabolism of cortisol occurs and may lead to a relative deficiency, treatment with glucocorticoids may be helpful, particularly in the presence of hyperpyrexia and shock. Hydrocortisone 200 mg/m²/day can be given. Propranolol given IV may be required to control adrenergic signs.

Euthyroid Sick Syndrome in Patients With Hyperthyroidism

Severely ill children and adolescents may have coexisting ESS in the presence of hyperthyroidism. These patients have *normal* or *subnormal* serum T_4 and T_3 levels as a result of their coexisting severe nonthyroidal illness. In the pediatric patient, diabetic ketoacidosis is one of the severe intercurrent nonthyroidal illnesses with which hyperthyroidism may occur with low or normal thyroid hormone levels. The prevalence of hyperthyroidism in insulin-dependent diabetes mellitus patients is much higher than in nondiabetic individuals. Inappropriately *normal* serum T_4 and T_3 concentrations in critically ill patients should raise the question of coexisting hyperthyroidism.

Triiodothyronine Toxicosis

The syndrome of T_3 toxicosis is a state of hyperthyroidism which appears to be a reflection of preferential T_3 secretion by a hyperstimulated thyroid gland.

The criteria for diagnosis are (1) clinical hyperthyroidism; (2) normal total T_4; (3) normal FT_4; (4) normal or increased ^{131}I thyroidal uptake which cannot be suppressed by administration of L-T_3; (5) increased total T_3; and (6) normal TBG binding capacity. T_3 toxicosis occurs in pediatric patients and can be due to a diffuse goiter or a thyroid nodule. Therapy is identical to that given in Graves' disease.

Thyroxine Toxicosis

Hyperthyroidism due to elevated serum T_4 levels and associated with normal T_3 levels has been called thyroxine toxicosis or T_4 toxicosis. T_4 toxicosis most commonly results from impairment of peripheral T_4 to T_3 conversion due to either intercurrent nonthyroidal illness or inadequate caloric intake.

Peripheral Resistance to Thyroid Hormones

The syndrome of generalized tissue resistance to the action of thyroid hormones was described in 1967.[56] The original family described consisted of three siblings of consanguineous parentage; they presented with goiter, were deaf and mute, had delayed bone ages, had epiphyseal stippling, and had hyperthyroxinemia. Both sporadic and familial cases of thyroid hormone resistance have been described. This disorder is transmitted as an autosomal dominant trait and is characterized by (1) elevated serum levels of FT_3 and FT_4; (2) absence of the usual symptoms and metabolic consequences of excess thyroid hormones; (3) goiter; and (4) normal TSH response to TRH.

Peripheral or pituitary resistance to thyroid hormones is associated with variable degrees of pituitary or peripheral tissue unresponsiveness, thus explaining the different clinical features exhibited by the patients. The normal negative feedback control of TSH secretion appears to be insensitive to thyroid hormones. Basal serum TSH levels and the TSH response to TRH are normal or increased in the presence of high endogenous T_3 and T_4 levels, and show a variable but incomplete suppression to exogenous thyroid hormone administration.

Indications for thyroid hormone therapy are not clear. It has been suggested that because the severity of peripheral refractoriness to thyroid hormone may vary from tissue to tissue, the compensatory increase in endogenous hormone production may not be sufficient to satisfy all peripheral tissues. In such patients administration of *pharmacologic* doses of thyroid hormone may be appropriate.

EUTHYROID HYPERTHYROXINEMIA

There are an increasing number of syndromes in which serum thyroid hormone concentrations are elevated in the absence of hyperthyroidism (Table 5–9). This has been called *euthyroid hyperthyroxinemia*. It is important to recognize these disorders in order that these patients not be treated for hyperthyroidism. The most common cause of euthyroid hyperthyroxinemia is *acquired* TBG excess.

The first inherited abnormality of serum thyroid hormone binding proteins to be described was familial TBG excess which was discussed earlier in this chapter. An autosomal dominant form of familial hyperthyroxinemia characterized by increased T_4 binding in the albumin region on serum protein electrophoresis has been described. This syndrome has been called *familial dysalbuminemic hyperthyroxinemia* and increased T_4 binding is due to an abnormal binding site with a much greater affinity for T_4 than that on the hormone binding site of TBG.[58] The abnormal albumin has little or no affinity for T_3; therefore, the serum T_3 concentration is normal as well as the T_3RU which does not reflect the abnormal T_4 binding. FT_4 is normal; however, the *FT_4 index*, which is derived from the product of serum T_4 and T_3RU, is elevated (Table 5–10).

A syndrome due to increased T_4-binding prealbumin has been described. Laboratory studies are similiar to those seen in familial dysalbuminemic hyperthyroxinemia because thyroid-binding prealbumin probably also binds T_4 but not T_3.

A normal serum TSH response to TRH excludes the possibility of hyperthyroidism in patients with euthyroid hyperthyroxinemia due to one of the inherited abnormalities of serum thyroid hormone binding proteins.

TABLE 5–9.

Causes of Euthyroid Hyperthyroxinemia

I. Increased thyroid hormone binding
   A. Acquired in thyroxine-binding globulin
      1. Physiologic
         a. Pregnancy
         b. Newborn
      2. Nonthyroidal illnesses
         a. Liver disease (e.g., infectious hepatitis)
         b. Acute intermittent porphyria
      3. Drug-induced
         a. Oral contraceptives, exogenous estrogens
         b. Heroin, methadone
   B. Inherited abnormalities of serum thyroid hormone binding proteins
      1. Increased thyroxine-binding globulin
      2. Excess albumin binding
      3. Increased thyroxine-binding prealbumin
II. Resistance to thyroid hormone (pituitary, peripheral)
III. Euthyroid sick syndrome (transient hyperthyroxinemia of acute medical illnesses)
IV. Transient hyperthyroxinemia of acute psychiatric illnesses
V. Drug-related hyperthyroxinemia (amphetamine)

TABLE 5–10.

Thyroid Function Tests in Euthyroid Hyperthyroxinemia Syndromes*

	Total T$_3$	FT$_4$ and FT$_3$	FT$_4$ Index	TSH Response to TRH
Increased TBG	↑	N	N	N
Excess albumin binding	N	N	↑	N
Increased TBPA	N	N	↑	N
Generalized resistance to thyroid hormone	↑	↑	↑	N
Anti-T$_4$ antibodies	N	N	↑	N or ↑
Euthyroid sick syndrome (high T$_4$ syndrome)	↓	↑	↑	N or ↓

*T$_3$ = triiodothyronine; FT$_4$ = free thyroxine; FT$_3$ = free T$_3$; TSH = thyroid-stimulating hormone; TRH = thyrotropin-releasing hormone; TBPA = thyroxine-binding prealbumin; N = normal; ↑ = increased; ↓ = decreased.

SYNDROMES OF INAPPROPRIATE TSH SECRETION

The syndromes of inappropriate TSH secretion represent a heterogeneous group of disorders in which patients have normal to elevated circulating levels of TSH in the presence of elevated thyroid hormone concentrations.[74] There are two types: neoplastic production of TSH with or without concomitant hypersecretion of other anterior pituitary hormones; and nonneoplastic production of TSH.

Neoplastic hypersecretion of TSH takes in the larger group of patients. These patients are hyperthyroid and may have signs of pituitary tumors such as headaches or visual field defects. The TSH level is variably elevated and usually does not increase after TRH administration. Elevation of serum level of the alpha subunit of TSH and a high alpha subunit–total TSH ratio is a frequent finding.[74] Almost all of the tumors can be detected by CT or MRI studies of the pituitary gland. Therapy is surgery or pituitary irradiation, or both.

In patients without tumors, inappropriate secretion of TSH is a consequence of resistance to the effects of thyroid hormone. When the resistance is restricted to the pituitary, the persistent secretion of TSH and thyroid hormones leads to clinical hyperthyroidism. When the resistance is general, the patient is euthyroid even though serum TSH, T$_4$, and T$_3$ levels are elevated. Various agents have been used as therapy including T$_4$, T$_3$, steroids, bromocriptine, and somatostatin.

GOITERS

A goiter is any enlargement of the thyroid gland. It is difficult to find criteria in the literature to determine what constitutes a goiter in the pediatric patient. In one series all thyroid glands that were both visible and palpable were *not* considered to be abnormal, while in another series, those children having a palpable but only minimally enlarged thyroid isthmus were considered to be normal. In a third series a normal gland was described as one which was not visible and either nonpalpable or barely palpable.

The precise incidence of goiter is unknown. A 3.9% incidence in 5,179 children 11 to 17 years of age in Arizona, Utah, and Nevada was found between 1965 and 1971.[53]

The causes of euthyroid goiters in pediatrics are listed in Table 5–11. The two most common causes are CLT, or Hashimoto's thyroiditis, and simple or colloid goiter.

Chronic Lymphocytic Thyroiditis

The most common cause of euthyroid goiters is CLT and it is now the single most frequent thyroid disorder seen in pediatrics.[18] In several series of patients referred to medical centers for evaluation, CLT accounted for 55% to 65% of the causes of euthyroid goiters.

CLT is an autoimmune disease. It is now generally accepted that a very close relationship exists between Graves' disease and CLT and the two disorders may have a common etiologic basis (see above discussion of etiology of Graves' disease). CLT is characterized histologically by epithelial cell abnormalities and lymphocytic infiltration.

CLT is seen more frequently in females than in males. The common clinical findings are listed in Table 5–12. The thyroid gland may be symmetric or asymmetrically enlarged, firm, lobulated or nodular, and is usually nontender (Fig 5–5). Rarely, the thyroid gland may be tender and painful. Occasionally a patient may have signs of hyperthyroidism and have both CLT and Graves' disease, a syndrome known as *hashitoxicosis*.

Characteristic laboratory features include elevated serum TSH level; presence of circulating antithyroid antibodies; elevated ^{131}I thyroidal uptake; defective binding of inorganic iodide; and asymmetric uptake of radioisotope on thyroid scintiscanning.[18] Figure 5–6 is a thyroid scan showing asymmetric uptake of the radioisotope. Ultrasonography of the thyroid gland is extremely accurate in differentiating between CLT and colloid goiter.[18]

TABLE 5–11.

Causes of Euthyroid Goiter

Thyroiditis	Adenomatous
Chronic lymphocytic	Hyperplasia of the thyroid
Acute suppurative	Diffuse nodular nontoxic
Acute nonsuppurative or subacute	Carcinoma
Colloid or simple	Iodide excess

TABLE 5–12.

Clinical Features of Chronic Lymphocytic Thyroiditis

Asymptomatic goiter	Hoarseness, dysphagia
Nervousness and irritability	Cough
Fatigue	Pressure in neck
Headache, dizziness	Increased sweating

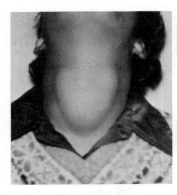

FIG 5–5.
Patient with goiter due to chronic lymphocytic thyroiditis.

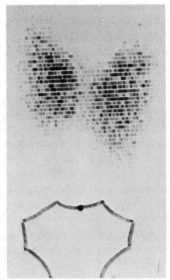

FIG 5–6.
Thyroid scintiscan in chronic lymphocytic thyroiditis, showing asymmetric uptake of radioisotope.

Four types of thyroid autoantibodies have been demonstrated:

1. An antithyroglobulin antibody (ATG) directed against thyroglobulin, the thyroid hormone precursor.
2. An antibody directed against thyroid cell membrane antigens-antimicrosomal antibodies (AMA). Recently shown to be directed against predominately membrane-bound thyroid peroxidase enzyme—antithyroid peroxidase antibodies (anti-TPO).
3. An antibody directed against a colloid antigen distinct from Tg, demonstrable by the fluorescent antibody technique using fixed thyroid tissue.
4. An antibody reacting with a nuclear component of thyroid cells detectable by the fluorescent antibody technique using unfixed thyroid tissue.

The ATG and anti-TPO determinations are those most readily available to the clinician. Detectable antithyroid antibodies are present in 56% to 76% of children and adolescents with clinical CLT. Only 25% to 58% of patients with biopsy-proven CLT have detectable serum antithyroid antibodies.[41]

In normal functioning or hyperfunctioning thyroid glands, oxidation of iodine and organic binding are fairly rapid so that relatively little free iodide is present in the thyroid gland. Consequently, there is little loss of iodide from the normal thyroid following administration of agents such as perchlorate that inhibit iodide transport and thereby discharge accumulated iodide. With defective binding of inorganic iodide, substantial accumulation of iodide occurs, and significant discharge follows inhibition of iodide transport. One test of the integrity of the organic binding mechanism is the iodide-perchlorate discharge test. An acute load of stable iodide, potassium iodide 300 $\mu g/m^2$ of body surface, is administered with ^{131}I.

One to 2 hours after administration of the tracer dose of ^{131}I, potassium perchlorate 200 mg/m^2 is given orally, resulting in inhibition of iodide transport and discharge of accumulated iodide.[18] A "discharge" of more than 10% of ^{131}I within 1 hour after administration of potassium perchlorate is indicative of defective binding of inorganic iodide. An abnormal perchlorate test is seen in other thyroid disorders in addition to CLT.

A definitive diagnosis of CLT may require a biopsy. However, the diagnosis may be made with reasonable certainty by use of the laboratory tests described above together with the clinical picture.

There is no general agreement as to the therapy of CLT. It is the most common cause of goiters and acquired hypothyroidism in children and adolescents. Some believe that CLT in most patients will eventually lead to hypothyroidism and therefore recommend full replacement doses of thyroid hormone indefinitely in order to prevent further enlargement of the thyroid, the occurrence of hypothyroidism, and to relieve accompanying complaints. Others believe that CLT may be self-limiting, that spontaneous remissions occur, and that thyroid therapy is indicated only in those patients who are hypothyroid or have large goiters. Thyroid hormone therapy does not affect the antithyroid antibody titers. The reported association of CLT and neoplasia of the thyroid may provide another rationale for thyroid hormone therapy (see below). We believe that if the thyroid gland does not decrease in size after 3 months of adequate therapy, a biopsy should be performed to rule out the possibility of a malignancy being present.

A number of studies have pointed to a relationship between thyroid autoimmunity and chromosomal disorders such as Turner and Down syndromes. There is a suggestion that patients with Noonan syndrome may have a predisposition to thyroid autoimmunity. The association of CLT with other diseases considered to be of autoimmune origin has been recognized and includes Addison disease, pernicious anemia, idiopathic hypoparathyroidism, and primary ovarian failure.

CLT and Graves' disease are usually separate and distinct clinicopathologic entities although the occurrence of both disorders in the same patient is well documented.[17] CLT presenting with hyperthyroidism (hashitoxicosis) is associated with normal or elevated ^{131}I thyroid uptake, elevated serum T_4 and T_3 levels, and high titers of antithyroid antibodies. It has been suggested that the serum T_3/T_4 ratio might be useful in differentiating patients with Graves' disease from those with hashitoxicosis. Patients with Graves' disease have a T_3/T_4 ratio greater than 20 $ng/\mu g$ while almost all patients with hashitoxicosis have a T_3/T_4 ratio of less than 20. Patients with hashitoxicosis have an increased tendency for remission of the hyperthyroidism and subsequent development of hypothyroidism. During the hyperthyroid phase, antithyroid therapy may be necessary. A variant of this syndrome is the occurrence of CLT, hyperthyroidism, and a low thyroidal uptake of ^{131}I. It is important to recognize this syndrome because its course is short and self-limited, and the usual therapeutic measures for Graves' disease are contraindicated.

The relationship between CLT and neoplasia of the thyroid gland is controversial. It has been suggested that CLT predisposes the gland to the development of lymphoma and follicular and papillary carcinoma. This association has not been substantiated but has been reported in adolescent patients. We believe that all patients with CLT and a nodule of the thyroid gland should have the nodule biopsied to rule out the presence of a malignancy.

Simple or Colloid Goiter

Simple or colloid goiters constitute the second most common cause of euthyroid goiters in pediatrics. Almost all patients have no symptoms. The physical examination, in most instances, does not allow the clinician to differentiate between colloid goiter and CLT. Firmness and diffuse nodularity can occur in colloid goiters. Laboratory studies may also not allow differentiation. Very low or negative antithyroid antibody titers and symmetric uptake of radioisotope on thyroid scintiscanning are seen in colloid goiters. It has been suggested that ultrasonographic study of the thyroid gland will differentiate between CLT and colloid goiter.

The course of a colloid goiter is unpredictable. It has been postulated and supported by ^{131}I radioautography studies that simple diffuse enlargement of the thyroid gland in a young patient can lead to a large multinodular goiter in the older individual. This is the rationale for the use of thyroid hormones in the therapy of a large colloid goiter.

Adenomatous goiter and hyperplasia of the thyroid gland require histologic examination in order to make a definitive diagnosis. The chief importance of adenomatous goiter arises from the need to differentiate it from carcinoma. Hyperplasia of the thyroid gland is rarely seen in euthyroid children or in adolescents who do not live in an endemic goiter area. Thyroid function studies are usually normal in patients with either adenomatous goiter or hyperplasia of the thyroid gland, with the exception of patients with hyperplasia of the thyroid gland secondary to an inborn error of thyroid hormone synthesis. The preferred treatment of adenomatous goiter and hyperplasia of the thyroid gland is surgical. Removing most of the goiter does not alter the underlying pathologic mechanism. To insure euthyroidism and to attempt to prevent recurrence of the goiter, the patient should be placed on lifelong thyroid therapy.

Thyroiditis

Acute suppurative and nonsuppurative or subacute thyroiditis are uncommon problems in pediatrics. Subacute thyroiditis is more common than acute suppurative thyroiditis. Acute suppurative thyroiditis is usually preceded by an upper respiratory infection. The most common bacteria causing suppurative thyroiditis are hemolytic streptococcus, *staphylococcus aureus,* and pneumococcus. There is usually a sudden onset with chills, fever, dysphagia, hoarseness, and pain, erythema of the overlying skin, and tenderness of the thyroid.[68] The white blood cell count and sedimentation rate are elevated while thyroid function studies are usually normal. In less typical cases, differentiation from subacute thyroiditis can be difficult.

The management necessitates a vigorous approach. Antibiotics are essential. Incision and drainage of any thyroid abscess should be performed early to prevent complications. Normal thyroid function usually follows.

Nonsuppurative or subacute thyroiditis is rare in pediatric patients and is generally considered to be viral in origin. It often follows an upper respiratory illness. The mumps virus has been implicated in some cases and there is some evidence suggesting that echovirus, influenza, coxsackievirus, and adenovirus may be etiologic agents. Subacute nonsuppurative thyroiditis is usually a benign, self-limited disease characterized primarily by local thyroid tenderness, pain, and systemic symptoms of inflammation. The pain may radiate to the jaw or ears. Characteristic histologic findings include giant cells, granuloma, and pseudotubercles. During the acute phase of the disease, a sufficient amount of thyroid hormones may be released to produce symptoms of hyperthyroidism. This acute phase may be followed by a period of hypothyroidism which is usually temporary.

The results of thyroid function tests are variable, depending on the stage of the disease. The sedimentation rate is usually markedly elevated and the T_4 may be elevated at this time. At the same time there is a marked *decrease* in ^{123}I thyroidal uptake. With recovery, thyroid function may be *subnormal* with an increase in serum TSH concentration. Ultimately, thyroid function studies return to normal.

The course may vary from a few days to 3 months or longer. Therapy with aspirin is generally adequate to control the symptoms. In severe cases, glucocorticoids will alleviate the clinical complaints rapidly but will not influence the basic disease process. The usual therapeutic measures for Graves' disease are contraindicated during the phase of the disease when the patient may be clinically hyperthyroid and have an elevated T_4 level.

Nodular Goiters

A thyroid nodule is a discrete, palpable, or localized enlargement of the thyroid. It is of diagnostic importance to distinguish a nodule that is part of a lobe from an enlarged thyroid itself. Furthermore, masses adjacent to the thyroid, such as lymph nodes, must be differentiated from thyroid nodules. Thyroid nodules may be single or multiple.

A palpable nodule in the thyroid gland in an otherwise normal euthyroid patient may represent: (1) an adenoma, (2) a cyst, (3) lobulation of normal thyroid tissue, (4) lobulation of the gland with CLT, (5) a primary malignant lesion, (6) an adenoma or malignancy associated with CLT, (7) an autonomous nodule, (8) hypertrophy of one lobe due to congenital absence of the other lobe, or (9) nonthyroid disease such as dermoid cyst. The presence of a solitary nodule of the thyroid in a child or adolescent is uncommon and raises the strong possibility of malignancy. Carcinoma has been reported in 14% to 50% of pediatric patients with a palpable nodule of the thyroid gland.[30]

The precise diagnosis of nodules in the thyroid is not easy. A careful history should be taken, especially to determine if the patient has ever had irradiation to the head, neck, or chest and to determine if the patient has received any goitrogens.

The palpable features of a nodule in the thyroid may reflect its nature (Fig 5–7). A soft, well-circumscribed nodule is not likely to be malignant; it probably represents a cyst or cystic adenoma. A hard or firm nodule found in an otherwise normal gland would suggest a malignant lesion. Malignant lesions, however, seldom occupy the entire gland without extension and fixation to adjacent structures. A firm nodule in a gland that is equally firm may represent lobulation of the gland, CLT, adenoma associated with CLT, or a malignant lesion. A tender nodule may represent an inflammatory process or hemorrhage into the gland.

Laboratory studies are necessary to establish a presumptive diagnosis. These studies include T_4, FT_4, TSH, and antithyroid antibodies. A thyroid scintiscan is essential. Radioactive iodine uptake studies, TSH stimulation, T_3 suppression test, and an ultrasonic examination may also be necessary.

Thyroid nodules may be classified as "functioning" or "nonfunctioning." A functioning thyroid nodule can accumulate iodine and synthesize thyroid hormones. A nonfunctioning thyroid nodule is usually unable to concentrate iodine or to adequately synthesize thyroid hormones. Thyroid nodules may be further differentiated on the basis of thyroid scintiscanning into three categories: warm, hot, or cold nodules. The thyroid scan will detect a nodule smaller than 1 cm in diameter.

The hot or hyperfunctioning nodule is commonly referred to as an *autonomous functioning thyroid nodule* (AFTN) because it is presumed to be independent of TSH stimulation for growth and function. The autonomous nature of the nodule is evaluated by a T_3 suppression test. AFTNs can be classified as toxic or nontoxic on the basis of the usual clinical and laboratory criteria for hyperthyroidism. Malignancy occurs in AFTNs in children and adolescents. Hyperthyroidism may develop in an AFTN

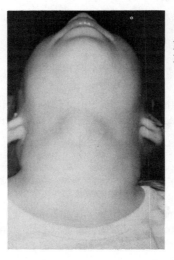

FIG 5–7.
Patient with solitary nodule of the thyroid gland.

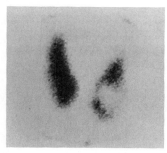

FIG 5–8.
Thyroid scintiscan with cold nodule in the left lobe due to papillary carcinoma.

and should be removed surgically. In one series of AFTNs in children and adolescents, there was a 25% incidence of hyperthyroidism, and carcinoma was present in 11% of patients.[12] Thyroid lobectomy has been recommended for nontoxic AFTNs.

A nodule classified as functional or warm indicates that the tissue within the nodule is capable of concentrating the isotope in a normal or nearly normal fashion. Although malignancy can occur in a warm nodule, it is rare because normal or toxic thyroid tissue has a greater affinity for the isotope than does neoplastic tissue. Another variant of the warm nodule is seen in patients with congenital absence of a thyroid lobe. All of the radioactivity is confined to one side. The presence or absence of a contralateral lobe should be determined by repeating the thyroid scan after TSH stimulation. Warm nodules are seldom of surgical importance and usually regress with adequate thyroid replacement therapy.

A cold or nonfunctioning nodule does not trap any administered radioisotope and is devoid of functioning thyroid tissue (Fig 5–8). It is in patients with cold nodules that the greatest variation is seen and in which the delineation of the potentially dangerous from the completely innocuous lesion is most difficult. The reported incidence of malignancy in cold nodules in the pediatric age group has decreased. The decreased incidence may reflect the fact that children with benign lesions of the head and neck no longer receive therapeutic irradiation.

It has been recommended that thyroid suppression should be attempted for a 4- to 6-month period in patients who have no findings suggestive of malignancy.[19] If during this period the nodule grows, or if over a 1-year period the nodule does not decrease 50% in size, surgery is then recommended. We believe that either fine-needle aspiration of the nodule with cytologic examination by an experienced cytopathologist be performed or that a open biopsy be done in order to establish a definitive histopathologic diagnosis. This recommendation is made because of the significant incidence of carcinoma.

THYROID CANCER

The incidence of thyroid cancer in children and adolescents has increased greatly since 1951 when Winship was able to find 93 cases in the world's literature, to which he added four personally observed cases and 95 cases gathered from a survey of hospitals throughout the world.[76] In his final report in 1970, Winship had collected 878 known cases of childhood thyroid cancer[77]; approximately 60% of the patients were female.

Etiology

In 1949, Quimby and Werner suggested the possibility of a relationship between radiation to the head and neck and the subsequent development of thyroid cancer.[52] Since then numerous investigations have verified that *low-dose* external irradiation to the head and neck results in an increased incidence of benign and malignant thyroid tumors. Most patients had irradiation to the thymus in infancy, but many were treated for enlarged tonsils and adenoids, hemangioma, nevi, acne, eczema, or cervical adenitis. In the Childhood Thyroid Cancer Registry, an attempt was made to obtain a history of previous radiation to the head and neck from only 476 of the 878 cases.[30] Of these, 76% had received radiation from 3½ to nearly 14 years before the diagnosis of thyroid cancer was made.

High-dose external radiation (>2000 rads) has most often been associated with hypothyroidism and *not* thyroid cancer. However, patients have been reported who developed thyroid cancer years after exposure to radiation to the head and neck in excess of 2,000 rads.

Histologic Classification

All of the various histologic types of thyroid cancer that occur in adults are found in children, but fortunately with a slightly higher proportion of differentiated carcinomas. Table 5–13 shows the classification of 606 of the 878 cases from the Childhood Thyroid Cancer Registry. Papillary carcinomas often contain follicular elements, and these may be described as mixed papillary and follicular adenocarcinomas.

Clinical Data

In approximately three-fourths of the patients the first sign of disease was one or more firm, painless nodules in the neck. Hoarseness, dyspnea, and dysphagia are uncommon initial complaints. Pulmonary metastases may be the first evidence of disease. These metastases have been misinterpreted as miliary tuberculosis or his-

TABLE 5–13.

Histologic Classification of Thyroid Cancer From the Childhood Thyroid Cancer Registry (n = 606)*

Cancer Type	%
Papillary	17.6
Follicular	17.6
Medullary	2.6
Undifferentiated	2.6
Unclassified	5.4

*Data from Winship T, Rosvoll RV: *Clin Proc Child Hosp DC* 1970; 26:327.

toplasmosis. In Winship's series[76] pulmonary metastases were present in 14.4% (103/878) of patients on initial examination and appeared in 5.2% (37/878) of other patients at a later time. Osseous metastases may occur but these are uncommon. The well-differentiated cancers in children are noted for their slow growth.

Diagnosis

Surgical biopsy is essential for diagnosis. Roentgenographic soft tissue examination of the neck in suspected cases of thyroid cancer in children may be helpful. Criteria have been established to allow separation of calcified malignant and benign lesions of the thyroid on the basis of the characteristics of the calcification. Calcifications in malignant lesions are poorly marginated, not dense, hazy, and are of about equal size. Calcifications in benign lesions are well marginated, sharply defined, dense, and vary in size. The presence of psammoma bodies in thyroid cancers is apparently responsible for the calcifications seen on radiographs. Psammoma bodies are seen histologically in over 50% of thyroid cancers in children. Radioiodine ablation of presumed *normal* thyroid tissue in patients who have had surgery for follicular and papillary thyroid cancer has gained wide acceptance despite the absence of controlled prospective studies to confirm its effectiveness. One of the reasons given in support of radioiodine ablation of presumed normal thyroid tissue is the high incidence of multicentricity in patients with thyroid cancer.

Radiotherapy is indicated in all patients with nonresectable cancers that show no uptake on scanning. Full suppressive doses of thyroid hormone should be given after surgery or ^{131}I ablation but its effectiveness in controlling the growth of thyroid cancer by suppression of TSH is debatable. Chemotherapeutic drugs, such as doxorubicin hydrochloride (Adriamycin), have been used in the therapy of metastatic thyroid cancer. Patients should be followed carefully, with chest films periodically, and, if indicated, ^{131}I scans of the neck and chest.

Debate continues over the frequency of intraglandular metastases and their future malignant potential. The reported incidence of cancer in both lobes ranges from 18% to 80%.[5] Unilateral lobectomy, followed later by surgical removal of the opposite lobe, reveals cancer in the opposite lobe in 66% of patients.[5] Unilateral lobectomy without subsequent excision of the opposite lobe is associated with recurrence in the opposite lobe in approximately 4% of patients only. Childhood thyroid carcinoma is frequently associated with lymphocytic infiltration. It has been suggested that lymphocytic infiltration around the thyroid carcinoma is an immunologic reaction induced by antigens from the carcinoma and may be a good prognostic sign.[34] Serum Tg determination is of limited value in the preoperative assessment for possible carcinoma since serum Tg levels may be elevated in a variety of thyroid disorders, including carcinoma. Persistent elevation of serum Tg, however, following treatment for differentiated thyroid carcinoma, suggests the presence of residual or recurrent tumor.

Therapy

The treatment of thyroid cancer in children and adolescents is primarily surgical but is controversial because of differences in criteria for diagnosis, the variable and usually prolonged course of the disease, and the lack of controlled studies of surgical and adjuvant types of therapy. The main controversy is over the extent of surgery, whether the cancer has extended beyond the capsule or to the regional lymph nodes, requiring total thyroidectomy and prophylactic node dissection. There is seldom an indication for radical surgery in children.

Iodine 131 scans should be obtained 5 to 6 weeks postoperatively to detect areas of residual neoplasm and metastases. Thyroid hormone therapy should be withheld in order to obtain the maximal amount of concentrations of radioactivity. If residual disease or metastases are found, these should be treated with therapeutic doses of [131]I. At times, the metastatic nodules from mixed papillary and follicular tumors contain more follicles than the primary cancer. Since few papillary carcinomas spontaneously incorporate ^{131}I, they may be stimulated to do so by administration of bovine TSH intramuscularly daily for 3 days.

Children with papillary tumors have a long survival time even with lymph node and lung metastases. The mortality of childhood thyroid cancer matches that for adults as shown in the Childhood Thyroid Cancer Registry.[76] During the 20-year study 17% of the 878 patients had died. More than half of all the mortality was caused by local extension to vital structures in the neck and the remainder by metastases and dissemination.

Secondary Thyroid Neoplasms

Survival rates for many pediatric malignancies have improved recently. Those patients who undergo successful therapy of their cancer are at increased risk for development of thyroid tumors. A recent study revealed a 4.6% incidence of secondary thyroid neoplasm.[70] The primary malignancies included leukemia, Wilms' tumor, Hodgkin's disease, rhabdomyosarcoma, and ganglioneuroblastoma. Careful attention should be given to the thyroid gland during follow-up evaluations of pediatric patients who survive malignancies.

Medullary Thyroid Carcinoma

Medullary thyroid carcinoma (MTC) originates in the parafollicular thyroid cell which is derived from the ultimobranchial body. It is a solid nonfollicular tumor with amyloid in the stroma. The finding of amyloid interspersed among the neoplastic cells is diagnostic. MTC may occur either sporadically or as an autosomal dominant in some families. MTC is a feature of multiple endocrine neoplasia type IIA (MEN-IIA) and type IIB (MEN-IIB) (Table 5–14). As such, it may occur alone or in association with pheochromocytoma; mucosal or subcutaneous neuromas or neurofibromas; tumors or hyperplasia of the parathyroid glands; and Cushing's syndrome. The association of MTC and pheochromocytoma (MEN-IIA) is known as Sipple's syndrome.[63] Approximately half of the cases of Sipple's syndrome have been familial.

MTC elaborates calcitonin, which can be detected in the primary tumor, metastatic lesions, blood, and urine. Immunohistochemical studies have demonstrated the presence of carcinoembryonic antigen (CEA) in normal and in malignant C cells.

TABLE 5–14.

Components of Multiple Endocrine Neoplasia (MEN) Syndromes*

	Components	Approximate Involvement in Affected Patients (%)
I	Parathyroid hyperplasia	90
	Islet cell tumors	80
	Pituitary adenomas	65
	Others: adrenal adenomas, thyroid abnormalities, thymomas, carcinoid tumors, multiple lipomas	Variable
IIA	Parathyroid hyperplasia	40
	Medullary thyroid carcinoma	95
	Pheochromocytoma	50
IIB	Mucosal neuromas	100
	Medullary thyroid carcinoma	95
	Pheochromocytoma	50

*Data from references 61, 64, 78.

TABLE 5–15.

Clinical Features in Multiple Mucosal Neuroma Syndrome and Medullary Thyroid Carcinoma

Marfanoid habitus	Pes cavus
Thick bumpy lips	Slipped femoral epiphyses
Prominent jaw	Pectus excavatum
Thickened eyelids	Diarrhea
Mucosal neuromas of lips and tongue	Hypertrophic corneal nerves
Single or multiple nodules of thyroid	Intestinal ganglioneuromas
Scoliosis	

Elevated plasma CEA levels have been reported in some patients with MTC. The tumor also produces other humoral substances, including prostaglandins, serotonin, histaminase, and ACTH-like substances.

The prognosis of MTC lies between that of well-differentiated tumors and anaplastic cancers.

Clinical Presentation

Most frequently, MTC presents as single or multiple neck masses, nodule(s) of the thyroid, or associated with cervical adenopathy.[24] In advanced disease, hoarseness, dysphagia, or symptoms of systemic spread may be prominent. In some patients diarrhea is severe and both prostaglandin and serotonin have been suggested as possible causes of the diarrhea. Pediatric patients may present with the distinctive features listed in Table 5–15.[24] It is important to remember that the distinctive features of MEN-IIB, which include characteristic facies, marfanoid habitus, and mucosal neuromas, are often not present at birth. The mucosal neuromas appear first on the tongue, eyelids, and lips and are usually present by 3 years of age. The importance of early clinical suspicion, diagnosis, and thyroidectomy in MEN-IIB has been stressed.[24] MEN-IIB can be a cause of neonatal feeding difficulties and failure to thrive.

Laboratory Findings

The single or multiple nodules of MTC appear as cold thyroid nodule(s) on thyroid scintiscanning. An elevated basal plasma calcitonin level and an enhanced calcitonin response to pentagastrin infusion (0.5 µg/kg) is pathognomonic of MTC. Elevated plasma levels of CEA are present in patients with MTC but are not a sensitive marker for early diagnosis. Other diagnostic studies should include radiographs of the thyroid for calcification and of the lungs for metastatic lesions. Plasma or urinary catecholamines should be determined even if the patient is normotensive. If catecholamines are increased, further studies for a pheochromocytoma must be performed since surgical excision of a pheochromocytoma must precede thyroid surgery. Serum parathyroid hormone and calcium concentrations should be obtained to evaluate parathyroid status.

Therapy

Surgery is the treatment for MTC. MTC is generally unresponsive to external radiation, chemotherapy, or administration of thyroid hormones. Iodine 131 has no value as adjunct therapy in the management of MTC. Postoperatively, the completeness of excision of the MTC may be confirmed by the serum calcitonin level. A return of elevated serum calcitonin levels may be the earliest sign of recurrence. Measurement of plasma CEA has been suggested as a better prognostic marker than the serum calcitonin level. Since MTC frequently occurs as a familial disease, the patient and all family members should be carefully followed and reevaluated for years.

Multiple Endocrine Neoplasia Syndromes

Medullary thyroid cancer is an integral part of MEN-IIA. MEN syndromes consist of three distinct disease entities. They have in common adenomatous, carcinomatous, or hyperplastic involvement of a variety of endocrine glands, and an autosomal dominant inheritance. MEN-I includes hyperparathyroidism, islet cell, and pituitary tumors.[78] The components of MEN-IIA are hyperparathyroidism, MTC, and pheochromocytoma.[64] MEN-IIB or MEN-III includes multiple neuromas, MTC, and pheochromocytoma.[61] The components of the MEN syndromes are listed in Table 5–14. Because MEN syndromes involve an autosomal dominant inheritance, parents, siblings, and offspring of affected patients should be screened. Effective tests are available for the early detection of components of the syndromes in potentially affected patients.[64,78]

A number of theories have been offered to account for the MEN syndromes, but none is completely satisfactory. The one that has the largest number of adherents at the present time invokes a genetic disturbance in neural crest cell differentiation. This theory attempts to tie together embryologically all the cells in both the endocrine and the paracrine systems via a common characteristic, namely, the ability to secrete peptide hormones (the APUD [amine precursor uptake and decarboxylation system] concept).[50]

REFERENCES

1. Abbassi V, Aldige C: Evaluation of sodium L-thyroxine (T_4) requirement in replacement therapy of hypothyroidism. *J Pediatr* 1977; 90:298.
2. Alves C, et al: Changes in brain maturation detected by magnetic resonance imaging in congenital hypothyroidism. *J Pediatr* 1989; 115:600–603.
3. Ballabio M, et al: Maturation of thyroid function in normal human foetuses. *Clin Endocrinol* 1989; 31:565–571.
4. Barnes HV: Treatment of hyperthyroidism in children and adolescents. *Pharmacol Ther C* 1976; 1:12.
5. Black BM, Kirk TA Jr, Woolner LB: Multicentricity of papillary adenocarcinoma of the thyroid: Influence on treatment. *J Clin Endocrinol Metab* 1960; 20:130.
6. Bliddal H, et al: The relationship between T_3 index, thyroid volume and thyroid stimulating, TSH receptor binding, and thyroid growth stimulating antibodies in untreated Graves' disease. *Clin Endocrinol* 1987; 27:75.
7. Bode HH, Vanjonack WJ, Crawford JD: Mitigation of cretinism by breast feeding. *Pediatrics* 1978; 62:13.
8. Brown Al, et al: Racial differences in the incidence of congenital hypothyroidism. *J Pediatr* 1981; 99:934.
9. Buchanan BD, Hagen GA: Elevated thyroxine-binding globulin with X-chromosome linked inheritance. *Clin Endocrinol* 1979; 11:665.
10. Buchanan CR, et al: Gonadotrophin, growth hormone and prolactin secretion in children with primary hypothyroidism. *Clin Endocrinol* 1988; 29:427–436.
11. Cooper DS: Antithyroid drugs. *N Engl J Med* 1984; 311:1353.
12. Croom RD, et al: Autonomously functioning thyroid nodules in childhood and adolescence. *Surgery* 1987; 102:1101.
13. DeGroot LJ, Quintans J: The causes of autoimmune thyroid disease. *Endocr Rev* 1989; 10:537.
14. DeGroot LJ, et al: The molecular basis of thyroid hormone action. *J Endocrinol Invest* 1989; 12:843.
15. Delange F, et al: Increased risk of primary hypothyroidism in preterm infants. *J Pediatr* 1984; 105:462.
16. Farooki ZQ, et al: Myocardial dysfunction in hypothyroid children, *Am J Dis Child* 1983; 137:65–68.
17. Fatourechi V, McConahey WM, Woolner LB: Hyperthyroidism associated with histologic Hashimoto's thyroiditis. *Mayo Clin Proc* 1971; 46:682.
18. Fisher DA: Advances in the laboratory diagnosis of thyroid disease. Part I. *J Pediatr* 1973; 82:1–9.
19. Fisher DA: Thyroid nodules in childhood and their management. *J Pediatr* 1976; 89:866.
20. Fisher DA: Thyroid physiology in the perinatal period and during childhood, in Ingbar SH, Braverman LE (eds): Werner's The Thyroid, ed 5. Philadelphia, JB Lippincott Co, 1986.
21. Fisher DA, Klein AH: Thyroid development and disorders of thyroid function in the newborn. *N Engl J Med* 1981; 304:702.
22. Fisher DA, et al: Screening for congenital hypothyroidism: results of screening 1 million North American infants. *J Pediatr* 1979; 94:700.
23. Francis G, Riley W: Congenital familial transient hypothyroidism secondary to transplacental thyrotropin-blocking autoantibodies. *Am J Dis Child* 1987; 141:1081–1083.

24. Frank K, et al: Importance of early diagnosis and follow-up in multiple endocrine neoplasia (MEN II B). *Eur J Pediatr* 1984; 143:112.

25. Franklin R, O'Grady C, Carpenter L: Neonatal thyroid function: Comparison between breast-fed and bottle-fed infants. *J Pediatr* 1985; 106:124.

26. Freitas JE, et al: Iodine-131: Optimal therapy for hyperthyroidism in children and adolescents. *J Nucl Med* 1979; 20:847.

27. Hollingsworth DR, Mabry CC: Congenital Graves' disease: Four familial cases with long-term follow-up and perspective. *Am J Dis Child* 1976; 130:148.

28. Howard CP, Hayles AB: Hyperthyroidism in childhood. *Clin Endocrinol Metab* 1978; 7:127.

29. Hung W, Fitz CR, Lee EDH: Pituitary enlargement in a newborn due to a lingual thyroid gland and primary hypothyroidism. *Pediatr Neurol* 1990; 6:60–62.

30. Hung W, et al: Solitary thyroid nodules in children and adolescents. *J Pediatr Surg* 1982; 17:225.

31. Ivarsson SA, Persson PH, Ericsson UB: Thyroid gland volume as measured by ultrasonography in healthy children and adolescents in a non-iodine deficient area. *Acta Pediatr Scand* 1989; 78:633–634.

32. Jacobson DH, Gorman CA: Endocrine ophthalmopathy: Current ideas concerning etiology, pathogenesis and treatment. *Endocr Rev* 1984; 5:200.

33. Jenkins MB, Steffes MW: Congenital thyroxine binding globulin deficiency: Incidence and inheritance. *Hum Genet* 1987; 77:80.

34. Kamma H, Fujii K, Ogata T: Lymphocytic infiltration in juvenile thyroid carcinoma. *Cancer* 1988; 62:1988.

35. Kay C, Abraham S, McLain P: The weight of normal thyroid glands in children. *Arch Pathol* 1966; 82:349.

36. Klein RZ: Infantile hypothyroidism then and now: The results of neonatal screening, *Curr Probl Pediatr* 1985; 15:1.

37. Lever EG, Medeiros-Neto GA, DeGroot LJ: Inherited disorders of thyroid metabolism. *Endocr Rev* 1983; 4:213.

38. Levy WJ, Schumacher OP, Gupta M: Treatment of childhood Graves' disease: A review with emphasis on radioiodine treatment. *Cleve Clin J Med* 1988; 55:373.

39. Lewander WJ, et al: Acute thyroxine ingestion in pediatric patients. *Pediatrics* 1989; 84:262.

40. Lippe EM, Landaw EM, Kaplan SA: Hyperthyroidism in children treated with long term medical therapy: Twenty-five percent remission every two years. *J Clin Endocrinol Metab* 1987; 64:1241.

41. Loeb PB, Drash AL, Kenny FM: Prevalence of low-titer and "negative" antithyroglobulin antibodies in biopsy-proved juvenile Hashimoto's thyroiditis. *J Pediatr* 1973; 82:17.

42. Maenpaa J: Congenital hypothyroidism: Etiological and clinical aspects. *Arch Dis Child* 1972; 47:914.

43. Mancuso AA, Dillon WP: The neck. *Radiol Clin North Am* 1989; 27:407–434.

44. Martino E, et al: Human serum thyrotrophin measurement by ultrasensitive immunoradiometric assay as a first-line test in the evaluation of thyroid function. *Clin Endocrinol* 1986; 24:141–148.

45. McFarland KF, et al: Thyrotrophin-releasing hormone test: An adverse reaction. *Arch Intern Med 1982; 142:132.*

46. Miki K, et al: Transient infantile hyperthyrotrophinemia. *Arch Dis Child* 1989; 64:1177–1182.

47. Muir A, et al: Thyroid scanning, ultrasound, and serum thyroglobulin in determining the origin of congenital hypothyroidism. *Am J Dis Child* 1988; 142:214–216.

48. New England Congenital Hypothyroidism Collaborative: Elementary school performance of children with congenital hypothyroidism. *J Pediatr* 1990; 116:27.
49. Nocross-Nechay K, Richards GE, Cavallo A: Evoked potentials show early and delayed abnormalities in children with congenital hypothyroidism. *Neuropediatrics* 1989; 20:158–163.
50. Pearse AG, Polak JM: Neural crest origin of the endocrine polypeptide (APUD) cells of the gastrointestinal tract and pancreas. *Gut* 1971; 12:783.
51. Penny R: Cord serum thyroid-stimulating hormone and thyroglobulin levels decline with increasing birth weight in newborns. *J Clin Endocrinol Metab* 1984; 59:979.
52. Quimby EH, Werner SC: Late radiation effects in roentgen therapy for hyperthyroidism. *JAMA* 1949; 140:1046.
53. Rallison ML: Thyroid disease in children. *Am J Med* 1974; 567:457.
54. Redmond GP, Soyka LF: Abnormal TSH secretory dynamics in congenital hypothyroidism. *J Pediatr* 1981; 98:83.
55. Refetoff S: Inherited thyroxine-binding globulin abnormalities in man. *Endocr Rev* 1989; 10:275–293.
56. Refetoff S, DeWind LT, DeGroot LJ: Familial syndrome combining deaf-mutism, stippled epiphyses, goiter and abnormally high PBI: Possible target organ refractoriness to thyroid hormone. *J Clin Endocrinol Metab* 1967; 27:279.
57. Rivkees SA, Bode HH, Crawford JD: Long-term growth in juvenile acquired hypothyroidism: The failure to achieve normal adult stature. *N Engl J Med* 1988; 318:599–602.
58. Ruiz M, Rajatanavin R, Young RA, et al: Familial dysalbuminemia hyperthyroxinemia. *N Engl J Med* 1982; 306:635.
59. Safa AM, Schumacher OP, Rodeiques-Antunez A: Long-term follow-up results in children and adolescents treated with radioactive iodine (^{131}I) for hyperthyroidism. *N Engl J Med* 1975; 292:167.
60. Sakaguchi M, et al: Longitudinal study of free thyroxine in low-birth-weight infants by paper disk method. *J Pediatr* 1983; 103:793.
61. Schimke RN: Genetic aspects of multiple endocrine neoplasia. *Ann Rev* Med 1984; 35:25.
62. Singer PA, et al: Transient TRH deficiency after prolonged thyroid hormone therapy. *J Clin Endocrinol Metab* 1978; 47:512.
63. Sipple JH: The association of pheochromocytoma with carcinoma of the thyroid gland. *Am J Med* 1961; 31:163.
64. Sizemore GW, Heath H, Carney JA: Multiple endocrine neoplasia type 2. *Clin Endocrinol Metab* 1980; 9:299.
65. Smith DW, Blizzard RM, Wilkins L: The mental prognosis in hypothyroidism of infancy and childhood. *Pediatrics* 1957; 19:1011.
66. Smith DW, et al; Congenital hypothyroidism: Signs and symptoms in the newborn period. *J Pediatr* 1975; 87:958.
67. Surks MI, et al: American Thyroid Association guidelines for use of laboratory tests in thyroid disorders. *JAMA* 1990; 263:1529.
68. Szabo SM, Allen DB: Thyroiditis: Differentiation of acute suppurative and subacute. *Clin Pediatr* 1989; 28:171.
69. Trent JM, et al: Localization of the human thyroxine-binding globulin gene to the long arm of the X chromosome (Xq21-22). *Am J Hum Genet* 1987; 41:428.
70. Vane D, King DR, Boles ET: Secondary thyroid neoplasms in pediatric cancer patients: Increased risk with improved survival. *J Pediatr Surg* 1984; 19:855.
71. Viscardi RM, et al: Hyperthyroxinemia in newborns due to excess thyroxine-binding globulin. *N Engl J Med* 1983; 309:897.

72. Walter RM, Bartle WR: Rectal administration of propylthiouracil in the treatment of Graves' disease. *Am J Med* 1990; 88:69.
73. Weinblatt ME, et al: Polycythemia in hypothyroid infants. Am J Dis Child 1987; 141:1121–1123.
74. Weintraub BD: Inappropriate secretion of thyroid-stimulating hormone. *Ann Intern Med* 1981; 95:339.
75. Wilson DM, et al: Serum free thyroxine values in term, premature and sick infants. *J Pediatr* 1982; 101:113.
76. Winship T: Carcinoma of the thyroid in children. *Trans Am Goiter Assoc* 1951; 364.
77. Winship T, Rosvoll RV: Thyroid carcinoma in childhood. Final report on a 20 year study. *Clin Proc Child Hosp DC* 1970; 26:327.
78. Yamaguchi K, Kameya T, Abe K: Multiple endocrine neoplasia type 1. *Clin Endocrinol Metab* 1980; 9:261.
79. Zakarija M, McKenzie JM: Pregnancy-associated changes in the thyroid-stimulating antibody of Graves' disease and the relationship to neonatal hyperthyroidism. *J Clin Endocrinol Metab* 1983; 57:1036.

Chapter 6

Adrenal Cortex and Medulla

Selma F. Siegel
Peter A. Lee

EMBRYOLOGY OF THE ADRENAL GLAND

The adrenal gland in man and higher vertebrates is formed by the coalescence of two distinct glands which retain separate identities in fish and other primitive vertebrates. Histologic and functional characteristics distinguish these two components into cortex and medulla. The cortex is identifiable in the fetus at 6 weeks of gestation as a groove in the coelom near the mesonephros. Over the next 2 weeks, the cells enlarge into cords near the developing urogenital structures, become encapsulated by connective tissue, and lose the connection with the coelomic mesothelium.

Gonadal and adrenocortical cells share a common primordium. Thus, the synthesis of steroids by cells in both organs involves the same steroidal enzymes (Fig 6–1) under similar genetic control and subject to similar enzymatic defects. Since primitive adrenocortical cells may migrate along with gonadal steroid–producing cells, accessory adrenal tissue may be found both adjacent to the adrenals and near or within the gonads.

The medulla and sympathetic ganglia are derived from the neural crest. Neural crest cells are classified as chromaffin cells because of the brown color produced after treatment with chromic acid. During the seventh and eighth weeks of gestation, some of these cells migrate along the adrenal vein, penetrate the cortex, and become the adrenal medulla. Small masses of these cells also remain along the developing spinal column and become paraganglia.

The fetal adrenal cortex contains an inner, distinct fetal zone, which is larger but involutes within days of birth, and an outer zone, which persists and later differentiates into the three zones of the adult adrenal cortex. During gestation, the adrenal glands

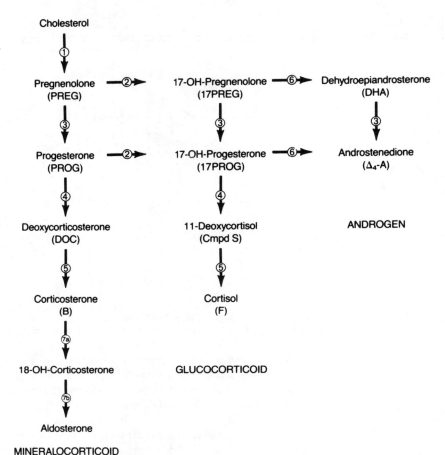

FIG 6–1.
Schematic representation of synthetic steps of adrenal mineralocorticoid, glucocorticoid, and androgen steroids. Numbers denote enzymatic steps: (*1*) 20,22-desmolase, P-450$_{scc}$; 20-hydroxylase, 22-hydroxylase; (*2*) 17-hydroxylase, P-450$_{c17}$; (*3*) 3β-hydroxysteroid dehydrogenase; (*4*) 21-hydroxylase, P-450$_{c21}$; (*5*) 11-hydroxylase, P-450$_{c11}$; (*6*) 17,20-desmolase 17,20-lyase, P-450$_{c17}$; (*7a*) 18-hydroxylase corticosterone methyloxidase I, P-450$_{c11}$; (*7b*) 18-dehydrogenase, corticosterone methyloxidase II, P-450$_{c11}$.

are relatively much larger than in adult life. The fetal adrenal synthesizes steroids, especially dehydroepiandrosterone (DHEA) and its sulfated form (DHEA-S), which are substrates for conversion to estrogens by the placenta.

STRUCTURE

The paired adrenal glands are located at the cranial pole of the kidneys. At birth, the combined weight is approximately 7 g. Adult adrenal glands weigh 3.5 to 5.0 g each. Accessory adrenal tissue may occur adjacent to the main glands, near the gonads, or within the gonads. The cortex is subdivided into three zones: an outer zona glomerulosa, a middle zona fasciculata, and an inner zona reticularis. Zona glomerulosa cells, located in nests of cells about the periphery of the cortex, produce aldosterone and are principally responsive to angiotensin and potassium. Zona fasciculata cells, clear cells, and zona reticularis cells, compact cells, are responsive to adrenocorticotropic hormone (ACTH) and primarily synthesize and secrete glucocorticoids and C-19 steroids, the so-called adrenal androgens, respectively.

ADRENAL STEROIDOGENESIS

Adrenal steroidogenesis involves the synthetic pathways through which cholesterol is converted into mineralocorticoids (zona glomerulosa), glucocorticoids (zona fasciculata), and adrenal androgens (zona reticularis).[52] Steroidogenesis is dependent on the activity of the hypothalamus through the release of corticotropin-releasing hormone (CRH) as well as the pituitary via ACTH secretion.

CRH is a 41-amino-acid polypeptide secreted by the hypothalamus which stimulates ACTH secretion from the anterior lobe of the pituitary. ACTH, a 39-amino-acid-peptide, is secreted by the pituitary corticotrophs and stimulates steroidogenesis within the adrenal cortex (see Fig 6–1). ACTH is synthesized as part of a larger molecule (Fig 6–2), proopiomelanocortin (POMC). In the anterior pituitary, CRH stimulates increased ACTH secretion as well as increased transcription of pre-POMC which undergoes posttranslational modification yielding, principally, ACTH and β-lipotropin. In contrast, in the intermediate lobe of the pituitary, pre-POMC is processed differently to yield α-melanocyte-stimulating hormone (α-MSH), corticotropin-like intermediate lobe peptide (CLIP), β-endorphin, and γ-lipotropin. Vasopressin is also able to stimulate ACTH release from the pituitary.

CRF, ACTH, and cortisol secretion occur in an episodic pattern. This is superimposed upon an overall pattern of diurnal variation of plasma ACTH, cortisol, and other adrenocortical steroid levels. With the usual sleep-awake cycle, hormone levels

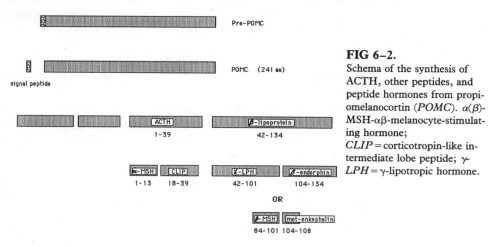

FIG 6–2.
Schema of the synthesis of ACTH, other peptides, and peptide hormones from propiomelanocortin (*POMC*). α(β)-MSH-αβ-melanocyte-stimulating hormone; *CLIP* = corticotropin-like intermediate lobe peptide; γ-*LPH* = γ-lipotropic hormone.

rise after midnight to reach peak levels at approximately 6 A.M. Such diurnal variation is absent in the neonate, develops at approximately 6 months of age,[46] and thereafter adjusts to the hours of sleep. Additional regulatory mechanisms include negative feedback control and stress-induced release of these hormones. Morphologic and functional heterogeneity of pituitary corticotrophes has suggested that intrapituitary paracrine interactions involving CRF and vasopressin may modulate ACTH synthesis and secretion.

Cholesterol, the initial substrate for steroid hormone biosynthesis, is taken up into adrenal cells (Fig 6–3) through low-density lipoprotein (LDL) receptors or synthesized by 3-hydroxy-3-methylglutaryl coenzyme A reductase (HMG-CoA). Cholesterol may also be stored as cholesterol esters within intracellular vesicles. The first step in steroidogenesis, common to all steroids, is side-chain cleavage resulting in the formation of pregnenolone (Fig 6–4). The enzyme responsible for this activity is a specific cytochrome P-450, named P-450$_{scc}$ (side-chain cleavage), which is located on the inner aspect of the mitochondrial membrane. The gene encoding this enzyme is located on chromosome 15.[11] Three other ancillary proteins located in the mitochondrial membrane shift reducing equivalents sequentially from mitochondrial NADPH to adrenodoxin reductase to adrenodoxin to P-450$_{scc}$. Adrenodoxin reductase, loosely bound to the mitochondrial membrane, has been cloned. Adrenodoxin shuttles electrons for adrenodoxin reductase to P-450$_{scc}$; the functional gene for adrenodoxin is located on chromosome 11.[52]

Pregnenolone moves to the endoplasmic reticulum (see Fig 6–3) where it is converted to progesterone by 3β-hydroxysteroid dehydrogenase. This enzyme, the only noncytochrome enzyme in this pathway, has also been cloned.[42] In the endoplasmic reticulum of fasciculata cells, pregnenolone or progesterone undergo 17α-hydroxylation to form 17-hydroxypregnenolone or 17-hydroxyprogesterone, respectively. These 17-hydroxylated steroids subsequently may be converted through 17,20-lyase activity to DHEA and androstenedione, respectively (see Fig 6–4). A single enzyme, P-450$_{c17}$ (17α-hydroxylase/17,20-lyase) mediates both activities. Since the adrenal and testicular complementary DNA (cDNA) nucleotide sequences for this gene, located on chromosome 10, are identical, the same gene is apparently expressed in both tissues.[12] In the zona glomerulosa, P-450$_{c17}$ is not expressed so that further progesterone metabolism is limited to the mineralocorticoid pathway.

Progesterone, or 17-hydroxyprogesterone, is converted to 11-deoxycorticosterone, or 11-deoxycortisol, respectively, by 21-hydroxylase, P-450$_{c21}$. The gene for P-450$_{c21}$ is located on chromosome 6; the enzyme is located in the endoplasmic reticulum.[52]

Deoxycorticosterone (DOC) and 11-deoxycortisol reenter the mitochondria where 11β-hydroxylase, P-450$_{c11}$ (see Fig 6–3), converts DOC to aldosterone and 11-deoxycortisol to cortisol. The conversion of DOC to aldosterone also involves 18-hydroxylation and 18-oxidation. It appears that P-450$_{c11}$ possesses all three enzyme activities. The gene encoding these activities is located on chromosome 8.[52]

Regulation of adrenal steroidogenesis is temporally biphasic. The acute response, occurring within minutes, provides a rapid increase in cortisol secretion, typically in response to stress. This response is initiated by ACTH and further mediated by cyclic adenosine monophosphate (cAMP). The conversion of cholesterol to pregnenolone is

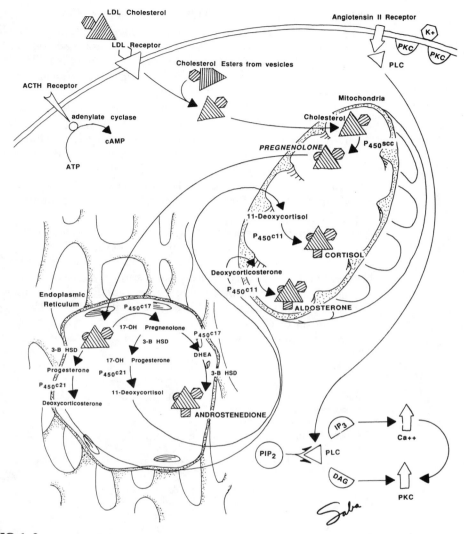

FIG 6–3.
Diagram of adrenal steroid synthesis of cortisol, aldosterone, and androstenedione within a composite adrenal cell showing location of enzymatic and receptor actions on the cell membrane, in the mitochondrion, and the endoplasmic reticulum. See text.

the rate-limiting step. The two limiting factors are the availability of substrate, cholesterol, and the ability of the cholesterol to cross to the inner mitochondrial membrane where the necessary enzyme, $P\text{-}450_{scc}$, is located. Cholesterol ester hydrolase acts upon cholesterol esters stored in lipid vesicles to produce free cholesterol which can then be transported across the mitochondrial membrane. Cycloheximide pretreatment, which inhibits protein synthesis, interferes with steroidogenesis in cultured bovine adrenocortical cells, suggesting a requirement for a labile protein.[81] However, cAMP can induce $P\text{-}450_{scc}$ gene transcription rapidly and independently of protein synthesis.[56]

The chronic action of ACTH is to maintain optimal levels of the steroidogenic enzymes.[53] ACTH induces increased synthesis of messenger RNA (mRNA) and proteins for $P-450_{scc}$, $P-450_{c11}$, $P-450_{c21}$, $P-450_{c17}$, adrenodoxin, and adrenodoxin reductase.[81] Since dibutyl cAMP mimics these actions of ACTH, it is presumed that increased cellular cAMP levels initiate a cascade of intracellular events which regulate steroid gene transcription.[81]

Additional proteins necessary for steroidogenesis include LDL receptors which take up cholesterol from circulating lipoproteins, the major source of cholesterol for steroidogenesis in humans. The important role of LDL cholesterol in steroidogenesis is demonstrated by the occurrence of normal basal cortisol levels but decreased cortisol response to ACTH in a patient with homozygous hypobetalipoproteinemia.[34] HMG-CoA is the rate-limiting enzyme for cholesterol biosynthesis and is subject to negative feedback inhibition. Sterol carrier protein 2 is involved in the transport of cholesterol into the mitochondria.

Tissue-specific regulation of steroidogenic enzymes accounts for the inability of the gonads to produce mineralocorticoids and glucocorticoids; the enzymes $P-450_{c11}$ and $P-450_{c21}$ are not expressed in ovarian or testicular tissues.[81] Other intracellular second messengers may be involved in adrenal steroidogenesis. For example, protein kinase C and calcium may influence the function of the zona glomerulosa and aldosterone production, perhaps through inhibition of $P-450_{c17}$ activity.[29]

Control of aldosterone secretion in the zona glomerulosa is multifactorial with several regulatory factors.[69] Increased renin, secreted in response to decreased blood

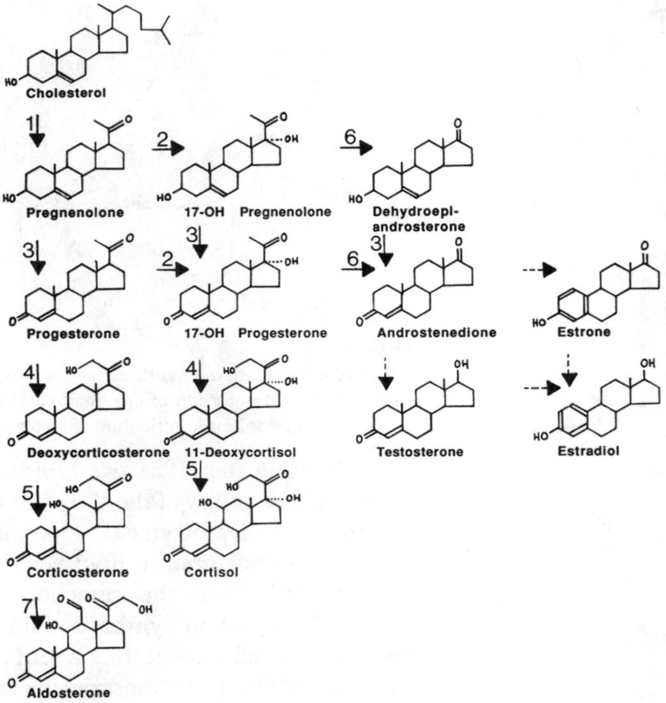

FIG 6–4.
Biosynthetic pathways of the adrenal cortex showing the structural formulas of the steroids. The enzymatic steps are as noted in the legend to Figure 6–1.

volume or sodium depletion, leads to increased activity of converting enzyme on angiotensinogen substrate resulting in increased levels of angiotensin II. Angiotensin II, a potent stimulus for aldosterone secretion, binds to specific adrenocortical plasma membrane receptors initiating the hydrolysis of phosphatidylinositol-4, 5-bisphosphate (PIP_2) into inositol trisphosphate (IP_3) and 1,2-diacylglycerol (DAG) through the action of phospholipase C. IP_3 acts to increase cytosolic free calcium. DAG increases the activity of protein kinase C.

Potassium is another potent regulator of aldosterone secretion. Indeed, potassium levels may influence responses to other secretagogues. ACTH acutely stimulates aldosterone secretion, probably through increased intracellular cAMP, but tachyphylaxis occurs. Because mineralocorticoid replacement therapy is generally unnecessary in patients with ACTH deficiency, ACTH apparently plays a minor role in the overall regulation of aldosterone secretion. Dopamine appears to inhibit aldosterone secretion through a direct action on glomerulosa cells.

The glucocorticoids are excreted primarily in the urine. The traditional method for the measurement of the urinary metabolites has been the Porter-Silber reaction which measures the glucuronide and tetrahydro derivatives of cortisol, cortisone, and deoxycortisol. Because of decreased glucuronyl-transferase activity in the neonatal period, these derivatives are not formed and, therefore, 17-hydroxycorticoids are not indicative of cortisol secretion in the neonatal period. The method for 17-ketogenic steroids can be used since a broader range of metabolites are measured with this method. Both procedures, however, are an indication of total glucocorticoid secretion and excretion. The measurement of urinary free cortisol provides a better indication of cortisol secretory rate because it is a better index of non–protein-bound cortisol in circulation.

MECHANISM OF ACTION

Following secretion, cortisol circulates in both protein-bound and free forms. Most cortisol is bound to corticosteroid-binding globulin (CBG) while a small amount is bound to albumin. The active hormone is the free or unbound form. CBG is synthesized in the liver; sex steroids, particularly estrogen therapy,[25] produce increased levels. CBG shares structural similarities with serine protease inhibitor proteins which are cleaved by elastase, an enzyme released by neutrophils at local sites of inflammation. Increased free cortisol levels at sites of inflammation may occur because CBG has decreased affinity for cortisol after cleavage by elastase. In addition, CBG may have other functions which are not yet well characterized.[74] Familial CBG deficiency has been reported.

Free cortisol binds to its intracellular (cytoplasmic, nuclear) receptor which has three domains. At the C-terminal, there is a steroid-binding domain. In the midportion, there is a DNA-binding domain. At the N-terminal, there appears to be a gene-activating domain. Binding of cortisol to its receptor causes dissociation of an inhibitory protein to form an "activated steroid-receptor complex" which binds to specific glucocorticoid response elements on DNA to enhance transcription of specific mRNAs.[50] Metal ions appear to be important in maintaining the proper tertiary structure of the receptor. While a small mutation in the steroid binding domain leads to a nonfunctional receptor, deletion of the entire steroid binding domain results in a constitutively active receptor.[6] Primary cortisol resistance, attributed to abnormal glucocorticoid receptors, has been described. These patients have hypercortisolism without Cushing's syndrome. A male child with primary cortisol resistance presented with isosexual precocious puberty due to ACTH-dependent overproduction of adrenal androgens.[43]

Glucocorticoid physiologic actions are multiple; some are generalized while some are organ-specific. The effects upon protein, carbohydrate, and fat metabolism are often counterregulatory to the effects of other hormones. Protein anabolism and utilization of glucose by muscle are inhibited, while gluconeogenesis is enhanced. In opposition to insulin effects, lipolysis is stimulated and lipogenesis is inhibited. Glucocorticoids antagonize the effects of vitamin D upon intestinal calcium absorption. Their hematologic effects include polycythemia, lymphocytopenia, monocytopenia, and eosinopenia. Neutrophilia occurs due to increased release from vascular walls, increased entry from bone marrow, and decreased vascular egress. Glucocorticoids have some salt-retaining activity and may induce hypertension also through potentiation of norepinephrine effects.

FETAL ADRENAL

The biosynthetic pathways in the fetal zone differ from those in postnatal life in that DHEA and DHEA-S are the principal products. DHEA-S is further metabolized to 16-OH-DHEA-S by the fetal liver. In the placenta, DHEA-S and 16-OH-DHEA-S are subsequently converted to estradiol and estriol, respectively. Low fetal zone levels of 3β-hydroxysteroid dehydrogenase favor the formation of DHEA over cortisol.[17]

Regulation of fetal adrenal steroidogenesis appears to be multifactorial involving the placenta, hypothalamic-pituitary axis, other peptide growth factors, and, perhaps, fetal adrenal cells themselves.[67] Comparison of fetal adrenals from anencephalic fetuses with those from normal fetuses has shown early involution of the fetal zone, decreased ability to synthesize DHEA-S, decreased concentration of LDL receptors, and decreased activity of HMG-CoA in anencephalic fetuses. Yet, comparable midgestation levels of the cytochrome P-450 adrenal steroidogenic enzymes in normal and anencephalic fetuses suggest that ACTH-independent regulatory mechanisms are also involved.

Cortisol is principally produced by the "adult" zone or transferred across the placenta from the mother. The placenta can reversibly oxidize cortisol to cortisone, an inactive metabolite, through the activity of 11β-hydroxysteroid dehydrogenase. Placental cortisol-cortisone metabolism may modulate fetal maturation by influencing fetal cortisol levels. For example, at approximately 35 weeks of gestation, cortisol levels increase inducing differentiation of type II pneumocytes with resultant increased surfactant production. Clinically, this glucocorticoid-induced maturation has been implemented as maternal betamethasone treatment to promote lung maturation in preterm (<32 weeks' gestation) infants.

NEONATAL ADRENAL

Except for the neonatal period, cortisol production rates are relatively constant in relation to body size rather than age. During the first few days of life, this rate is about 50% greater than in later life. Cortisol production rates gradually decline over the first several months of life to rates that persist relative to body size into childhood, adolescence, and adulthood. Circulating cortisol levels follow a similar pattern. Newborns that suffer unusual perinatal stress may demonstrate a stress response with higher circulating levels. Aldosterone levels are also relatively elevated in the neonatal period in relation to older children. Adrenal androgens are likewise higher during early infancy than later. However, urinary 17-ketosteroids, the excreted androgen metabolites, are low and not indicative of androgen secretion because of decreased glucuronide activity.

CONGENITAL ADRENAL HYPERPLASIAS

The congenital adrenal hyperplasias are inborn errors of metabolism secondary to deficiency of the adrenal steroidogenic enzymes. The manifestations of each type of congenital adrenal hyperplasia provide insight into steroid biosynthesis (Table 6–1). Inheritance appears to be autosomal recessive. In general, interference with cortisol synthesis leads to increased ACTH secretion which results in further secretion of precursor hormones proximal to the deficient enzyme in the biosynthetic pathway. The first description of this entity is attributed to de Crecchio who in 1865 reported autopsy results of an individual who had conducted "himself" as a man while having male external genitalia with first-degree hypospadias, cryptorchidism, normal female internal genitalia, and enlarged adrenal glands.[15]

21-Hydroxylase Deficiency

The most common form of congenital adrenal hyperplasia is 21-hydroxylase deficiency.[54] This enzyme converts progesterone into deoxycorticosterone in the mineralocorticoid pathway and 17-hydroxyprogesterone to 11-deoxycortisol in the glucocorticoid pathway. Enzyme deficiency results in deficient cortisol production resulting in excessive ACTH stimulation. Consequently, intermediate metabolites and adrenal androgens are synthesized and secreted in excess. The clinical manifestations are those suggesting excessive virilization, glucocorticoid deficiency if synthesis is not adequately compensated, and, among some, mineralocorticoid deficiency. It has become apparent that 21-hydroxylase deficiency is not only variable in severity but is one of the most frequent inborn errors of metabolism with a reported incidence of 1 in 5,000 to 1 in 15,000.[65] For comparison, the incidence of phenylketonuria is 1 in 10,000.

Signs and symptoms of the most severe forms of 21-hydroxylase deficiency (see Table 6–1) relate to sodium loss and hypocortisolism and include weight loss, anorexia, vomiting, and hypotension because of aldosterone and cortisol deficiencies. Since the enzyme deficiency exists prenatally, the female fetus is exposed to excessive

TABLE 6–1.

Clinical and Laboratory Features of the Congenital Adrenal Hyperplasia*

Enzyme Deficiency	Principal Elevated Steroid(s)	Prenatal Virilization (Females)	Incomplete Male Masculization	Postnatal Virilization
			Clinical Findings	
21-Hydroxylase				
Severe		+	N	+
Moderate	17-OH-Progesterone	+N	N	+
Mild		N	N	+
11β-Hydroxylase				
Severe		+	N	+
Mild–moderate	11-Deoxycortisol	+N	N	+
3β-Hydroxysteroid				
Severe		+	+	+
Mild–moderate	DHEA	+N	+N	+
17β-Hydroxylase/ 17,20-lyase	Progesterone, pregnenolone, 17-progesterone, 17-pregnanolone	N	+	N
Side-chain cleavage	Cholesterol	N	+	N
CMO-II	18-OH-Corticosterone	N	N	N

*DHEA = dehydroepiandrosterone; 17-KS = 17-ketosteroids; CMO-II = corticosterone methyloxidase type II; N = normal; + = present or excessive; − = absent or decreased.

amounts of adrenal androgens during the time of sexual differentiation. This may cause development of ambiguous external genitalia owing to adrenal androgen-induced masculinization of the external genitalia. Internal genital differentiation is unaffected because testicular antimüllerian hormone is absent. Male infants with severe 21-hydroxylase deficiency appear normal at birth with normal male genitalia, but present within the first 2 weeks of age with weight loss, vomiting, hyponatremia, and hyperkalemia. If not rapidly diagnosed, this most severe form can have a fatal outcome.

Less severe adrenal hyperplasia has been traditionally referred to as *simple virilizing adrenal hyperplasia*, characterized by prenatal virilization of the female child and virilization of both sexes in early childhood manifested by clitoral or penile enlargement and premature pubic hair. The extent of prenatal virilization varies. It may result in ambiguous genitalia in female infants, or simply posterior labial fusion without clitoromegaly,[99,100] which may go unnoticed in the neonate. Generally, these patients do not have hyponatremia. In fact, renin levels may be elevated, and aldosterone levels are either normal or elevated, suggesting a compensated status. It is now apparent that designations of salt-losing and simple virilizing forms are arbitrary categories. It is appropriate to consider a spectrum of degrees of severity and to realize that salt loss may become apparent in some patients previously considered to have simple virilizing adrenal hyperplasia if stress and sodium restriction are rigorous while others not subjected to such conditions are considered not to have compromise of mineralocorticoid secretion. Thus, complexities of intraadrenal influences on steroidogenesis may lead to apparent alterations in clinical phenotype over time such that the degree of mineralocorticoid deficiency may vary over time in the individual patient.[84]

Even milder degrees of 21-hydroxylase deficiency are frequently recognized and

Salt Wasting	Hyper-tension	Plasma Levels					Urinary Levels	
		17-OH-Progesterone	Andro-stenedione	DHEA	Testosterone	Renin	17-OH-Corticosterone	17-KS
+	N	+ + +	+ +	N+	+	+ +	+ +	−
−	N	+ +	+ +	N+	+	N+	+ +	−N
−	N	+	+	N+	N+	N	+	N
−	+	+	+ +	+	+	−	+ +	+ +
−	+N	N+	+	+	N+	−N	+	+
+	N	N+	N+	+ +	M	+	+	−
−	N	N+	N+	+	F	N	+N	−N
−	+	− /N+	−	− /N−	−	− /N	−	−N
+	N	−	−	−	N	+	−	−
+	−	N	N	N	N	+	N	N+

appear to be more common than the classic forms, especially in certain ethnic groups. Symptoms are premature sexual hair, peripubertal and postpubertal hirsutism, and menstrual irregularities. Peripheral tissue conversion of 17-hydroxyprogesterone to androgens has been implicated as a significant factor in the physical findings in these patients.

Untreated or inadequately treated children commonly have rapid somatic growth with advanced skeletal maturation. If this is accelerated enough, premature epiphyseal fusion occurs. Such patients may have short stature as adults. Postpubertal women may have menstrual irregularities, infertility, and polycystic ovaries. Precocious puberty may occur if skeletal maturation is significantly advanced even among patients receiving glucocorticoid therapy.

The gene for 21-hydroxylase deficiency (Fig 6–5) is located on the short arm of chromosome 6 in the class III region of the major histocompatibility complex in close linkage disequilibrium with the gene for the fourth component of serum complement.[7] There are two tandemly duplicated 21-hydroxylase genes; one gene (B) is functional while the other (A) is inactive owing to three separate mutations each of which leads to a premature stop codon: (1) 8–base pair deletion in exon 3; (2) single base insertion in exon 7; and (3) C to T mutation in exon 8.[55]

The close physical proximity of the 21-hydroxylase genes and the HLA markers has proved useful in family studies. In certain ethnic groups, specific combinations of HLA markers have been identified in 21-hydroxylase deficiency. For example, the rare haplotype HLA-Bw47, DR7 is associated with classic forms of 21-hydroxylase deficiency which appears to be due to a large deletion of the functional gene. In contrast, the supratype, HLA-B14, DR1, is associated with late-onset 21-hydroxylase

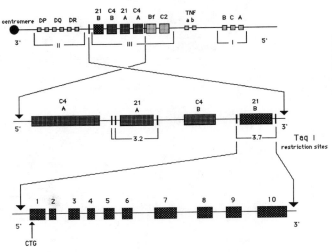

FIG 6–5.
Representation of 21-hydroxylase gene structure and location on the short arm of chromosome 6.

21-HYDROXYLASE GENE

deficiency, especially in Ashkenazi Jews, Hispanics, and Italians. However, these associations are not constant throughout the general population as the HLA-Bw47 haplotype is not associated with congenital adrenal hyperplasia in the Old Order Amish.[55]

Prenatal Diagnosis and Treatment

This association with HLA supratypes has improved former techniques of prenatal diagnosis which utilized amniotic fluid 17-hydroxyprogesterone concentrations. However, evaluation of HLA haplotypes still requires that an affected child must already have been born. In addition, the occurrence of recombination events involving chromosome 6 may lead to inaccurate diagnoses. Since genital differentiation begins by 8 weeks of gestation, effective prenatal treatment must be initiated early in the first trimester. Amniocentesis can only be performed relatively late in gestation whereas chorionic villus sampling allows for earlier detection. Prenatal treatment with dexamethasone of pregnancies at risk has decreased the degree of masculinization of female infants.[85] Current limitations of prenatal treatment are that a proband must exist; all pregnancies at risk must be treated before a prenatal diagnosis can be made, and the long-term effects of prenatal dexamethasone are unknown.[51]

Molecular Biology

Initial analysis of the gene and pseudogene was performed with restriction endonucleases. These bacterial enzymes recognize specific nucleotide sequences at which they cleave DNA. This results in DNA fragments that can be separated by size and recognized by labeled probes specific for the desired nucleotide sequence. One restriction endonuclease, *Taq*I, distinguishes between the functional gene and the pseudogene because it generates a 3.7-kb fragment that contains the functional gene and a 3.2-kb fragment that contains the pseudogene. Despite preliminary optimism regarding this technique, it has become apparent that gene conversion events alter the recognition site of the restriction endonucleases changing fragment lengths.[12,55] These frequent point mutations and conversion events complicate analysis based on fragment size. Additional distinguishing restriction endonuclease fragment polymorphisms for the functional gene are 11-kb *Bgl*II, 2.9-kb *Kpn*I, and 1.8-kb *Pvu*II while the comparable ones for the pseudogene are 12-kb *Bgl*II, 4.0-kb *Kpn*I, and 2.0 *Pvu*II.[55]

More detailed information regarding specific defects can be obtained through nucleotide sequencing. Enzyme activity can then be examined using forced gene expression in a heterologous system because adrenal tissue from affected individuals is ordinarily not available. While such expression provides insight into the structure-function relationships of 21-hydroxylase, it must be recognized that these expression systems bypass the physiologic tissue-specific regulatory mechanisms.

Sequencing and vector expression detected three patients with salt-losing 21-hydroxylase deficiency who had cytosine-to-thymidine conversions at nucleotide 1994 resulting in a stop codon at codon 318.[22] Point mutations changing Ile[172] to Asn and Arg[356] to Trp have also been recognized.[10] Transfection of cloned DNA in COS monkey kidney cells showed that the insertion of a codon (CTG) after nucleotide 28, mutation of nucleotide 453 from thymidine to cytosine, conversion of nucleotide 1586 from cytosine to guanine, and mutation of nucleotide 655 from cytosine to adenine are neutral mutations in that apparent enzyme activity appears to be unaffected. In contrast, conversion of nucleotide 655 from cytosine to guanine led to aberrant mRNA splicing resulting in a nonfunctional enzyme.[27,55]

Analysis of phylogenetically conserved DNA sequences allows speculation regarding the functional domains of the 21-hydroxylase gene. A substrate binding site is thought to be located at amino acids 342–358 while the heme binding site is thought to be at amino acids 421–440.[55] Deleterious mutations presumably alter protein function or affect mRNA translation through premature termination codons or aberrant mRNA splicing.[55]

While the tools of molecular biology are providing greater insight into the pathophysiology of this disorder, unanswered questions remain. ACTH-stimulated 17-hydroxyprogesterone levels in asymptomatic obligate heterozygotes can overlap with those in individuals with milder 21-hydroxylase deficiency.[60] Further, correlation of genotype and phenotype is complicated by variable individual end-organ responsiveness. Intraadrenal hormone levels may also influence steroidogenesis. It can be speculated that these steroidogenic defects make up a continuous spectrum of enzyme activity.[41]

Clinical and Laboratory Assessment

Ambiguous genitalia consistent with the result of excessive androgens in the female fetus (nonpalpable gonads with varying degrees of midline fusion) should alert the examiner to the possibility of adrenal hyperplasia. However, other causes of female pseudohermaphroditism and minor variations of normal (Fig 6–6) need to be considered. Thus, not only should ambiguous genitalia without palpable gonads suggest the possibility of congenital adrenal hyperplasia (Fig 6–7) but also the finding on physical examination of a "male infant" with bilateral undescended and nonpalpable testes. Other presenting symptoms and signs in infancy include poor feeding, poor

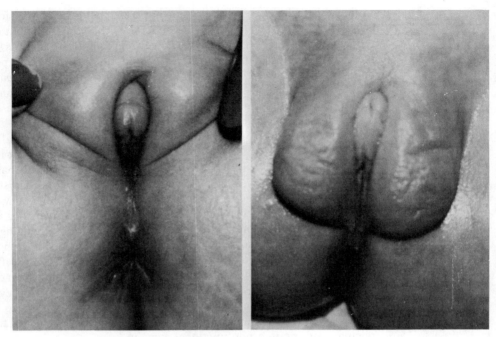

FIG 6–6.
External genitalia of two newborn 46,XX girls with minimal virilization but no evidence of abnormal steroidogenesis. The photo on the *left* shows a clitoris which appears somewhat large owing primarily to abundant prepuce. The *right* photo shows prominent labia minora and some scrotalization of the labia majora.

weight gain or excessive weight loss, vomiting, and irritability.

Findings among older patients include premature pubic hair (Figs 6–8 and 6–9), a mature body odor, penile growth, clitoromegaly (see Fig 6–9), tall stature, and acne. In adolescent girls, hirsutism, menstrual irregularities, and severe acne may be the presenting complaints; polycystic ovaries may be visualized on ultrasound examination in these girls. The frequency of mild, late-onset 21-hydroxylase deficiency as the cause of premature pubic hair is unclear. Scrotal masses due to hyperplastic adrenal rest tissue, which may be mistaken for testicular tumors, may occur in untreated or inadequately treated patients; they regress with glucocorticoid suppressive therapy. Lack of adequate suppression or patient noncompliance may also result in excessive virilization during childhood. Females may develop acne, sexual hair, and further clitoral growth. Precocious pseudopuberty may occur in males (see Fig 6–6).

Increased 17-hydroxyprogesterone levels in a newborn infant with hyponatremia and hyperkalemia are diagnostic of salt-losing 21-hydroxylase deficiency. In milder forms, the basal 17-hydroxyprogesterone level is usually elevated although some individuals may at times have levels within the normal range. Among these patients, ACTH stimulation testing, 0.25 mg intravenous (IV) or intramuscular (IM) synthetic ACTH with plasma hormone levels obtained at 0 and 30 or 60 minutes, may be necessary to detect compromised enzyme activity.[46] Indeed, through additional family studies, asymptomatic and mildly affected individuals have been detected.[55] The increased incremental 17-hydroxyprogesterone response following ACTH stimulation, noted in obligate heterozygotes (parents of affected individuals), is considered the most discriminating laboratory test for decreased 21-hydroxylase activity. Calculation of the combined incremental rise of 17-hydroxyprogesterone and progesterone has also been found helpful in distinguishing heterozygotes and mildly affected persons from normal individuals.

11β-Hydroxylase Deficiency

The enzyme 11β-hydroxylase, or $P-450_{c11}$, converts 11-deoxycortisol to cortisol in the glucocorticoid pathway. In the mineralocorticoid pathway, this enzyme converts deoxycorticosterone in three separate steps, 11-hydroxylation, 18-hydroxylation, and 18-oxidation, into aldosterone. Deficiency of each specific activity of this enzyme is characterized as a distinct disorder. The true incidence of 11β-hydroxylase deficiency is unknown, but it reportedly accounts for 5% to 8% of patients with congenital adrenal hyperplasias.[100] Deficient 18-hydroxylation is termed *corticosterone methyloxidase type I* (CMO-I), whereas deficient 18-oxidation is termed *corticosterone methyloxidase type II* (CMO-II).

As predicted from the biochemical pathways, glucocorticoid deficiency due to

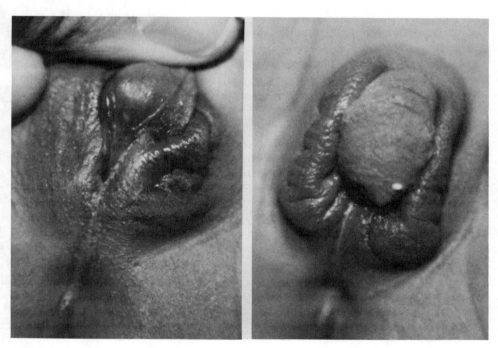

FIG 6–7.
External genitalia of a 46,XX infant with severe 21-hydroxylase ($P-450_{c21}$) deficiency. Clitoromegaly and partial labioscrotal fusion are evident.

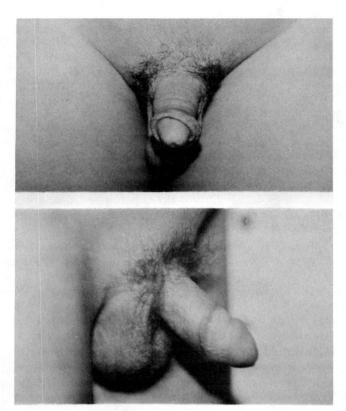

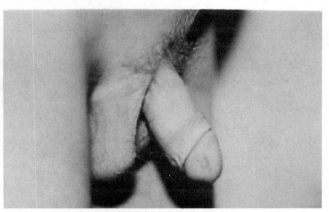

FIG 6–8.
Premature postnatal virilization in three boys resulting from adrenal androgen excess. *Top*: 7-year-old boy with premature sexual hair and mild 21-hydroxylase (P-450$_{c21}$) deficiency. *Middle* and *bottom*: genitalia of twin 10-year-old males with severe 21-hydroxylase deficiency diagnosed in infancy. Noncompliance resulted in early genital maturation as well as height and bone age acceleration while testes remained prepubertal.

decreased 11β-hydroxylase activity leads to increased ACTH and adrenal androgen production. Prenatal and postnatal virilization may occur. Gynecomastia, as the presenting complaint, has been reported. Excessive ACTH stimulation leads to increased levels of DOC resulting in adequate or excessive mineralocorticoid activity and suppressed plasma renin levels. Thus, mineralocorticoid excess rather than deficiency may be present and patients may be hypertensive (Table 6–2). However, apparent enzyme activity as suggested by hormone levels does not correlate with the degree of hypertension, virilization, or hypokalemia. Indeed, it is controversial as to whether DOC is the sole mineralocorticoid produced. Milder forms of this enzyme deficiency are also recognized.

In 11β-hydroxylase deficiency, elevation of 11-deoxycortisol, DOC, and adrenal androgens with decreased secretion of corticosterone, 18-hydroxydeoxycorticosterone, and cortisol are typical. Following ACTH stimulation, elevated levels of DOC and deoxycortisol may be found in affected individuals. Elevated urinary metabolites include tetrahydro-11-deoxycortisol, tetrahydro-11-DOC, and 17-ketosteroids. Prior to treatment, renin levels are suppressed owing to the mineralocorticoid effects of the overproduced precursor hormones. However, salt loss may occur in the untreated neonate with relatively low DOC levels leading to insufficient mineralocorticoid activity, as well as in treated patients with adrenal suppression. Unlike heterozygotes carrying the 21-hydroxylase gene, ACTH stimulation tests may not be useful in

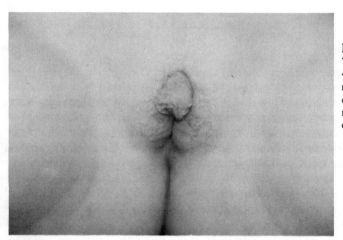

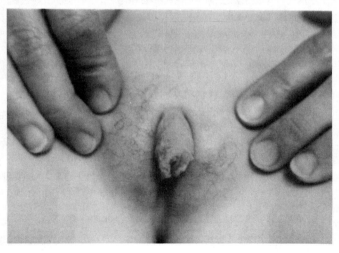

FIG 6–9.
Virilization of the genitalia of a 46,XX girl at age 6 years with mild 21-hydroxylase deficiency. Clitoromegaly and premature sexual hair are apparent.

TABLE 6–2.

Endocrine Hypertension*†

	K$^+$	PRA	Aldosterone	ACTH	Postural
Pheochromocytoma	N, ↓	N, ↑	N, ↑	N	
Aldosterone-secreting adenoma	↓	↓	↑	N	No response
Hyperplasia	↓	↓	↑	N	↑ When upright
Renovascular	N	↑	↑	N	
11β-Hydroxylase	↓	↓	↓	↑	
17α-Hydroxylase/ 17,20 lyase	↓	↓	↓	↑	
DSH	↓	↓	↑	N	
AME	↓	↓	N	N	
Renin-secreting tumors	↓	↑	↑	N	
Cushing syndrome					
Cushing disease	N/↓	↓	↑ or ↓	↑	
Adrenal	↑ or ↓	↓	↑ or ↓	↓	
Ectopic	↑ or ↓	↓	↑ or ↓	↑	

*Data from references[33,54]
†N = normal; ↑ = increased; ↓ = decreased.

distinguishing 11β-hydroxylase heterozygosity because obligate heterozygotes for 11β-hydroxylase deficiency have inconsistent hormone responses following ACTH stimulation.

Decreased 18-oxidative activity (CMO-II) has been described most frequently in Iranian Jews, and is presumably due to a "founder" effect. Hyponatremia, hyperkalemia, hypotension without virilization, and increased ratios of 18-hydroxycorticosterone to aldosterone have been found in affected individuals and obligate heterozygotes. Hyperreninemia and increased urinary ratio of 18-hydroxy-11-dehydrotetrahydrocorticosterone (18-OH-THA) to tetrahydroaldosterone are typical.

A specific restriction fragment length polymorphism detected with a cDNA probe corresponding to the midportion of the mRNA encoding P-450$_{c11}$ is associated with clinical findings of CMO-II deficiency in families of similar ethnic background. This suggests that point mutations in P-450$_{c11}$ may affect one activity, 18-oxidation, without affecting the other two enzymatic activities, 11β-hydroxylation and 18-hydroxylation.

17α-Hydroxylase/17,20-Lyase Deficiency

This single enzyme, P-450$_{c17}$, has two activities.[52] Through 17α-hydroxylation, it converts mineralocorticoids to glucocorticoids. It also converts glucocorticoids to the sex steroids. Thus, this autosomal recessive enzyme deficiency is characterized by decreased secretion of glucocorticoids and sex steroids. The decreased cortisol level leads to increased ACTH which results in the overproduction of DOC leading to hypertension (see Table 6–2) and hyperkalemic alkalosis.

Decreased production of sex steroids leads to decreased testosterone secretion resulting in incomplete formation of the external genitalia in male infants. Since testicular antimüllerian hormone secretion is unaffected, internal genital ducts are poorly developed, if present at all. Because of normal female external genitalia, females may not be diagnosed until adolescence when they present with delayed puberty, primary amenorrhea, and hypertension. Hypergonadotropic hypogonadism occurs because of decreased secretion of sex steroids. One specific action of this enzyme may be more affected than the other activity, i.e., apparent isolated 17,20-lyase activity.

The gene encoding this enzyme is located on chromosome 10.[45] The same gene is expressed in both the adrenals and the gonads. While the amino acid homology is less than 30% for P-450$_{c17}$ and P-450$_{c21}$, structural similarities as well as similar hydropathy patterns suggest that there is a selective evolutionary pressure to maintain sequence homology in the presumed functional domains of these proteins.[68] This enzyme catalyzes important branch points in steroid biosynthesis suggesting that changes in 17α-hydroxylase/17,20-lyase activities may regulate the pattern of steroid secretion. Indeed, levels of 17α-hydroxylase/17,20-lyase mRNA appear to be more responsive to ACTH and cAMP stimulation than are the other steroidogenic enzymes.

Genomic libraries prepared from two affected families showed identical four-base pair duplications which shifted the reading frame of the C-terminal amino acid sequence of the protein resulting in decreased enzyme activity.[35,94] A Japanese patient has been found to have a stop codon due to a point mutation in the first exon resulting in the absence of a functional enzyme.[96] Partial combined 17α-hydroxylase/17,20-lyase deficiency was attributed to the deletion of a codon for phenylalanine in the N-terminal region of the gene.[97] A seven–base pair duplication in exon 3 was reported in an XY individual with hypertension, hypokalemia, female external genitalia, and delayed puberty.[98]

Administration of ACTH leads to increased incremental elevation of progesterone, 18-hydroxydeoxycorticosterone, 18-hydroxycorticosterone, and corticosterone. Heterozygote responses to ACTH stimulation are variable.[72]

3β-Hydroxysteroid Dehydrogenase Deficiency

This enzyme, 3β-hydroxy-5-ene-steroid dehydrogenase/Δ^5-Δ^4-ene isomerase, catalyzes the conversion of pregnenolone to progesterone. This step is crucial to the formation of all adrenal and gonadal steroids. Thus, deficient enzyme activity affects synthesis of mineralocorticoids, glucocorticoids, and sex steroids. However, as in 21-hydroxylase deficiency, both salt-wasting and non–salt-wasting forms are apparent.

Ambiguous external genitalia occur in neonates of both sexes (Fig 6–10). In males, inadequate amounts of testosterone are produced such that ambiguous external genitalia due to inadequate masculinization of the fetus occurs.[5] In females, increased secretion of DHEA, which can undergo peripheral conversion to more potent androgens, may cause prenatal virilization and postnatal clitoromegaly. In older girls premature pubic hair, acne, amenorrhea, or hirsutism may occur. Since this enzyme deficiency can affect both the adrenals and gonads, pubertal development in females may rarely be delayed due to inadequate estrogen production.

Elevated levels of 17-hydroxypregnenolone or DHEA, or both, in addition to an increased ratio of Δ^5 to Δ^4 steroids, of 17-hydroxypregnenolone to 17-hydroxyprogesterone, and of DHEA to androstenedione, are diagnostic of this disorder. Since

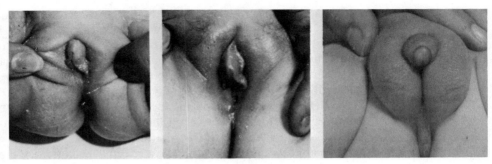

FIG 6–10.
Three patients with 3β-hydroxysteroid dehydrogenase deficiency. The two photos at the *left* show virilized genitalia of genetic females (46,XX). At the *right* are the undervirilized genitalia of a male (46,XY) patient.

basal plasma hormone levels may be normal in patients who are mildly affected, ACTH stimulation may be necessary to detect mild enzyme deficiencies.

Lipoid Adrenal Hyperplasia

Conversion of cholesterol to pregnenolone, also known as side-chain cleavage, 20,22-desmolase, or P-450$_{scc}$, is the rate-limiting step in steroidogenesis. Deficiency results in decreased mineralocorticoid, glucocorticoid, and sex steroid production. External genitalia are normal in female infants while appearing as female or minimally masculinized in male infants. Hyperpigmentation of skin creases, nipples, and genitalia with signs and symptoms of adrenal insufficiency occur in the neonatal period.[54] Defects in the ancillary cellular proteins necessary for this step, adrenodoxin, adrenodoxin reductase, and cholesterol ester hydrolase, among others, would have similar effects.

Decreased activity of this enzyme has been found in hypertrophied foam-filled adrenal cells obtained from the autopsy of a phenotypic female infant with hyponatremia, mild hyperkalemia, and 46,XY karyotype.

Treatment of Congenital Adrenal Hyperplasias

The goal of treatment is suppression of the excessive ACTH stimulation and the replacement of the specific hormone deficiencies. Since cortisol is the hormone which suppresses ACTH through negative feedback inhibition, physiologic glucocorticoid replacement dosage is the basis of treatment. Glucocorticoid therapy replaces deficient or compensated cortisol secretion resulting in suppression of excessive ACTH secretion which, in turn, results in decreased adrenal androgen secretion in the virilizing forms of congenital adrenal hyperplasia and reduction of the secretion of precursors with mineralocorticoid activity. Such therapy is followed by remission of the hypertension in the hypertensive forms. In the adequately suppressed patient, other hormones that are insufficient, such as mineralocorticoid, are supplemented.

Oral hydrocortisone (cortisol), administered in three daily divided doses, is the most commonly used glucocorticoid therapy in children with adrenal hyperplasias. Physiologic replacement for parenteral therapy is based on cortisol production rate of 7 to 12 mg/m^2/day in children and adults.[41] Despite knowledge of these production rates, the precise guidelines for oral replacement remain indefinite. However, clinical experience has shown that most patients are adequately replaced on a dosage between 12 and 20 mg/m^2/day. The initial dosage should be within this range except when the patient has acute adrenal insufficiency and requires higher doses. Subsequent dosage adjustments should be based upon clinical and hormonal indices of suppression, titering the dosage for adequate suppression while avoiding oversuppression and glucocorticoid excess. With inadequate suppression, growth and maturation tend to be excessive while oversuppression results in the retarded growth velocity characteristic of Cushing syndrome.

In 21-hydroxylase deficiency, adequacy of treatment can be assessed by a combination of growth velocity data, physical findings, and laboratory tests. Appropriate therapy in the prepubertal child is suggested by the lack of progressive virilization, normal growth rate for age, normal skeletal maturation, and hormone levels appropriate for age and indicative of adequate adrenal androgen suppression. Hormone secretion can be evaluated using measurements of androstenedione, plasma renin activity, and urinary 17-ketosteroids. In girls and prepubertal boys, testosterone levels can be useful. Mineralocorticoid administration to patients who have not presented with salt-losing crises but who have elevated renin levels may improve hormonal control.

During times of stress, such as fever, persistent vomiting, significant trauma, or surgery, increased glucocorticoid dosage is necessary. Generally two to three times the usual dose is sufficient, but higher doses may be necessary for surgical procedures. Families should have injectable hydrocortisone (Solu-Cortef) available for emergencies. Recommended doses are 50 mg for children less than 4 years old and 100 mg for older patients. During surgical procedures, hydrocortisone can be administered with the IV fluids. IV hydrocortisone must be given as a continuous infusion rather than by bolus injections because of its rapid half-life.

For mineralocorticoid replacement therapy, fludrocortisone (Florinef) is generally used. It can be administered once daily. The usual daily dose is 0.1 mg. Because normal aldosterone production rates are greater in infancy, neonates and infants may require as much as 0.2 to 0.3 mg/day. Plasma renin levels can be used to monitor adequacy of therapy. When oral medications are not tolerated, IV isotonic saline may be necessary because parenteral DOC is generally unavailable.

Forms of congenital adrenal hyperplasia that result in excessive fetal adrenal androgen production can cause ambiguous genitalia in the female fetus while those which interfere with testosterone synthesis lead to ambiguous genitalia in males. In both 17α-hydroxylase/17,20-lyase and cholesterol desmolase deficiencies, male infants are undervirilized while female infants have normal female external genitalia. In 3β-hydroxysteroid dehydrogenase deficiency, male infants are undervirilized while female infants are excessively virilized because of increased DHEA secretion. Overproduction of adrenal androgens leads to virilization of the female fetus in both 21-hydroxylase and 11β-hydroxylase deficiency.

The occurrence of ambiguous external genitalia is a social emergency as well as a potential medical emergency. Virilized female infants have normal female internal genitalia with good potential for fertility if properly treated. Treatment includes appropriate hormone replacement and genital reconstructive surgery. Prenatal androgen "imprinting," postnatal body image and environmental cues of sexual identity, and inadequate vaginal introitus secondary to prenatal virilization are factors which potentially complicate development of a healthy sexual identity.[82] Gender assignment in undervirilized male infants depends on whether the penis can be adequately surgically reconstructed to allow for urination in the standing position and for normal adult sexual activity.

Sex steroid replacement consistent with sex of rearing is indicated in patients with deficient sex steroid production during adolescence and adulthood, i.e., 17α-hydroxylase/17,20-lyase deficiency, males with 3β-hydroxysteroid dehydrogenase deficiency, and cholesterol side-chain cleavage deficiency. Innovative infertility treatment offers hope of fertility such as exogenous hormone treatment–induced ovarian follicular development in a woman with 17α-hydroxylase/17,20-lyase deficiency.[70]

ADRENARCHE

Adrenarche, the onset of increased secretion of DHEA and DHEA-S by the zona reticularis of the adrenal gland, occurs prior to gonadarche, the pubertal reactivation of the hypothalamic-pituitary-gonadal axis. Pubarche, the appearance of pubic hair, follows adrenarche and results from the gradually increasing levels of DHEA, DHEA-S, and androstenedione during puberty.[31] These so-called adrenal androgens are primarily androgenic precursor hormones which undergo conversion by peripheral tissues to more potent androgens. DHEA-S, secreted almost exclusively by the adrenal gland, is often considered an indicator of the activity of the zona reticularis.

While an adrenal androgen-stimulating factor has been postulated to cause adrenarche, no such factor has been found. During adrenarche, steroidogenic enzyme activity appears to change such that there is decreased activity of 3β-hydroxysteroid dehydrogenase and increased 17,20-lyase activity leading to increased DHEA production. Indeed, intraadrenal androgen levels may influence these biosynthetic pathways. However, the precise mechanism for increased adrenal androgen production is unknown. Prolactin appears to have no significant role in this process. Importantly, adrenarche and gonadarche are independent events.[14]

Premature adrenarche is the occurrence of the pubertal increase in adrenal androgen production at an earlier-than-usual age. The characteristic clinical manifestation is the appearance of pubic hair—coarse, dark hair on the labia majora, mons pubis, or base of the penis—prior to 8 years of age in girls and 9½ years in boys. Premature adrenarche occurs more commonly in girls and may occur at any age during childhood. Additional features can include axillary hair, acne, slightly accelerated skeletal maturation, and mature-type body odor. The development of pubic hair is usually slowly progressive. Dynamic luteinizing hormone (LH) and follicle-stimulating hormone (FSH) responses to luteinizing hormone–releasing hormone (LHRH) stimulation are prepubertal. Gonadarche occurs at a normal age. While glucocorticoid suppression is generally not indicated or necessary to make the diagnosis, dexamethasone treatment suppresses hormone levels. Obesity and central nervous system abnormalities may be noted in affected individuals. Final adult height is not compromised.

DHEA, DHEA-S, and androstenedione levels are increased over prepubertal levels and are appropriate for early puberty. Since there are no unique clinical features, premature adrenarche is a diagnosis of exclusion in the evaluation of premature pubic hair or other signs of virilization during childhood. In particular, mild congenital adrenal hyperplasias and true precocious puberty are the most frequent diagnoses to be excluded. Exogenous medications, androgen-secreting tumors, primary cortisol resistance, mixed gonadal dysgenesis, and familial testotoxicosis are rarer causes of premature pubarche.

HYPERCORTISOLISM

Patients with Cushing's syndrome, irrespective of the cause, exhibit the clinical findings of hypercortisolemia, excessive glucocorticoid levels. Cushing syndrome is rare in childhood when those cases secondary to iatrogenic exogenous administration of hydrocortisone or other glucocorticoids are excluded. Etiologies can be classified as ACTH-dependent or ACTH-independent. The eponym *Cushing disease* is reserved for ACTH-dependent hypothalamic-pituitary disease, due to basophilic pituitary adenomas in the cases originally described by Harvey Cushing. Ectopic CRH or ACTH secretion can be considered within the ACTH-dependent category. Neoplastic autonomous adrenal cortisol secretion represents ACTH-independent Cushing syndrome.

Cushing disease is ascribed to ACTH-secreting pituitary microadenomas although pituitary adenomas or microadenomas may or may not be radiologically demonstrable. Because excessive ACTH stimulation may persist or recur after excision of adenomas, the underlying pathophysiology may involve excessive CRH secretion leading to adenomatous changes in the pituitary. Indeed, analysis of episodic cortisol secretion in patients with Cushing disease suggests that some patients have primarily pituitary ACTH oversecretion while others may have oversecretion of, or increased pituitary responsiveness to CRH.

After age 7 years, most cases of Cushing syndrome are due to Cushing disease. Prior to 7 years of age, adrenal tumors are the most common cause. Congenital adrenocortical tumors have been reported. Both adenomas and carcinomas occur. Virilization commonly occurs with childhood adrenocortical tumors. The increased adrenal androgen production which causes the virilization may also lead to increased growth velocity despite hypercortisolism. In some instances, hemihypertrophy and the Beckwith-Wiedemann syndrome have also been present.

Tumors that produce ectopic ACTH or CRH can cause Cushing syndrome. Such tumors are rare in children; Leyton reported the first case with autopsy findings of oat cell carcinoma of the thymus and bilateral adrenal cortical hyperplasia.[40] Cushing syndrome due to ACTH production by a Wilms' tumor has been described.

Hypercortisolism due to macronodular adrenocortical hyperplasia is characterized by bilateral macroscopic yellowish nodules. Patients with pituitary-dependent Cushing syndrome and unilateral macronodular adrenocortical hyperplasia have been reported. It has been suggested that this disease represents long-standing Cushing disease with increasing adrenocortical autonomy.

Primary pigmented nodular adrenocortical disease is identified by ACTH-independent hypercortisolism with multiple bilateral adrenocortical nodules most typically in adolescent patients.[61] The histologic findings are black-to-yellow nodules composed of large eosinophilic or clear cells with or without lipofuscin granules. These nodules are located in the inner cortical zones, but may extend beyond the adrenal capsule into the periadrenal adipose tissue. Histochemical staining of these nodules is consistent with active steroidogenesis. Familial cases are reported. An autoimmune mechanism has been suggested because of the finding of serum immunoglobulins that stimulate in vitro adrenocortical DNA and cortisol synthesis.[87] However, the exact pathophysiologic mechanism remains unknown. These patients may have Carney's complex with associated findings of myxomas (cutaneous or cardiac), spotty cutaneous pigmentation, and other endocrine disorders.

Clinical Findings

Signs and symptoms of Cushing syndrome include obesity, decreased muscle mass and muscle weakness, fatigue, hypertension (see Table 6–2), and increased bruising with ecchymoses over the abdomen, arms, and thighs. Protein wasting results in thin skin and purple striae. Findings unique to childhood are growth failure and premature sexual hair. Indeed, growth failure may be the only sign. Hirsutism and amenorrhea may be the presenting complaints in adolescent girls. The extremities are not markedly thin because of decreased subcutaneous fat, but an altered distribution of fat leads to a rounded or moon facies (Fig 6–11) and hypertrophy of supraclavicular and dorsocervical fat ("buffalo hump") on the upper back. Because the manifestations are due to cortisol, mineralocorticoid, or androgen excess, the symptoms may suggest, but do not indicate, the underlying etiology. Delayed skeletal maturation is usually present, although it may not be significantly retarded if excessive androgen secretion is occurring simultaneously.

Additional findings are impaired carbohydrate tolerance and decreased free water

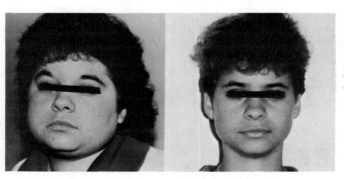

FIG 6–11.
Pre- and posttreatment photos of an adolescent girl with Cushing's disease.

TABLE 6–3.
Assessment for Cushing Syndrome

I. *Document hypercortisolism*
    Increased plasma cortisol with or without loss of diurnal variation
    Elevated urinary free cortisol
    Elevated urinary 17-hydroxycorticoids
    Lack of suppression by:
        Overnight dexamethasone suppression
        Low-dose dexamethasone suppression
II. *Differentiate etiology of primary lesions**

	Pituitary	Adrenal	Ectopic
Plasma ACTH	+	−	+ +
High-dose dexamethasone suppression	Yes	No	No
Corticotropin-releasing hormone	+	±	±
Metapyrapone	+ +	NC	+
Urinary 17-ketosteroids	+	+ +	+

III. *Localization of lesion*
    Petrosal sinus sampling of ACTH source
    Ultrasound, CT, MRI
    Adrenal vein catheterization

*+ = Elevated; − = decreased; NC = no change.

---

clearance. Psychiatric symptoms may occur. Osteoporosis is frequently present. Hypertension, which is usually present, may be due to multiple factors.[75]

Hormone Assessment

For diagnosis (Table 6–3), persistent hypercortisolism must first be confirmed either by measurement of urinary free cortisol, 17-hydroxycorticosteroids, or an overnight dexamethasone test. Typically, there is a loss of diurnal variation in cortisol levels and elevated urinary free cortisol levels. Measurement of urinary hydroxycorticoids is less reliable. Further procedures are required to identify the underlying cause, particularly to differentiate Cushing disease from other causes of Cushing syndrome. Low- and high-dose dexamethasone suppression tests and metyrapone testing may be helpful in the differentiation between pituitary, adrenal, and ectopic disease. If the baseline studies do not show unequivocal elevation of cortisol levels in patients with clinical features suggestive of Cushing syndrome, overnight or low-dosage dexamethasone tests may corroborate the presence of autonomous hormone secretion. Overnight dexamethasone tests using 1 mg (low-dose) and 8 mg (high-dose) taken at 11 P.M. with determination of morning cortisol and ACTH levels are reliable screening tests.

    The standard methods for dexamethasone suppression include pretreatment 24-hour urine collections for the determination of 17-hydroxycorticoids, urinary free cortisol, and creatinine. Dexamethasone 0.5 mg every 6 hours (20 μg/kg/day in children) is administered for 2 days followed by a dosage of 2 mg every 6 hours (80 μg/kg/day in children) for 2 more days. Throughout the test, 24-hour urine collections and morning plasma cortisol and ACTH levels are obtained. Decline of urinary free cortisol levels by 50% or of plasma cortisol levels to less than 5 μg/dL on the low dosage suggest normal suppression. Elevated cortisol levels in patients with pituitary lesions should decrease on high-dose dexamethasone, but not on low-dose. Autonomous adrenal lesions show no suppression. Elevated cortisol levels secondary to ectopic hormone production are generally unaffected by dexamethasone treatment, although in some cases of ectopic hormone production, high-dose dexamethasone may suppress or even paradoxically increase cortisol levels. Such dissimilar responses may be due to altered intracellular processing of POMC mRNA in the neoplastic tissue.[2]

Additional laboratory studies include the determination of ACTH levels and ovine CRH stimulation testing (oCRH).[99] ACTH levels are suppressed in primary adrenal disease and generally very elevated in ectopic disease. Use of oCRH stimulation testing provides more consistent results than with human CRH because of its longer half-life. In general, patients with Cushing disease show increased ACTH and cortisol after oCRF whereas those with ectopic ACTH production or primary adrenal hypercortisolism do not. However, the overlap between normal individuals and those with Cushing disease makes this test most useful to differentiate pituitary from adrenal causes of Cushing syndrome once hypercortisolism is confirmed. Another complicating factor is that response to oCRH has been reported in patients with ectopic ACTH.

Combined use of the high-dose dexamethasone test and the oCRH test improves diagnostic accuracy. Recently, better discrimination has been reported using a 7-hour continuous dexamethasone infusion.[3]

These procedures may also be useful in differentiating depressed patients from those with Cushing syndrome. Both may have similar subjective complaints, obesity, hirsutism, and elevated basal cortisol values, so it may be difficult to distinguish between the two. Responses to oCRH may differentiate patients with Cushing disease from those with depression; patients with Cushing disease have increased ACTH responses to oCRH while depressed patients can be expected to have attentuated peak ACTH responses.

The metyrapone test is seldom indicated in the assessment of glucocorticoid excess because ACTH levels can be measured directly. Metyrapone inhibits 11-hydroxylase, decreasing cortisol production which leads to increased ACTH secretion in the normal individual. This results in increased secretion of 11-deoxycortisol which can be measured directly in the plasma or in urine as 17-hydroxycorticoids. Glucocorticoid excess as a result of excessive ACTH stimulation will be stimulated to even greater levels if an intact feedback component is operative, while no change is expected if there is an autonomous adrenal tumor or if there is an ectopic source of ACTH.

Adrenocortical lesions are usually detectable on computed tomography (CT) or magnetic resonance imaging (MRI) and adrenal ultrasonography as an initial study and adrenal vein catheterization for localization of steroid synthesis excess may be helpful in certain instances. Adrenal scintigraphy can aid in the localization and verification of abnormal adrenal function. Increased use of radiographic techniques has revealed the occurrence of "nonfunctioning adrenal masses," usually in older adults. Epidemiologic data suggest that screening for pheochromocytomas and primary aldosteronism is appropriate for all patients with incidentally discovered adrenal masses while additional laboratory evaluation should depend on the clinical assessment of the individual patient.

Many pituitary microadenomas are not visualized on CT. MRI appears to improve their detection. In cases where discrimination between pituitary and ectopic ACTH is difficult, simultaneous measurement of ACTH (before and after oCRH) from peripheral vein and both inferior petrosal sinuses in the untreated adult patient has proved helpful.[62]

Treatment

Therapy of patients with adrenal tumors is surgical excision. For most patients, children or adults, with Cushing disease, transsphenoidal microsurgery is the recommended treatment.[48] The presence of ACTH or cortisol responses to oCRH testing in the immediate postoperative period may indicate an increased risk of recurrence. While hypopituitarism or recurrence may develop following pituitary irradiation, it may be a useful secondary therapy in patients that fail to respond to transsphenoidal surgery. Treatment with bilateral adrenalectomy may be necessary if other options fail; this necessitates long-term replacement therapy and may be complicated by Nelson syndrome. Nelson syndrome, characterized by the development of hyperpigmentation, sellar enlargement, and visual field abnormalities, is reported to occur in 25% of pediatric patients.

Pharmacologic agents have also been used, generally as adjunctive rather than as the sole therapy. In Cushing disease, cyproheptadine, a serotonin antagonist, and bromocriptine, a dopamine agonist, are of limited utility. Inhibitors of steroid biosynthesis have been used. Metyrapone inhibits the β-hydroxylase activity of $P-450_{c11}$ while aminoglutethimide inhibits $P-450_{scc}$; both are associated with side effects. Increased ACTH secretion may occur, which overcomes the adrenal blockade. Gastrointestinal upset and hirsutism may occur with the use of metyrapone; drowsiness, skin rashes, nausea, and vomiting are associated with aminoglutethemide. Combined use of these agents has been proposed as adjunctive therapy in treatment of Cushing syndrome. Ketoconazole, which interferes with steroidogenesis, has been used. An adrenolytic agent, mitotane, which causes necrosis of the zona reticularis and zona fasciculata, has been used in the treatment of adrenal carcinoma.

ADRENOCORTICAL TUMORS

The adrenal carcinomas that present with Cushing syndrome have a poor prognosis whether or not they have concomitant androgen production. Tumors which present with virilization may produce increased glucocorticoids and mineralocorticoids in addition to androgen hypersecretion. Virilizing adrenal tumors occurring during child-

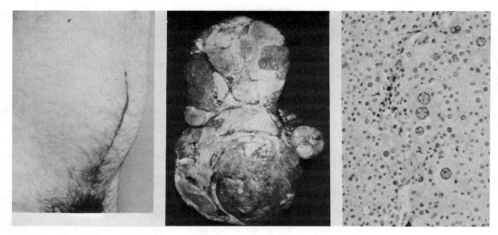

FIG 6–12.
Androgen-producing adrenal tumor in a 6-year-old female. Photos show sexual and abdominal hair (*left*), massive tumor with growth through the capsule (*middle*), and microscopic appearance of tumor (*right*).

hood present with inappropriate growth acceleration and development of sexual characteristics. These characteristics may include sexual hair and excessive body hair (Fig 6–12), excessive muscle development, voice change, and acne, with clitoral growth in females and genital, but not testicular, growth in males. These tumors are difficult to classify on a pathologic basis as adenomas or carcinomas. The clinical course cannot be predicted by the usual microscopic features of malignancy (see Fig 6–12). Those which have not invaded the capsule or metastasized at the time of surgical removal generally have a good prognosis. Those that are metastatic or have invaded the capsule (see Fig 6–12) at the time of surgery have a poor prognosis.

Virilizing tumors must be differentiated from virilizing congenital adrenal hyperplasia, and in males from other causes of sexual precocity. While females with more severe forms of adrenal hyperplasia can be expected to have abnormal differentiation of genitalia and virilization at birth, those with milder forms and males may present with postnatal virilization, as do children with virilizing adrenal tumors.

Rarely, tumors secrete estrogens as well as androgens. In males the presenting findings include gynecomastia; in girls, sexual precocity. Even more rarely, adrenal tumors may be only feminizing.

Hormonal assessment will confirm or identify the autonomous steroid secretion. Circulating levels of adrenal androgens, androstenedione and DHEA, are elevated, although this elevation may be episodic so DHEA-S levels, which have a prolonged half-life, are useful. Testosterone levels are elevated as well, in part as a result of peripheral conversion from adrenal androgens in addition to direct secretion. Urinary 17-ketosteroid levels may be markedly elevated. Among the patients with feminizing tumors, estrogen levels are markedly elevated. The autonomy of this secretion is indicated by the lack of suppression after high-dosage dexamethasone testing. Treatment is surgical, and if complete excision is not possible, chemotherapy using mitotane has been used.

ADRENAL INSUFFICIENCY

Symptoms of adrenal insufficiency are anorexia, vomiting, malaise, weight loss, and fatigue. Hypoglycemia and hypotension may occur. Hyperpigmentation, particularly of the extensor surfaces, skin creases, scars, and gingiva, may occur in primary adrenal insufficiency because of increased ACTH and β-lipotropin secretion.

The eponym *Addison disease* refers to chronic hypocortisolism resulting from any infectious, infiltrative, or destructive process that obliterates the adrenal gland. The processes which cause atrophy or destruction of the adrenal cortex, primary adrenal insufficiency (Table 6–4), generally result in both glucocorticoid and mineralocorticoid deficiency. In the original description by Thomas Addison, in 1855, infiltrative tuberculosis of the adrenal led to adrenal insufficiency. Other fungal agents including histoplasmosis, sarcoidosis, amyloidosis, neoplastic infiltration, or hemochromatosis can also destroy the adrenal gland. Bilateral adrenalectomy leads to insufficiency. Hypoadrenalism may be due to congenital adrenal hyperplasia, congenital adrenal hypoplasia, adrenal leukodystrophy, Wolman disease, and bilateral adrenal hemorrhage with (Waterhouse-Friderichsen syndrome) or without septicemia. Glucocorticoid deficiency without mineralocorticoid deficiency occurs in the ACTH unresponsiveness syndrome and in adrenal atrophy due to exogenous glucocorticoid suppression of ACTH. Currently, the most common cause of acquired primary adrenal insufficiency is autoimmune disease. Some of these patients have serologically detectable antiadrenal antibodies and some have additional manifestations of autoimmune disease.

TABLE 6–4.

Etiology of Hypoadrenalism

Primary	Secondary
ACTH unresponsiveness	Anorexia nervosa
Adrenalectomy (bilateral)	Hypothalamic or pituitary defects
Adrenoleukodystrophy	Corticotropin-releasing hormone deficiency
Amyloidosis	ACTH deficiency
Autoimmune	Idiopathic hypopituitarism
Congenital adrenal hyperplasia	Organic hypopituitarism
Congenital adrenal hypoplasia	Craniopharyngioma
Granulomatosis (tuberculosis, histoplasmosis, sarcoidosis)	Other tumors
Hemochromatosis	Radiation
Hemorrhage (bilateral, with or without fulminant infection—Waterhouse-Friderichsen syndrome)	Sarcoidosis
Neoplastic infiltration	Trauma
Wolman disease (lysosomal acid lyase deficiency)	Hypophysectomy
Xanthomatosis	Pituitary aplasia
	Ectopic posterior pituitary
	Starvation
	Temporary suppression
	After withdrawal of glucocorticoid therapy
	After removal of autonomously secreting adrenal tumor

Adrenal insufficiency is a component of both polyglandular autoimmune endocrine syndromes (Table 6–5). The type I polyglandular syndrome is characterized by mucocutaneous candidiasis, hypoparathyroidism, and adrenal insufficiency. Onset is generally in childhood with a consistent progression of findings; mucocutaneous candidiasis followed by hypoparathyroidism followed by adrenal insufficiency.[59] Chronic active hepatitis, gonadal failure, alopecia, pernicious anemia, malabsorption syndromes, and vitiligo may develop. Rarely, hypothyroidism or insulin-dependent diabetes mellitus occurs. Inheritance appears to be autosomal recessive without any HLA associations. Patients should be monitored with liver function tests to detect the development of chronic active hepatitis.

Adrenal insufficiency, hypothyroidism, and insulin-dependent diabetes mellitus define type II polyglandular autoimmune endocrinopathy, or Schmidt's syndrome. While the peak age at onset tends to middle age, there is a broader range of age at onset than in type I. Multiple generations of a family may be affected. There is an association with HLA-B8, DR3. Vitiligo and primary hypogonadism may be associated findings.[59]

Acute adrenal insufficiency can be precipitated by bilateral adrenal hemorrhages, generally associated with intrapartum complications or overwhelming infections. In the neonate, typical signs and symptoms are pallor, anorexia, vomiting, lethargy, and abdominal masses. Radiographic studies are helpful in demonstrating adrenal enlargement and hemorrhage; adrenal calcifications are subsequently found. The pathophysiologic mechanism may involve adrenal vein stasis leading to adrenal vein thrombosis resulting in adrenal corticomedullary necrosis and hemorrhage. Despite adrenal hemorrhages in the neonatal period, adrenal function may apparently be normal.

Congenital hypoplasia of the adrenal gland has been described. Both sex-linked and autosomal recessive inheritance have been described.[64,93] Characteristic neonatal

TABLE 6–5.

Autoimmune Polyglandular Syndromes*

	Type I	Type II
Mucocutaneous candidiasis	+	−
Autoimmune thyroid disease	Rare	+
Hypoparathyroidism	+	−
Diabetes mellitus	Rare	+
Addison's disease	+	Rare
Associated with HLA-B8, DR3	−	+
Chronic active hepatitis	+	−
Gonadal failure	+	Possible
Pernicious anemia	±	±
Alopecia	±	±
Vitiligo	±	±
Peak incidence (age)	<10 yr	20–60 yr
Female-male ratio	4:3	2:1
Family affected	Siblings	Multiple generations

*+ = present; − = absent; ± = present or absent.

symptoms include poor feeding, vomiting, failure to gain weight, hypoglycemia, cyanosis, and hypotension.

Unresponsiveness to ACTH is characterized by glucocorticoid deficiency, hyperpigmentation, elevated ACTH levels, and normal serum electrolytes. Aldosterone levels are maintained as a result of the renin-angiotensin system. Achalasia and alacrima have been reported in association with unresponsiveness to ACTH. One such patient demonstrated increased cortisol levels after administration of theophylline, which presumably increased intracellular cAMP, thus implicating a primary receptor defect as the pathophysiologic mechanism for this disorder.[83]

Adrenoleukodystrophy is a fatal peroxisomal disorder associated with progressive central demyelination and adrenocortical insufficiency. Serum very long-chain fatty acid levels (C_{26-28}) are elevated. The childhood form is X-linked recessive while the neonatal form is autosomal recessive. Characteristic cytoplasmic inclusions are found on microscopic examination of the adrenal cortex. Additional findings in neonatal adrenoleukodystrophy are severe hypotonia, seizures, retinitis pigmentosa, and optic atrophy.[36] Neurologic deterioration is not prevented by glucocorticoid replacement therapy.

Signs and symptoms typical of adrenal insufficiency are common in acquired immunodeficiency syndrome (AIDS). Indeed, microscopic adrenal findings extend from mild lesions of questionable clinical significance to necrotizing inflammation, hemorrhage, and infarction.[24] Impaired 17-deoxysteroid response to ACTH stimulation was observed in patients with AIDS. However, evaluation of nine children with AIDS showed normal cortisol responses to ACTH stimulation in all except one child receiving ketoconazole, a known inhibitor of steroidogenesis.[39] Thus, the frequency of adrenal insufficiency in AIDS is uncertain.

The most common cause of adrenal insufficiency is suppression of the hypothalamic-pituitary-adrenal axis owing to exogenous glucocorticoid therapy. If the duration of such therapy is less than 1 week, the hypothalamic-pituitary-adrenal axis is generally not suppressed. Patients receiving glucocorticoids for a longer period may require stress coverage for as long as 1 year after the discontinuation of therapy.

Causes of secondary adrenal insufficiency (see Table 6–4) include the hypothalamic-pituitary conditions traditionally referred to as *hypopituitarism*. These are idiopathic or due to tumor, irradiation, surgery, or trauma and include the temporary conditions seen after steroid withdrawal of exogenous steroid therapy or removal of an autonomously glucocorticoid-secreting tumor.

Congenital panhypopituitarism and developmental anomalies of the central nervous system such as septo-optic dysplasia or ectopic posterior pituitaries are associated with anterior pituitary hormone deficiencies.[73] Craniopharyngiomas and infiltrative lesions of the hypothalamus or pituitary such as histiocytosis X, sarcoidosis, or autoimmune diseases have been associated with secondary adrenal insufficiency. Therapeutic radiation therapy of the head and neck is associated with acquired hypopituitarism. Anterior and posterior pituitary hormone deficiencies were reported in a neonate who had group B meningitis. Isolated ACTH deficiency appears to be a rare cause of secondary adrenal insufficiency. CRH stimulation may be helpful in distinguishing between pituitary and hypothalamic causes of hypoadrenalism.

Hormone Assessment

Acute adrenal insufficiency is secondary to glucocorticoid and mineralocorticoid deficiencies. Clinical signs and symptoms include anorexia, dehydration, fever, vomiting, lethargy, and hypotension. Laboratory findings include hyponatremia, hyperkalemia, hypoglycemia, increased plasma renin activity, and biochemical evidence of dehydration. Serum cortisol, urinary free cortisol, and 17-hydroxycorticosteroid are low.

Once the patient is stabilized, the diagnosis of primary adrenal insufficiency can be confirmed by subnormal cortisol response to synthetic ACTH (α^{1-24}-corticotropin; syntropin; Cortrosyn) administered as an IV bolus or by IM injection with samples obtained at 0, 30, and 60 minutes. A dose of 0.25 mg provides maximal adrenocortical stimulation. Cortisol should increase by 10 μg/dL or to a value greater than 15 μg/dL.

The presence of hyperpigmentation or elevated ACTH levels with poor cortisol response establishes a diagnosis of primary adrenal insufficiency. To confirm a diagnosis of secondary adrenal insufficiency, ACTH stimulation, insulin-induced hypoglycemia, or metyrapone testing may be indicated. While metyrapone testing is seldom necessary since ACTH assays have become reliable, failure to respond to metyrapone or insulin-induced hypoglycemia in a patient with an inadequate response to ACTH indicates a pituitary or hypothalamic deficiency. To verify that the adrenal gland has been destroyed rather than severely atrophied with potential recovery, a long-acting form of ACTH, Acthar gel, must be administered for several days.

Treatment

For patients with acute adrenal insufficiency who are often hypotensive, glucocorticoid treatment and volume replacement with IV saline are urgently required. In children less than age 4 years, 50 mg hydrocortisone sodium hemisuccinate (Solu-Cortef), should be administered parenterally. Older children should receive 100 mg. Patients and their parents must understand the need for stress glucocorticoid dosage. Parents should be instructed on how to administer an IM injection; Solu-Cortef Mix-O-Vial is convenient for home use. Patients should wear Medic-Alert or other similar identification.

Glucocorticoid Therapy

Glucocorticoid and mineralocorticoid replacement therapy (Table 6–6) are necessary for patients with primary adrenal insufficiency. Parenteral glucocorticoid therapy is based on normal secretion rates and ranges from 6 to 12 mg/m^2/day.[41] Oral replacement is about twice this amount such that oral cortisol at 10 to 15 mg/m^2/day in three doses is generally adequate. Patients with secondary adrenal insufficiency usually require only glucocorticoid replacement therapy. The dose should be low enough so as to not interfere with growth if other pituitary hormone deficiencies are also present.

Patients require increased glucocorticoids when stressed. Stress may comprise fever greater than 101°F, significant trauma, surgery, and or repeated vomiting.

TABLE 6–6.

Commonly Used Adrenocorticosteroid Pharmaceutical Preparations

Generic Name	Brand Name	Oral	Parenteral
Fludrocortisone acetate	Florinef acetate	0.1 mg	—
Cortisone acetate	Cortone acetate	Tablets: 25 mg	Vials: 25 mg/mL, 20 mL; 50 mg/mL, 10 mL
Cortisol (hydrocortisone)	Cortef Hydrocortone	10 mg/5 mL Tablets: 5, 10, 20 mg	
Hydrocortisone sodium succinate	Solu-Cortef		Mix-O-Vial: 100, 200, 500 mg
Prednisone base	Pediapred		
Prednisone		5 mg/5 mL Tablets: 5, 10, 20, 50 mg	
Methylprednisolone	Medrol	Tablets: 2, 4, 8, 16, 32 mg	
Methylprednisolone sodium succinate	Solu-Medrol		Act-O-Vial: 40, 125, 1000 mg Vials: 500, 1,000 mg Powders: 40–2,000 mg
Dexamethasone	Decadron	Elixir: 0.5 mg/5 mL Tablets: 0.25, 0.5, 0.75, 1.5, 4, 6 mg	
Dexamethasone sodium phosphate	Decadron phosphate		4 mg/mL 24 mg/mL, IV only

Patients who cannot retain oral medications should be given IV or IM glucocorticoid replacement. A typical dosing regimen would be 50 mg every 6 hours as long as parenteral therapy is required. If given IV, a continuous infusion is preferable because an intermittent bolus will be rapidly metabolized. Cortisone acetate suspension is an excellent IM medication to provide a depot of parenteral drug. It cannot be used for immediate glucocorticoid effect but may be given 12 to 24 hours before the coverage is needed. Therefore, it is useful in the preparation of patients for surgery, when illness or stress is ongoing, or when the IV route is difficult or unsure. Absorption occurs over the first 24 hours after the injection and is maintained for 24 to 48 hours. For maintenance, injections can be given every three days. For stress, triple dosages can be given daily. The maintenance dosage is about 25% greater than cortisol, so may range from 10 to 16 mg/m^2/24 hr. The dosage should be tripled for stress so the daily dosage would be 30 to 45 mg/m^2.

The relative glucocorticoid and mineralocorticoid potency and the duration of action of the glucocorticoid preparation must be considered whether these drugs are to be used as replacement therapy for cortisol insufficiency, to suppress the adrenal cortex as in adrenal hyperplasia, or for other physiologic or pharmacologic effect. Glucocorticoid potency correlates with glucocorticoid receptor activity. In general, for glucocorticoid effect, cortisone is 80% as potent as cortisol, prednisone 4 times more potent, prednisolone 5 times, methylprednisolone 5 to 6 times, triamcinolone 6 to 10 times, and dexamethasone 25 to 50 times more potent. Therefore, approximate equivalent dosages are 5 mg of cortisol, 1 mg of prednisone and 0.25 mg or less of dexamethasone. Mineralocorticoid potency of cortisol and cortisone is about 50% that of 9α-fluorohydrocortisone on a weight basis while the mineralocorticoid potency of prednisone and prednisolone is 25%. The most potent forms have minimal or no mineralocorticoid effect. It is difficult to provide only physiologic replacement without excessive glucocorticoid therapy when the more potent forms are used in small children. Also, changing the type of glucocorticoid medication may require modification of mineralocorticoid supplementation.

In addition to glucocorticoid replacement therapy as described above, glucocorticoids are often utilized for their anti-inflammatory and immunosuppressive actions (see Table 6–6). Asthma, collagen-vascular diseases, juvenile rheumatoid arthritis, some types of chronic renal disease, some skin diseases, and prevention of organ transplant rejection are examples of nonendocrine indications for glucocorticoid therapy.

Most likely, the anti-inflammatory activities of glucocorticoids are effected through the traditional model of steroid hormone action with resultant synthesis of regulatory proteins. Mechanisms for this action include interference with the production of lymphokines including interleukin-1 and tumor necrosis factor-α (TNF-α) and the cellular response to lymphokines.[16] Indeed, glucocorticoids may induce protein intermediates, i.e., lipocortin, which may influence plasma membrane phospholipase A_2 activity.[66] Indeed, such anti-inflammatory activities may be physiologic characteristics as well as pharmacologic actions.[58]

Glucocorticoids help maintain blood glucose principally through regulatory influences on gluconeogenic enzymes and glucose uptake. Glucagon and epinephrine are the primary counterregulatory hormones for acute hypoglycemia. The importance of cortisol in carbohydrate metabolism is indicated by the occurrence of hypoglycemia in hypocortisolism. However, hypercortisolemia also affects carbohydrate metabolism through decreased glucose utilization, increased hepatic glucose output, and effects on glucagon and insulin secretion such that hyperglycemia may occur.[47]

Induction of the hepatic microsomal enzymes by phenytoin, barbiturates, or rifampin may accelerate glucocorticoid metabolism such that higher glucocorticoid doses may be necessary. Since glucocorticoids may increase salicylate metabolism, higher doses of salicylates may be needed. Higher insulin doses may be needed in diabetic patients that require glucocorticoid treatment, e.g., patients with diabetes and asthma.

Withdrawal of Glucocorticoid Therapy

The administration of supraphysiologic dosages of glucocorticoids at a frequency that causes continuous suppression may be followed by prolonged suppression if the duration of treatment is greater than 1 month. Suppression for a week or less can be followed by acute cessation of such therapy if the underlying indication will tolerate it. If the suppression has been from 1 to 4 weeks, a more gradual taper may be indicated. If the hypothalamic-pituitary-adrenal axis has been suppressed continuously for a month or longer, normal secretion may not resume for as long as 6 to 12 months thereafter. Therefore, withdrawal from pharmacologic glucocorticoid therapy must be done slowly, not only to prevent a possible potential exacerbation of the underlying disorder but also to prevent hypocortisolism secondary to suppression of the hypothalamic-pituitary-adrenal axis. Stress glucocorticoid dosage may be required for 1 year following discontinuation of pharmacologic glucocorticoid treatment. Tests which can be helpful to assess recovery of normal hypothalamic-pituitary-adrenal function include insulin-induced hypoglycemia, ACTH stimulation, and metyrapone administration. A reasonable dosage reduction schedule, assuming that the underlying disorder allows it, is to decrease the dosage by half at 2- to 3-day intervals until physiologic replacement (equivalent to cortisol at 12–18 mg/m^2/day) is reached. Thereafter the dosage can be decreased by one-half at weekly intervals. The dosage reduction schedule may also include a regimen which switches to alternate-day administration. During this period, or for several months up to 1 year after dosage reduction, stress dosages of glucocorticoids should be given for any major illness or stress significant enough to demand such dosage. Care must be exercised, however, to avoid giving glucocorticoid for minor illnesses or short-term stress. Once the period of stress has passed, the taper can be resumed or the drug discontinued.

HYPERALDOSTERONISM

Elevated secretion of aldosterone can be due to increased adrenal production (primary) or to increased plasma renin activity leading to increased aldosterone secretion (secondary). Primary hyperaldosteronism is rare in children. The signs and symptoms—nocturia, polyuria, weakness, parathesias, and tetany—are due to the potassium deficiency. However, most patients are asymptomatic. Glucose intolerance may occur. Persistent hypokalemia and urinary potassium excretion in hypertensive patients on sodium replete diets and who are not on diuretics indicate primary hyperaldosteronism.

Differentiation between the possible causes of primary hyperaldosteronism, adrenal adenomas, idiopathic hyperaldosteronism, and glucocorticoid-suppressible hyperaldosteronism, is important because appropriate treatment is dependent on the specific etiology. Surgical excision of an adenoma is curative. In primary hyperaldosteronism, plasma renin activity is suppressed and hypokalemia occurs. With adenomas, aldosterone secretion is autonomous. Thus, there is no increased aldosterone response to postural changes as there is in normal individuals or those with bilateral hyperplasia. Following saline infusion, ratios of aldosterone to cortisol and 18-hydroxycorticosterone to cortisol greater than 3 are suggestive of an adenoma.[1]

Idiopathic hyperaldosteronism, characterized by micro- or macronodular hyperplasia, which is usually bilateral, often exhibits exaggerated responses to physiologic stimuli.[4] Other secretagogues such as angiotensin II, potassium, and ACTH may be important in the pathogenesis of this disorder.[49] Indeed, the existence of a non-ACTH pituitary aldosterone-stimulating glycoprotein has been suggested. Bilateral adrenalectomy generally fails to completely correct the associated hypertension.

Adrenal ultrasound, CT and MRI scans, and catheterization of the adrenal veins with determination of aldosterone and cortisol may be helpful in differentiating these entities. Adrenal scintigraphy with I-6β-iodomethyl-19-nor-cholesterol (NP-59) has also been utilized to distinguish adenomas from hyperplasia.[4] Surgical excision of an aldosterone-secreting adenoma is curative. Bilateral hyperplasia generally does not respond to surgery; use of spironolactone, which antagonizes aldosterone at the receptor, may be effective. Amiloride, a potassium-retaining diuretic, may be useful in patients that cannot tolerate spironolactone.

In secondary hyperaldosteronism, renin levels are elevated leading to increased aldosterone levels. Hypertension is also present in cases of renovascular hypertension or renin-secreting tumors. Sodium or volume depletion, as in diuretic use, severe diarrhea, and vomiting, or laxative abuse can lead to increased renin secretion followed by increased aldosterone secretion. Both nephrotic syndrome and hepatic cirrhosis with ascites result in hypoalbuminemia leading to decreased effective blood volume due to decreased oncotic pressure; compensatory activation of the renin-angiotensin system can occur producing secondary hyperaldosteronism. Decreased effective blood volume in congestive heart failure also leads to the activation of the renin-angiotensin system resulting in secondary hyperaldosteronism.

Bartter's Syndrome

Bartter's syndrome is characterized by normotensive secondary hyperaldosteronism. Hypertrophy of the renal juxtaglomerular apparatus can be seen. Hypochloremic, hypokalemic alkalosis and decreased growth velocity are associated findings. Blood pressure does not increase during infusion of pressor agents such as angiotensin II or norepinephrine.[9] Increased urinary prostaglandin excretion may occur.

While the exact pathogenetic mechanism is unclear, one hypothesis is that decreased chloride reabsorption in the ascending loop of Henle leads to potassium wasting with the resultant hypokalemia causing increased activity of the renin-angiotensin-aldosterone system. Another proposed mechanism is a primary defect in membrane electrolyte transport since increased intracellular sodium and decreased cellular sodium efflux from red blood cells has been observed.

Treatment involves supplemental potassium. Triamterene 5 to 10 mg/kg/day in divided doses may be added if hypokalemia persists. Ibuprofen or indomethacin have also been used.

Hypokalemic metabolic alkalosis suggestive of Bartter's syndrome has been described in association with cystic fibrosis,[37] Kearns-Sayre syndrome,[23] and cystinosis. Chronic ingestion of chloride-deficient formula has been associated with a clinical pattern reminiscent of Bartter's syndrome.

Glucocorticoid-Suppressible Hyperaldosteronism

Glucocorticoid or dexamethasone-suppressible hyperaldosteronism is a rare autosomal dominant cause of low renin hypertension. This disorder is characterized by elevated aldosterone levels which are easily suppressed by low doses of dexamethasone. Aldosterone levels increase after ACTH stimulation but are unchanged during angiotensin II infusin.[19] Elevated levels of 18-hydroxycortisol and 18-oxocortisol are found. Indeed, urinary metabolites of C-18 oxygenated corticosteroids are elevated in the untreated state and promptly decrease with the initiation of glucocorticoid therapy.[90]

It has been suggested that hyperaldosteronism is not the sole cause of the associated hypertension; the presence of additional mineralocorticoids, e.g., 18-oxocortisol, has been suspected. The role of ACTH and other POMC-related peptides is unclear; elevated blood γ-MSH were detected in one family while in another family all POMC-related peptides, including ACTH, were normal.[21,92]

These findings suggest that the zona glomerulosa is less responsive to angiotensin II or that the zona fasciculata acquires the ability to produce aldosterone. It has been suggested that there is an increase in the "transitional zone" between the glomerulosa and fasciculata such that aldosterone, cortisol, 18-hydroxycortisol, and 18-oxocortisol are produced within the same cell.[20] Another hypothesis of the pathogenesis of this disorder is a mutation of P-450$_{c11}$, the enzyme involved in the last steps of aldosterone and cortisol biosynthesis, allowing aldosterone synthesis to occur in the zona fasciculata.[90]

APPARENT MINERALOCORTICOID EXCESS

Apparent mineralocorticoid excess, characterized by hypokalemia and severe hypertension, occurs primarily in children. Renin and aldosterone levels are suppressed. Such patients appear to have defective oxidation of cortisol to cortisone owing to decreased 11β-hydroxysteroid dehydrogenase activity.[86] The hypertension, hypokalemia, and suppressed renin-angiotensin system seen after ingestion of the active components of licorice, glycyrrhizic acid, and glycyrrhetinic acid may also be due to inhibition of 11β-hydroxysteroid dehydrogenase activity. Further, it is speculated that decreased 11-dehydrogenase activity leads cortisol to act upon the renal mineralocorticoid receptor. Urinary free cortisol excretion is increased.

HYPOALDOSTERONISM

Type 4 renal tubular acidosis is characterized by hyperkalemic, hyperchloremic metabolic acidosis with secondary hypoaldosteronism. Hyporeninemic hypoaldosteronism can be due to intrinsic renal disease with damage to the interstitial tissue and juxtaglomerular apparatus. Such disorders include obstructive uropathies, pyelonephritis, interstitial nephritis, glomerulonephritis, and diabetes mellitus.[71]

Pseudohypoaldosteronism is a rare disorder manifesting in infancy with dehydration, hyponatremia, and hyperkalemia. Aldosterone and renin levels are elevated. Defective mineralocorticoid end-organ responsiveness is presumed to be the pathophysiologic mechanism. In addition to the kidneys, salivary glands, sweat glands, and colonic mucosa may also be affected. Therapy requires supplemental sodium.

ADRENAL MEDULLA

Neural crest cells invade the developing adrenal cortex at 6 to 7 weeks of gestation to become the adrenal medulla. The medulla is innervated by preganglionic sympathetic fibers from splanchnic nerves. Owing to its vascular supply, it has a high concentration of glucocorticoids draining from the adrenal cortex.

Epinephrine, norepinephrine, and dopamine, the principal catecholamines in humans, are derived from similar precursors. Tyrosine (Fig 6–13) is hydroxylated by tyrosine hydroxylase forming dihydroxyphenylalanine (dopa) which can pass across the blood-brain barrier. In the cytoplasm, dopa is decarboxylated by aromatic amino acid dehydrogenase forming dopamine. Next, within storage granules, dopamine is hydroxylated by dopamine β-oxidase forming norepinephrine. In the adrenal medulla, norepinephrine returns to the cytoplasm where it is converted to epinephrine by phenylethanolamine-*N*-transferase. The activity of this enzyme is enhanced by glucocorticoids making epinephrine synthesis tissue-specific.[95] After release through exocytosis, catecholamines are either chemically inactivated or taken up to be recycled intracellularly.

Norepinephrine, secreted from sympathetic neurons which innervate almost all peripheral tissues, is widely distributed throughout the body. Epinephrine is released from the adrenal medulla. Since both substances have plasma half-lives of less than 1 minute, they are rapidly eliminated. The three major degradative pathways are monamine oxidase, or aldehyde reductase (MAO), catechol-*o*-methyltransferase (COMT), and conjugation (sulfation or glucuronidation) at the ring hydroxyl group. Such sulfated or glucuronidated metabolites are not substrates for MAO or COMT systems.[26] MAO is a mixed function oxidase found in all tissues while COMT, a cytosolic enzyme, is not found in nerves. Kidney and liver are significantly involved in the further metabolism of the catecholamines. Dopamine undergoes similar degradative metabolism to its major metabolite, homovanillic acid (HVA). Norepinephrine and epinephrine are converted to normetanephrine and metanephrine, respectively, and finally to 3-methoxy-4-hydroxymandelic acid (vanillylmandelic acid, VMA).

Since catecholamines are easily oxidized at neutral and basic pHs, blood and

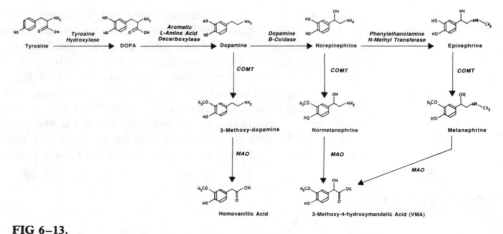

FIG 6–13.
Schematic illustration of pathways of catecholamine biosynthesis and metabolism. *COMT* = catechol-*o*-methyltransferase; *MAO* = monamine oxidase.

urine samples must be handled with great care to avoid degradation prior to analysis.[26] Radioenzymatic assays and high-performance liquid chromatography with electrochemical detection of free catecholamines and metabolites provide the most reliable results. These techniques are less significantly affected by diet (e.g., licorice). While plasma levels are useful, 24-hour urine collections may be the most desirable method to assess catecholamine production. Practical limitations to plasma levels are that venipuncture may elevate catecholamine levels and that meticulous handling of the sample is necessary. Timed urine samples, either overnight or during paroxysmal episodes, have been successfully utilized.

Catecholamine action is mediated through α, β, and dopamine receptors. Norepinephrine is principally an α-adrenergic agonist while epinephrine acts at both α- and β-receptors. Catecholamines affect vascular tone, cardiac output, glycogenolysis, and lipolysis for the proverbial "fight-or-flight" response. Phentolamine and phenoxybenzamine specifically block the α-receptor while propranolol is a specific β-receptor antagonist. Considerable knowledge of the pharmacology of these receptors exists because of their importance in cardiopulmonary function (hypertension, asthma).

PHEOCHROMOCYTOMA

Pheochromocytomas are biogenic amine–secreting tumors arising from chromaffin tissues. Most are found in the adrenal medulla, generally on the right side, but they can be located anywhere along the sympathetic chain from the pelvis to the brain. Common extraadrenal sites are the organ of Zuckerkandl, renal hilus, bladder wall, and cervical sympathetic chain.[28] Bilateral adrenal and extraadrenal tumors occur, especially in patients with multiple endocrine neoplasia syndrome type IIA (MEN-IIA). Familial pheochromocytomas have been described. Malignant tumors, by definition tumor cells in sites where chromaffin tissues are generally not located, are rare. Analysis of DNA in tumor tissue suggests an association between malignancy and abnormal DNA ploidy.[30]

The clinical manifestations are related to the effects of the secreted biogenic amines. Headaches, described as severe, diffusely located, and of short duration, are frequent and may be associated with nausea and vomiting. Headaches from pheochromocytomas differ from migraine in that the patients with pheochromocytomas are generally anxious rather than subdued and there is generally no preceding visual aura.[26] Diaphoresis, palpitations with or without tachycardia, pallor, weakness, fatigue, nervousness, chest or abdominal pain, and orthostatic hypotension are common symptoms. In children, weight loss, constipation, polyuria, polydipsia, and enuresis also occur.[32] While sustained hypertension is more common in children than adults, labile hypertension can also occur.[91] Carbohydrate intolerance may occur because catecholamines antagonize insulin action. Cardiomyopathy and acute myocardial infarction can occur; the direct cardiotoxic effects of pheochromocytomas cause significant morbidity and mortality. Chronic increased vascular tone results in vasoconstriction, ultimately leading to decreased vascular volume. Paroxysmal symptoms are interspersed with symptom-free periods which helps to differentiate pheochromo-cytoma from an anxiety attack.

Certain associations should prompt further evaluation for pheochromocytoma. MEN syndromes, neurofibromatosis, von Hippel-Lindau syndrome, cerebellar hemangioblastoma, and Cushing syndrome have been associated with pheochromocytoma. Persistent unexplained hypertension in pregnant adolescents should arouse suspicion of a pheochromocytoma. Differences between children and adults are the lower incidence of malignant pheochromocytomas as well as the increased frequency of bilateral tumors and MEN syndromes in children.[8] A two-mutation model, with one of the mutations occurring in the germ cells, may be involved in the pathogenesis in familial pheochromocytoma and neuroblastoma.[38]

The definitive diagnosis is documentation of a quantitative elevation of catecholamine levels. Timed urine collection with analysis for VMA and normetanephrine-metanephrine is a good screening test.[79] Determination of urinary excretion of free catecholamines may be helpful if the urinary metabolites are nonspecific. Elevated epinephrine levels suggest that the tumor is intraadrenal.

Since "normal values" vary with the analytic techniques, one must be aware of the technique utilized and the normal values of the laboratory used. Additionally, physiologic stresses may increase endogenous catecholamine secretion. Methyldopa, nose drops, cold remedies, and appetite suppressants may affect the laboratory values.

Provocative tests (histamine, glucagon, and tyramine) were used in the past, but are today largely of historical interest because of the inherent danger of such tests provoking a hypertensive crisis. Clonidine suppression tests have been used to differentiate essential hypertension from pheochromocytoma since plasma catecholamines decline after administration of clonidine in essential hypertension but not in pheochromocytoma. Levels of chromogranin A, a soluble 436-amino-acid protein often oversecreted by neoplastic neuroendocrine cells and found in catecholamine storage granules, may be elevated in patients with pheochromocytoma, but are not diagnostic. Since platelets concentrate catecholamines, measurement of platelet catecholamine concentrations may prove useful if this technique becomes more readily available.

Localization of the tumors can be challenging. Ultrasound is helpful, but has inherent technical limitations because of the retroperitoneal location of the adrenal glands. Adrenal CT scanning is the procedure of choice. If the lesion is not visualized, CT and MRI of possible extraadrenal sites are indicated.[57] Scintigraphy with α^{131}I-metaiodobenzylguanidine (MIBG), which is concentrated in sympathomedullary tissues, is also helpful in localizing lesions. Better availability of this noninvasive test may make it the procedure of choice in localizing pheochromocytomas.[78]

Surgical excision is the definitive treatment, but the patient must be adequately prepared by preoperative adrenergic blockade. Phenoxybenzamine hydrochloride is generally well tolerated and used to control hypertension. In the young child, 5 mg every 12 hours is an appropriate starting dose. Older children may need 10 mg every 12 hours. Propranolol is often administered, but should not be started until adequate α-adrenergic blockade exists. α-Methyltyrosine inhibits tyrosine hydroxylase and may be useful to further control symptoms; the starting dose is 5 to 10 mg/kg divided every 6 hours. For acute management of hypertension, phentolamine 1 mg per dose or 5 mg/kg/day is given every 4 to 6 hours. Propranolol 1 mg with continuous electrocardiographic (ECG) monitoring, or 5 to 10 mg every 6 to 8 hours, may be used for tachyarrythmias.

Careful intraoperative management of hypertension and fluid status is crucial. Glucocorticoid coverage is generally necessary since bilateral adrenalectomy is the usual procedure of choice. Persistent postoperative hypertension suggests residual tumor or renovascular disease. Because of the high incidence of tumor recurrence, catecholamine secretion should be monitored annually for at least 5 years.

NEUROBLASTOMA

Neuroblastoma is one of the most common extracranial solid tumors in childhood. Derived from primitive neuroblasts, this tumor may be found wherever sympathetic nervous tissue is located. The adrenal medulla or autonomic ganglia are common sites of origin. Prognosis is inversely related to age.

Signs and symptoms are variable depending on the location and substances secreted by the neoplasm. Detection of an abdominal mass is often the first sign. Abdominal pain, weight loss, fever, and anemia may be present. Other initial findings include Horner's syndrome (cervicothoracic disease), acute cerebellar ataxia, opsoclonus-myoclonus, and periorbital swelling and proptosis. Urinary catecholamine excretion is elevated in 85% to 90% of patients. Patients with a VMA/HVA ratio greater than 1, suggesting greater biologic maturity, tend to have a better prognosis. Elevated serum ferritin levels indicate a poor prognosis.[18] Radiographic studies, including ^{131}I-metaiodobenzylguanidine scan, aid in localizing the disease. Rearrangements and deletions of the short arm of chromosome 1 have been detected frequently by cytogenetic studies. More rapid progression of disease is associated with multiple copies of the N-*myc* oncogene.

Currently, in Japan, neonatal screening for neuroblastoma is being performed.[76] The cost-benefit ratio of such screening is unclear because of the heterogeneous biologic behavior of these tumors. Indeed, spontaneous regression of these tumors has been described in infants.[88,89]

Treatment depends upon staging at the time of diagnosis. Primary excision is the treatment of choice for localized disease. Chemotherapy and radiotherapy may also be necessary for more widespread disease.

Ganglioneuromas are benign tumors, often detected incidentally. These tumors may represent spontaneous maturation of neuroblastoma. Elevated catecholamine secretion may occur, but does not differentiate ganglioneuroma from neuroblastoma.

MULTIPLE ENDOCRINE NEOPLASIA SYNDROMES

Multiple endocrine neoplasia syndromes are autosomal dominant disorders with variable penetrance. Hyperplasia, carcinoma, endocrine hyperactivity, and ectopic hormone secretion occur variably. However, the clinical manifestations in an individual family tend to be consistent. Several distinct multiple endocrine adenomatoses or multiple endocrine neoplasias have been defined.

MEN-I is characterized by involvement of the pituitary, parathyroids, and pancreas. Hyperparathyroidism occurs in many affected patients. Both beta and non-beta islet cell tumors may occur. Zollinger-Ellison syndrome, peptic ulcer, and non-beta islet cell tumors are associated with MEN-I. A variety of pituitary abnormalities may occur, but hyperprolactinemia appears to be the most common.[80] Clinical manifestations of MEN-I are unusual in childhood.

Pheochromocytoma, medullary carcinoma of the thyroid, and hyperparathyroidism constitute MEN-II or Sipple's syndrome. Both sporadic and familial forms occur. Bilateral pheochromocytoma and multicentricity of the medullary thyroid carcinoma are commonly found in the familial form. Medullary thyroid carcinoma is generally the first clinical manifestation and may occur in childhood. Linkage analysis of several large affected families has shown a disease locus on chromosome 10.[44]

Measurement of basal calcitonin or following pentagastrin or calcium gluconate infusion allows for early detection of the medullary thyroid carcinoma. Affected patients should be screened for the presence of a pheochromocytoma prior to surgery. Annual screening, especially for medullary thyroid carcinoma, is recommended for affected families since early thyroidectomy is often curative.

Some families have mucosal neuromas with marfanoid habitus. This has been designated MEN-IIB. The mucosal neuromas frequently occur in the lips, giving them a "bumpy" patulous appearance. Diffuse ganglioneuromatosis of the gastrointestinal tract, café-au-lait lesions, and peripheral neurofibromas may also occur. The medullary thyroid carcinoma tends to progress more rapidly in these families.

ATRIAL NATRIURETIC FACTOR

Atrial natriuretic factor (ANF) is a 28-amino-acid peptide secreted principally by the cardiac atria which acts to promote natriuresis. It is secreted in response to increased vascular volume or atrial distention. Specific activities are decreasing renin and aldosterone secretion, vasorelaxation, and interference with the sodium-retaining action of aldosterone at the level of the kidney.[13]

Although the greatest levels of ANF are in the atria, it is found in other tissues such as hypothalamus, pituitary, gastrointestinal tract, and adrenal medulla. Its role in these other tissues is unknown. Increased levels of ANF mRNA were found in rat atria after dexamethasone treatment.

REFERENCES

1. Arteaga E, Klein RF, Biglieri EG: Use of saline infusion test to diagnose the cause of primary aldosteronism. *Am J Med* 1985; 79:722–729.
2. Bertagna X, de Keyser Y: Pro-opiomelanocortin gene expression, in Melmed S, Rob-

bins RJ (eds): *Molecular and Clinical Advances in Pituitary Disorders*. Boston, Blackwell Scientific Publications, 1991, pp 3–11.

3. Biemond P, de Jong FH, Lamberts SWJ: Continuous dexamethasone infusion for seven hours in patients with the Cushing syndrome. *Ann Intern Med* 1990; 112:738–742.

4. Biglieri EG, Irony I: Primary aldosteronism, in Biglieri EG, Melby JC (eds): *Endocrine Hypertension*. New York, Raven Press, 1990, pp 71–85.

5. Cara JF, Moshang T Jr, Bongiovanni AM, et al: Elevated 17-hydroxyprogesterone and testosterone in a newborn with 3-beta-hydroxysteroid dehydrogenase deficiency. *N Engl J Med* 1985; 313:618–621.

6. Carlstedt-Duke J, Gustafsson J-Å: The molecular mechanism of glucocorticoid action, in Lüdecke DK, Chrousos GP, Tolis G, (eds): *ACTH, Cushing's Syndrome, and Other Hypercortisolemic States*. New York, Raven Press, 1990, pp 7–14.

7. Carroll MC, Campbell RD, Porter RR: Mapping of steroid 21-hydroxylase genes adjacent to complement component C4 genes in HLA, the major histocompatibility complex in man. *Proc Natl Acad Sci USA* 1985; 82:521–525.

8. Caty MG, Coran AG, Geagen M, et al: Current diagnosis and treatment of pheochromocytoma in children. *Arch Surg* 1990; 125:978–981.

9. Chesney R: Clinical study of renal tubular disease, in Barakat AY (ed): *Renal Disease in Children: Clinical Evaluation and Diagnosis*. New York, Springer-Verlag, 1990, pp 185–206.

10. Chiou SH, Hu MC, Chung BC: A missense mutation at Ile^{172} to Asn or Arg^{356} to Trp causes steroid 21-hydroxylase deficiency. *J Biol Chem* 1990; 265:3549–3552.

11. Chung B, Matteson KJ, Voutilainen R, et al: Human cholesterol side-chain cleavage enzyme, P450scc: cDNA cloning, assignment of the gene to chromosome 15, and expression in the placenta. *Proc Natl Acad Sci USA* 1986; 83:8962–8966.

12. Chung B, Picado-Leonard J, Haniu M, et al: Cytochrome P450c17 (steroid 17α-hydroxylase/17,20 lyase): Cloning of human adrenal and testis cDNAs indicate the same gene is expressed in both tissues. *Proc Natl Acad Sci* 1987; 84:407–411.

13. Clinkingbeard C, Sessions C, Shenker Y: The physiological role of atrial natriuretic hormone in the regulation of aldosterone and salt and water metabolism. *J Clin Endocrinol Metab* 1990; 70:582–589.

14. Counts DR, Pescovitz OH, Barnes KM, et al: Dissociation of adrenarche and gonadarche in precocious puberty and in isolated hypogonadotropic hypogonadism. *J Clin Endocrinol Metab* 1987; 64:1174–1178.

15. DeCrecchio L. Sopra un caso di apparenze virili in una donna. *Il Morgagni* 1865; 7:151.

16. Dinarello CA, Mier JW: Lymphokines. *N Engl J Med* 1987; 317:940–945.

17. Doody KM, Carr BR, Rainey WE, et al: 3β-Hydroxysteroid dehydrogenase/isomerase in the fetal zone and neocortex of the human fetal adrenal gland. *Endocrinology* 1990; 126:2487–2492.

18. Evans AE, D'Angio GJ, Propert K, et al: Prognostic factors in neuroblastoma. *Cancer* 1987; 59:1853–1859.

19. Fallo F, Sonino N, Armanini D, et al: A new family with dexamethasone-suppressible hyperaldosteronism: Aldosterone unresponsiveness to angiotensin II. *Clin Endocrinol* 1985; 22:777–785.

20. Ganguly A: Glucocorticoid-suppressible hyperaldosteronism: An update. *Am J Med* 1990; 88:321–324.

21. Gillner HG, Nicholson WE, Gill JR, et al: Plasma immunoreactive propiomelanocortin-derived peptides with primary hyperaldosteronism, idiopathic hyperaldosteronism

with bilateral adrenal hyperplasia, and dexamethasone-suppressible hyperaldosteronism. *J Clin Endocrinol Metab* 1983; 56:853–855.

22. Globerman H, Amor M, Parker KL, et al: Nonsense mutation causing steroid 21-hydroxylase deficiency. *J Clin Invest* 1988; 82:139–144.

23. Gogo Y, Itami N, Kajii N, et al: Renal tubular involvement mimicking Bartter syndrome in a patient with Kearns-Sayre syndrome. *J Pediatr* 1990; 116:904–910.

24. Guenthner EE, Rabinowe SL, Vala Niel A, et al: Primary Addison's disease in a patient with the acquired immunodeficiency syndrome. *Ann Intern Med* 1984; 100:847–848.

25. Hammond GL: Molecular properties of corticosteroid binding globulin and the sex-steroid binding proteins. *Endocr Rev* 1990; 11:65–79.

26. Henry DP, Pratt JH: Pheochromocytoma from the biochemical, pharmacokinetic, and pathophysiologic point of view, in Biglieri EG, Melby JC (eds): *Endocrine Hypertension.* New York, Raven Press, 1990, pp 207–233.

27. Higashi Y, Tanae A, Inoue H, et al: Aberrant splicing and missense mutations cause steroid 21-hydroxylase [P-450(C21)] deficiency in humans: Possible gene conversion products. *Proc Natl Acad Sci* 1988; 85:7486–7490.

28. Hodgkinson DJ, Telander RL, Sheps SG, et al: Extra-adrenal intrathoracic functioning paraganglioma (pheochromocytoma) in childhood. *Mayo Clin Proc* 1980; 55:271–276.

29. Hornsby PJ: The mechanism of action of ACTH in the adrenal cortex, in Cooke BA, King RJB, van der Molen HJ, (eds): *Hormones and Their Actions*, part II. New York, Elsevier Science Publishers BV, 1988, pp 193–210.

30. Hosaka Y, Rainwater LM, Grant CS, et al: Pheochromocytoma: Nuclear deoxyribonucleic acid patterns studied by flow cytometry. *Surgery* 1986; 100:1003–1008.

31. Hubert GD, Carson SA: Adrenarche. *Adolesc Pediatr Gynecol* 1990; 3:3–14.

32. Hume DM: Pheochromocytoma in the adult and child. *Am J Surg* 1960; 99:458–496.

33. Hung W, August GP: Hyperreninemia and secondary hyperaldosteronism in pheochromocytomas. *J Pediatr* 1987; 94:215–217.

34. Illingworth DR, Kenny TA, Orwoll ES: Adrenal function in heterozygous and homozygous hypobetalipoproteinemia. *J Clin Endocrinol Metab* 1982; 54:27–33.

35. Kagimoto M, Winter JSD, Kagimoto K, et al: Structural characterization of normal and mutant human steroid 17α-hydroxylase genes: Molecular basis of one example of combined 17α-hydroxylase/17,20 lyase deficiency. *Mol Endocrinol* 1988; 2:564–570.

36. Kelley RI, Datta NS, Dobyns WB, et al: Neonatal adrenoleukodystrophy: New cases, biochemical studies, and differentiation from Zellweger and related peroxisomal polydystrophy syndromes. *Am J Hum Genet* 1986; 23:869–901.

37. Kennedy JD, Dinwiddie R, Daman-Williams C, et al: Pseudo-Bartter's syndrome in cystic fibrosis. *Arch Dis Child* 1990; 65:786–787.

38. Knudson AG Jr, Strong LC: Mutation and cancer: Neuroblastoma and pheochromocytoma. *Am J Hum Genet* 1972; 24:514–532.

39. Laue L, Pizzo PA, Butler K, et al: Growth and neuroendocrine dysfunction in children with acquired immunodeficiency syndrome. *J Pediatr* 1990; 117:541–545.

40. Leyton O: Multiglandular disease. *Lancet* 1934; 1:1221.

41. Linder BL, Esteban NV, Yergey AL, et al: Cortisol production rate in childhood and adolescence. *J Pediatr* 1990; 117:892–896.

42. Luu-The V, Lachance Y, Labrie C, et al: Full length cDNA structure and deduced amino acid sequence of human 3β-hydroxy-5-ene steroid dehydrogenase. *Mol Endocrinol* 1989; 3:1310–1312.

43. Malchoff CD, Javier EC, Malchoff DM, et al: Primary cortisol resistance presenting as isosexual precocity. *J Clin Endocrinol* Metab 1990; 70:503–507.

44. Mathew CGP, Chin KS, Easton DF, et al: A linked genetic marker for multiple endocrine neoplasia type 2a on chromosome 10. *Nature* 1987; 328:527–528.

45. Matteson KJ, Picado-Leonard J, Chung B, et al: Assignment of the gene for adrenal P450c17 (steroid 17α-hydroxylase/17,20 lyase) to human chromosome 10. *J Clin Endocrinol Metab* 1986; 63:789–791.

46. McLaughlin B, Barrett P, Finch T, et al: Late onset adrenal hyperplasia in a group of Irish females who presented with hirsutism, irregular menses and/or cystic acne. *Clin Endocrinol* 1990; 32:57–64.

47. McMahon M, Gerich J, Rizza R: Effects of glucocorticoids on carbohydrate metabolism. *Diabetes Metab Rev* 1988; 4:17–30.

48. Melby JC: Therapy of Cushing disease: A consensus for pituitary microsurgery. *Ann Intern Med* 1988; 109:445–446.

49. Melby JC: Endocrine hypertension. *J Clin Endocrinol Metab* 1989; 69:697–703.

50. Miesfeld R: Molecular genetics of corticosteroid action. *Am Rev Respir Dis* 1990; 141:S11–S17.

51. Migeon CJ: Comments about the need for prenatal treatment of congenital adrenal hyperplasia due to 21-hydroxylase deficiency (editorial). *J Clin Endocrinol Metab* 1990; 70:836–837.

52. Miller WL: Molecular biology of steroid hormone synthesis. *Endocr Rev* 198; 9:295–318.

53. Miller WL: Regulation of mRNAs for human steroidogenic enzymes. *Endocr Res* 1989; 15:1-16.

54. Miller WL, Levine LS: Molecular and clinical advances in congenital adrenal hyperplasia. *J Pediatr* 1987; 111:1–17.

55. Miller Wl, Morel Y: The molecular genetics of 21-hydroxylase deficiency. *Annu Rev Genet* 1989; 23:371–393.

56. Moore CCD, Brentano ST, Miller WL: Human P450scc gene transcription is induced by cyclic AMP and repressed by 12-*O*-tetradecanoylphorbol-13-acetate and A23187 through independent *cis* elements. *Mol Cell Biol* 1990; 10:6013–6023.

57. Moulton JS, Moutlon JS: CT of the adrenal glands. *Semin Roentgenol* 1988; 23:288–303.

58. Munck A, Guyre PM, Holbrook NJ: Physiological functions of glucocorticoids in stress and their relation to pharmacological actions. *Endocr Rev* 1984; 5:25–44.

59. Neufeld M, MacLaren N, Blizzard R: Autoimmune polyglandular syndromes. *Pediatr Ann* 1980; 9:43–53.

60. New MI, Lorenzen F, Lerner AJ, et al: Genotyping steroid 21-hydroxylase deficiency: Hormonal reference data. *J Clin Endocrinol Metab* 1983; 57:320–326.

61. Oelkers W, Bahr V, Hensen J, et al: Primary adrenocortical nodular hyperplasia: A rare case of Cushing syndrome in children and young adults, in Lüdecke DK, Chrousos GP, Tolis G (eds): *ACTH, Cushing's Syndrome, and Other Hypercortisolemic States.* New York, Raven Press, 1990, pp 91–96.

62. Oldfield EH, Chrousos GP, Schulte HM, et al: Preoperative lateralization of ACTH-secreting pituitary microadrenomas by bilateral and simultaneous inferior petrosal venous sinus sampling. *N Engl J Med* 1985; 312:100–104.

63. Onishi S, Miyazawa G, Nishimura Y, et al: Postnatal development of circadian rhythm in serum cortisol levels in children. *Pediatrics* 1983; 72:399–404.

64. Pakravan P, Kenny FM, Depp R, et al: Familial congenital absence of adrenal glands;

evaluation of glucocorticoid, mineralocorticoid, and estrogen metabolism in the perinatal period. *J Pediatr* 1974; 84:74–78.

65. Pang S, Wallace MA, Hofman L, et al: Worldwide experience in newborn screening for classical congenital adrenal hyperplasia due to 21-hydroxylase deficiency. *Pediatrics* 1988; 81:866–874.

66. Peers SH, Flower RJ: The role of lipocortin in corticosteroid actions. *Am Rev Respir Dis* 1990; 141:S18–S21.

67. Pepe GJ, Albrecht ED: Regulation of the primate fetal adrenal cortex. *Endocr Rev* 1990; 11:151–176.

68. Picado-Leonard J, Miller WL: Cloning and sequence of the human gene for P450c17 (steroid 17α-hydroxylase/17,20 lyase): Similarity with the gene for P450c21. *DNA* 1987; 6:439–448.

69. Quinn SJ, Williams GH: Regulation of aldosterone secretion. *Ann Rev Physiol* 1988; 50:409–426.

70. Rabinovici J, Blankstein J, Goldman B, et al: In vitro fertilization and primary embryonic cleavage are possible in 17α-hydroxylase deficiency despite extremely low intrafollicular 17β-estradiol. *J Clin Endocrinol Metab* 1989; 68:693–697.

71. Rodriguez-Soriano J, Vallo A, Sanjurjo P, et al: Hyporeninemic hypoaldosteronism in children with chronic renal failure. *J Pediatr* 1986; 109:476–482.

72. Rohmer V, Barbot N, Bertrand P, et al: A case of male pseudohermaphroditism due to 17α-hydroxylase deficiency and hormonal profiles in the nuclear family. *J Clin Endocrinol Metab* 1990; 71:523–529.

73. Root AW: Magnetic resonance imaging in hypopituitarism (editorial). *J Clin Endocrinol Metab* 1991; 72:10–11.

74. Rosner W: The functions of corticosteroid-binding globulin and sex-hormone-binding globulin: Recent advances. *Endocr Rev* 1990; 11:80–91.

75. Saruta T, Suzuki H, Handa M, et al: Multiple factors contribute to the pathogenesis of hypertension in Cushing syndrome. *J Clin Endocrinol Metab* 1986; 62:275–279.

76. Sawada T, Kidowaki T, Sakamoto I, et al: Neuroblastoma: Mass screening for early detection and its prognosis. *Cancer* 1984; 53:2731–2735.

77. Schwartz J: Evidence for intrapituitary intercellular control of adrenocorticotropin secretion. *Mol Cell Endocrinol* 1990; 68:77–83.

78. Shapiro B, Gross MD, Fig L, et al: Localization of functioning sympathoadrenal lesions, in Biglieri ED, Melby JC (eds): *Endocrine Hypertension*. New York, Raven Press, 1990, pp 235–255.

79. Sheps SG, Jiang NS, Klee GG, et al: Recent developments in the diagnosis and treatment of pheochromocytoma. *Mayo Clin Proc* 1990; 65:88–95.

80. Sherwood LM: Multiple endocrine neoplasia, in DeGroot LJ, Besser GM, Cahill GF Jr, et al (eds): *Endocrinology*, ed 2. Philadelphia, WB Saunders Co, 1989, pp 2599–2611.

81. Simpson ER, Mason JI, John ME, et al: Regulation of the biosynthesis of steroidogenic enzymes. *J Steroid Biochem* 1987; 27:801–805.

82. Slijper FME: Androgens and gender role behavior in girls with congenital adrenal hyperplasia (CAH). *Prog Brain Res* 1984; 1:417–422.

83. Smith EM, Brosnan P, Meyer WJ III, et al: An ACTH receptor on human mononuclear leukocytes. *N Engl J Med* 1987; 317:1266–1269.

84. Speiser PW, Agdere L, Ueshiba H, et al: Aldosterone synthesis in salt-wasting congenital adrenal hyperplasia with complete absence of adrenal 21-hydroxylase. *N Engl J Med* 1991; 324:145–149.

85. Speiser PW, Laforgia N, Kato K, et al: First trimester prenatal treatment and molecular genetic diagnosis of congenital adrenal hyperplasia (21-hydroxylase deficiency). *J Clin Endocrinol Metab* 1990; 70:838—848.

86. Stewart PM, Corrie JET, Shackleton CHL, et al: Syndrome of apparent mineralocorticoid excess: A defect in the cortisol-cortisone shuttle. *J Clin Invest* 1988; 82:340–349.

87. Teding Van Berkhout F, Croughs RJM, et al: Familial Cushing's syndrome due to nodular adrenocortical dysplasia is an inherited disease of immunological origin. *Clin Endocrinol* 1989; 31:185–191.

88. Tuchman M, Lemieux B, Auray-Blais C, et al: Screening for neuroblastoma at 3 weeks of age: Methods and preliminary results from the Quebec Neuroblastoma Screening Project. *Pediatrics* 1990; 86:765–773.

89. Tuchman M, Lemieux B, Woods WG: Screening for neuroblastoma in infants: Investigate or implement? *Pediatrics* 1990; 86:791–793.

90. Ulick S, Chan CK, Gill JR Jr, et al: Defective fasciculata zone function as the mechanism of glucocorticoid-remediable aldosteronism. *J Clin Endocrinol Metab* 1990; 71:1151–1157.

91. Voorhees ML: Disorders of the adrenal medulla, in Lifshitz F (ed): *Pediatric Endocrinology*, ed 2. New York, Marcel Dekker Inc, 1990, pp 413–434.

92. Weinberger MH, Ganguly A, Grim CE: Pituitary peptides in dexamethasone-suppressible hyperaldosteronism, in New MI, Borrelli P, (eds): *Dexamethasone-suppressible hyperaldosteronism*. Serono Symposia Review no. 10. Rome, Ares-Serono Symposia, 1986, pp 35–40.

93. Weiss L, Mellinger RC: Congenital adrenal hypoplasia—an X-linked disorder. *J Med Genet* 1970; 7:27–32.

94. Winter JSD, Couch RM, Muller J, et al: Combined 17-hydroxylase and 17,20-desmolase deficiencies: evidence for synthesis of a defective cytochrome $P450_{c17}$. *J Clin Endocrinol Metab* 1989; 68:309–316.

95. Wurtman RJ, Pohorecky LA, Baliga BS: Adrenocortical control of the biosynthesis of epinephrine and proteins in the adrenal medulla. *Pharmacol Rev* 1972; 24:411–426.

96. Yanase T, Kagimoto M, Matsui N, et al: Combined 17α-hydroxylase/17,20-lyase deficiency due to a stop codon in the N-terminal region of 17α-hydroxylase cytochrome P-450. *Mol Cell Endocrinol* 1988; 59:249–253.

97. Yanase T, Kagimoto M, Suzuki S, et al: Deletion of a phenylalanine in the N-terminal region of human cytochrome $P450_{17\alpha}$ results in a partial combined 17α-hydroxylase/17,20-lyase deficiency. *J Biol Chem* 1989; 264:76–82.

98. Yanase T, Sanders D, Shibata A, et al: Combined 17α-hydroxylase/17,20 lyase deficiency due to a 7-basepair duplication in the N-terminal region of the cytochrome $P450_{17\alpha}$(CYP17) gene. *J Clin Endocrinol Metab* 1990; 70:1325–1329.

99. Young WF, Zinsmeister AR, Twomey CK, et al: Ovine corticotropin releasing hormone stimulation test: Normal value study. *Mayo Clin Proc* 1990; 65:943–948.

100. Zachmann M, Tassinari D, Prader A: Clinical and biochemical variability of congenital adrenal hyperplasia due to 11β-hydroxylase deficiency. A study of 25 patients. *J Clin Endocrinol Metab* 1983; 56:222–229.

Chapter 7

Ovaries and Variants of Female Sexual Development

Wellington Hung

OVARY

Differentiation of the gonads is controlled by the genetic determinants of the sex chromosomes. Development of a normal ovary from the primitive gonad requires at least two chromosomes to be present. The presence of one X chromosome and the absence of a Y chromosome results in an undifferentiated fibrous streak. By the fourth week of fetal life a thickening of the coelomic epithelium in the genital ridges on both sides of the dorsal mesentery appears. This is the gonad which is undifferentiated, bipotential, and consists of a cortex and medulla. The germ cells migrate to these primordial gonads from the endoderm of the yolk sac. During ovarian development the cortex of the primitive gonad proliferates and the medulla regresses.

During fetal life primordial germ cells multiply in number. The majority of germ cells that migrate to the developing ovary will disappear during fetal life. Less than 1% of ova present at birth will eventually undergo ovulation.

During early development both wolffian and müllerian duct derivatives are present. The gonad controls ductal differentiation, which is completed by the third month of gestation. In the absence of testes, whether or not ovaries are present, the wolffian duct regresses and the müllerian duct derivatives differentiate, giving rise to the fallopian tubes, uterus, and the upper third of the vagina.[24]

Female external genital development occurs in the absence of androgens. The external genitalia of males and females differentiate from a common anlage.

The normal ovary in infancy and childhood is a dynamic organ which undergoes constant internal change. Growth is largely dependent upon an increase of stroma.

Simultaneously there is a tremendous decrease in the number of oocytes. The development of graafian follicles in infancy and childhood is comparable to that seen in adults.

Steroidogenesis is present from birth. Ovarian function is under the control of the hypothalamic-pituitary axis. See Chapter 3 for a discussion of the hypothalamus and anterior pituitary.

MENSTRUAL CYCLE AND HORMONAL REGULATION OF OVARIAN STEROIDOGENESIS

The hormonal events of the normal menstrual cycle leading to follicular development and, ultimately, ovulation involve interplay between gonadotropin levels and concentrations of ovarian steroid hormones. Gonadotropin-releasing hormone (GnRH), produced and secreted in a pulsatile manner by the hypothalamus, binds to gonadotrophs of the anterior pituitary, resulting in the synthesis and secretion of follicle-stimulating hormone (FSH) and luteinizing hormone (LH). The amplitude and frequency of GnRH pulses appear to be modulated by ovarian hormones and catecholamines, as well as by other neuropeptides. While initial follicular recruitment is independent of gonadotropin control, continued growth and development are dependent on the pulsatile release of FSH by the pituitary and estradiol (E_2) production by the granulosa cells of the developing follicle. The theca cells that surround the developing follicle produce androgens, which are converted to estrogens by the cytochrome P-450 enzyme aromatase in the granulosa cells. FSH initiates E_2 production in the granulosa cells by increasing the number of its own receptors and acting in concert with E_2 to stimulate the growth of granulosa cells. As the dominant follicle begins to grow, the pituitary responds by decreasing the release of FSH via a negative feedback system in the presence of increasing levels of E_2 and inhibin.[48] The decrease in FSH prevents the development and growth of other antral follicles, which then undergo atresia. The dominant follicle continues to grow despite decreasing FSH levels because of its enhanced number of granulosa cells, increased number of FSH receptors, and increased vascularization of the theca cells, allowing greater delivery of androstendione to the granulosa cells for aromatization.

During the late follicular phase, just prior to ovulation, there is a small but significant increase in basal production of progesterone that facilitates the positive feedback action of estrogen and augments the amplitude of the LH and FSH surge induced by estrogen. This is followed by a peak in estradiol and by a surge of LH approximately 14 to 24 hours later. The onset of the LH surge occurs 34 to 36 hours prior to ovulation. Prior to ovulation, LH initiates luteinization of the granulosa cells and secretion of progesterone, which continues throughout the luteal phase. The corpus luteum has a life span of approximately 14 days. If pregnancy does not occur, the corpus luteum involutes, with a subsequent drop in progesterone level and the onset of menstruation.

By convention, the first day of bleeding has been designated day 1 of the menstrual cycle. However, recently it has become more common to use the day of the serum

LH peak as the point of reference, i.e., as day 0 of the menstrual cycle. The menstrual cycle days before and after the LH peak are designated as minus or plus days, respectively. This method identifies more accurately the specific biochemical changes that precede or follow the LH surge and ovulation.

ESTROGENS AND PROGESTERONE

Estrogens

Estradiol is the major ovarian hormone secreted although estrone, androstenedione, testosterone, and other steroids are detected in ovarian venous blood. Umbilical artery levels of estrone (E_1) and E_2 are more than 100 times higher than in adult nonpregnant females[73] despite the fact that minimal estrogenization is seen in newborns. Levels in blood drawn during the first minutes and hours after birth display a rapid decrease.

Only a small fraction of the biologically active E_2 in circulation is free or non–protein-bound. It is the free E_2 which enters the cells to exert its hormonal effect. Free E_2 concentrations in females during the first 72 hours of life are approximately 2.5 times higher than those of adult females. The highest values are reached 2 to 6 hours after delivery. After 72 hours of life the percentage of free E_2 decreases and by 6 weeks of age is similar to those of older prepubertal children.[73]

Plasma levels of E_1 and E_2 remain at low levels until approximately 8 to 12 years of age, when E_2 increases in both sexes, but the levels are greater in females.

Estrone levels do not differ markedly between prepubertal females and males (Tables 7–1 and 7–2). Plasma levels of E_1 increase approximately four times during puberty in the female. E_1 levels are greater in females than in males at all stages of development following the onset of puberty.[73] In the adult female, approximately 75% of E_1 is secreted directly by the ovary and the adrenal with the remainder arising

TABLE 7–1.

Mean Serum Concentrations of Estrone, Estradiol, and Progesterone in Females*†

Age	Estrone (ng/dL)		Estradiol (ng/dL)		Progesterone (ng/dL)	
	Mean	Range	Mean	Range	Mean	Range
5–7 days	1.2	0–2.0	1.0	0–3.2		
8–60 days	1.2	0–2.0	1.5	0–5.0		
2–12 mo	1.0	0–1.6	1.1	0–7.5		
1–4 yr	3.0	1.9–4.6	1.1	0–2.0		
4–8 yr	2.7	1.7–4.4	0.5	0–1.7	5	3–23
8–10 yr	4.6	3.1–7.0	0.5	0–3.1	6	3–32
10–12 yr	4.4	2.8–6.8	1.6	0–6.3	8	3–55
12–14 yr	5.9	3.7–14	4.2	0.5–12.2	37	10–450
14–16 yr	8.9	2.1–14	8.6	1.0–25.2	189	5–1400
16–18 yr	6.7	1.4–14	8.4	1.0–28.4	161	23–1500

*Data from Winter JSD: Prepubertal and pubertal endocrinology, in Falkner F, Tanner JM (eds): *Human Growth*. New York, Plenum Press, 1979.
†Clinicians should obtain age-appropriate reference ranges for each hormone from their laboratory.

TABLE 7–2.

Mean Serum Concentrations of Estrone, Estradiol, and Progesterone in Males*

Age	Estrone† (ng/dL)		Estradiol† (ng/dL)		Age	Progesterone‡ (ng/dL)	
	Mean	Range	Mean	Range		Mean	Range
5–7 days	1.2	0–2.0	1.9	0–2.3	Cord blood	83,800	30,000–137,600
8–60 days	1.3	0–2.4	1	0–3.1	1 day	1,250	0–3,250
2–12 mo	1.0	0–1.6	1	0–1.9	7 days	50	0–130
1–4 yr	3.0	1.8–5.3	1	0–2.7	Prepubertal	13	
4–8 yr	2.9	1.7–4.8	0.5	0–0.9	9–11 years	34	10–58
8–10 yr	3.3	2.0–5.4	0.5	0–1.1	12 years	40	12–68
10–12 yr	3.2	2.1–4.9	0.5	0–1.5	13 years	33	5–61
12–14 yr	2.7	1.7–4.4	1.0	0–2.5	14 years	34	14–52
14–16 yr	3.9	2.1–7.0	1.5	0–2.4	15–18 years	56	0–124
16–18 yr	4.6	2.5–7.0	1.8	0.9–3.0			

*Clinicians should obtain age-appropriate reference ranges for each hormone from their laboratory.

†Data from Winter JSD: Prepubertal and pubertal endocrinology, in Falkner F, Tanner ED (eds): *Human Growth*. New York, Plenum Press, 1979.

‡Data from Nichols Institute Reference Laboratories, San Juan Capistrano, Calif.

from peripheral conversion of androstenedione and dehydroepiandrosterone (DHA). In the male, the adrenal is the principal secretory organ for E_1; there is approximately a twofold rise in plasma levels during puberty.

In females, E_2 levels increase approximately sevenfold during puberty while in males there is approximately a twofold rise in plasma levels during puberty.

Free E_2 concentrations also increase at 8 to 12 years of age and are associated with increasing serum levels of FSH and LH although there may be no clinical evidence of secondary sexual maturation. In both sexes the percentage of free E_2 rises during stages 2 and 3 of sexual maturation. The percentage levels off in girls but continues to increase in boys in stages 4 and 5. The percentage of free E_2 is therefore higher in adolescent boys than girls during the late stages of sexual maturation.

Plasma E_2 levels rise steadily during puberty in females. During the menstrual cycle, E_2 levels rise to a peak in the late follicular phase, followed by a smaller peak in the early luteal phase (Fig 7–1). In the male, E_2 levels rise during puberty. Most of the E_2 arises from peripheral conversion of E_1, DHA, and androstenedione, but approximately 25% of E_2 is secreted directly from the testes.

Serum E_2 levels related to bone age, stage of breast and pubic hair development, and phases of the menstrual cycle have been published.[2]

Progesterone

Plasma progesterone levels remain at prepubertal values in premenarchal females even if secondary sexual development has occurred (Table 7–3).[57] Plasma levels do not change until after menarche (see Table 7–1). Levels during the 2 years after the onset of menarche are significantly higher than during the 2 years prior to menarche.[58]

In males, the serum progesterone level increases significantly during stages 4 and

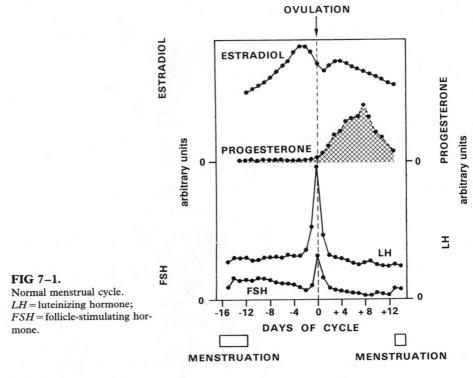

FIG 7–1.
Normal menstrual cycle.
LH = luteinizing hormone;
FSH = follicle-stimulating hormone.

TABLE 7–3.

Mean Serum Progesterone Concentrations in Males and Females*†

Age	Mean (ng/mL)	Range (ng/mL)
1 wk	0.20	0.03–2.13
2 wk–3 mo	0.34	0.03–0.99
3 mo–1 yr	0.24	0.03–1.26
1–3 yr	0.34	0.06–0.74
3–5 yr	0.20	0.03–0.95
5–7 yr	0.36	0.08–0.89
7–11 yr	0.10	0.03–0.96

*Data from Sippell WG, et al: *Pediatr Res* 1980; 14-39.
†Clinicians should obtain age-appropriate reference ranges for each hormone from their laboratory.

5 of sexual maturation (see Table 7–2).[58] Serum progesterone levels related to bone age, stage of breast development, and pubic hair growth and phase of the menstrual cycle are available.[2]

Effects of Estrogens and Progesterone

In the female estrogens are responsible for the growth and development of breasts; influence fat distribution; stimulate uterine, endometrial, and vaginal growth; and accelerate linear growth and skeletal maturation. Estrogens and gonadotropin interact synergistically in the ovary to effect development of the graafian follicle and subsequent ovulation. Estrogens also effect gonadotropin secretion, modulated through estradiol-binding protein receptors in the hypothalamus and pituitary gland. It is difficult to define progesterone concisely in terms of its physiologic effects since virtually none of its effects are exclusive. Progesterone becomes effective only after estrogen priming has occurred. Estrogens have mainly growth-stimulating effects, while the action of progesterone is directed more toward modification and differentiation. However, some growth must be present before progesterone can be effective.

MENARCHE

The age of menarche is not fixed but varies from population to population and changes with time. Physiologic puberty is initiated only after some unknown maturational process is completed in the central nervous system. The average age of menarche in North American girls is 12.5 years.[62] It is well known that most adolescent girls go through a length of time with irregular anovulatory cycles during the first 1 to 2 postmenarchal years. Progesterone is not secreted, because the corpus luteum is not formed and the endometrium is subjected to unopposed stimulation by estrogens which cause proliferative changes and increased vascularity.

DELAYED PUBERTY

Delayed puberty in girls may be considered to be present if breast development has not occurred by 13 years of age or if more than 5 years have elapsed between the beginning of breast development and menarche. Causes of delayed puberty are listed in Table 7–4. It is estimated to occur in 2% to 3% of adolescents. Constitutional delay in growth and pubertal development is the most common cause of delayed puberty, frequently is familial, and is more common in boys than in girls. The precise cause of constitutional delay in growth and pubertal development is not known, but most of the current evidence suggests that there is a physiologic delay in the maturation of the hypothalamic-pituitary-gonadal axis.[13] Constitutional delay in growth and pubertal development is a diagnosis of exclusion. The most difficult differential diagnosis lies in its distinction from isolated gonadotropin deficiency.

In most girls the diagnosis can be made from a detailed history, record of the patient's growth, physical examination, bone age radiographs, and a few selective laboratory studies (Table 7–5). The history should include the family history of times of onset and patterns of growth and sexual development, ability to smell (hyposmia or anosmia), and the presence of headaches or visual disturbances. Frequently, there is a family history of delayed onset of puberty. These girls are characterized by a growth pattern at or below the third percentile, but parallel to the third percentile.

TABLE 7–4.

Causes of Delayed Puberty in Girls

  I. Constitutional delay in growth and development
 II. Hypogonadotropic hypogonadism
     A. Central nervous system—hypothalamus/pituitary gland
        1. Congenital anomalies
        2. Tumors
        3. Postinflammatory
        4. Trauma
     B. Idiopathic and genetic forms of multiple pituitary hormone deficiencies
     C. Isolated idiopathic gonadotropin releasing-hormone deficiency
        1. Normal sense of smell
        2. Kallmann's syndrome
     D. Miscellaneous disorders
        1. Laurence-Moon-Biedl syndrome
        2. Prader-Willi syndrome
        3. Functional gonadotropin deficiency
           a. Chronic systemic diseases
           b. Anorexia nervosa
           c. Hypothyroidism
           d. Strenuous exercise
III. Hypergonadotropic hypogonadism
     A. Syndrome of gonadal dysgenesis and its variants (Turner's syndrome)
     B. Familial or sporadic XX and XY gonadal dysgenesis and its variants
     C. Other forms of primary ovarian failure
        1. Postbilateral oophorectomy
        2. Post-irradiation and post-chemotherapy for malignancies
        3. Autoimmune oophoritis
        4. Resistant ovary syndrome
        5. Toxic substances, e.g., galactose or its metabolites
     D. 17-Hydroxylase deficiency

TABLE 7–5.

Laboratory Tests in Some Causes of Delayed Puberty in Females*

	Hypogonadism		Hypogonadotropic Hypogonadism	
Tests	Constitutional Delayed Puberty	Gonadal Dysgenesis	Hypothalamic Abnormality	Pituitary Abnormality
Serum LH	N	↑	↓ /N	↓ /N
Serum FSH	N	↑	↓ /N	↓ /N
Serum estradiol	N	↓	↓ /N	↓ /N
Buccal smear	N	Abn	N	N
Karyotype	N	Abn/N	N	N
GnRH stimulation	N	↑ ↑	N	Abn
hCG stimulation	N	Abn	N	N
Clomiphene stimulation	N	N	Abn	Abn
Pubertal sleep-augmented LH secretion	N	N	0	0

*LH = luteinizing hormone; FSH = follicle-stimulating hormone; GnRH = gonadotropin-releasing hormone; hCG = human chorionic gonadotropin; N = normal; Abn = abnormal; ↑ = increased; ↑ ↑ = abnormally increased; ↓ = decreased; 0 = not present.

As the girls approach the age of puberty, however, their growth may deviate a little further away from the third percentile.

The bone age is delayed and is usually commensurate with the height age. Most patients with constitutional delay in growth and pubertal development have plasma dehydroepiandrosterone sulfate (DHEA-S) levels which are inappropriately low for their chronologic age but appropriate for their bone age.

Serum FSH and LH levels are usually in agreement with the bone age and the stage of sexual development and are therefore less than expected for the chronologic age. There may be difficulty in attempting to differentiate between normal and pathologically low serum gonadotropin levels by a single determination. Some studies have suggested that the GnRH stimulation test could be used to distinguish patients with constitutional delay in growth and pubertal development from those with isolated gonadotropin deficiency. Girls with delayed puberty and bone ages greater than 12 years have adult serum LH responses while patients with isolated gonadotropin deficiency have blunted or immature-type LH responses. However, the clinician should note that the LH response to GnRH may produce overlap values between prepubertal, hypogonadotropic, and early prepubertal patients and therefore the use of this test may be limited.[49] A GnRH agonist (nafarelin) stimulation test has recently been used and may be more sensitive in allowing differentiation between constitutional delay in growth and pubertal development and isolated gonadotropin deficiency in males. However, this test may not be as sensitive in females.[49]

The use of prolactin response to intravenous (IV) metoclopramide in combination with the GnRH test has been reported to allow distinction between patients with constitutional delay in growth and pubertal development and those with hypogonadotropic hypogonadism.[26] In the study of Lanes et al., all patients with constitutional delay in growth and pubertal development responded normally to both tests while patients with hypogonadotropic hypogonadism responded only to one or to neither of the tests.[26]

The following endocrine disorders may be necessary in the differentiation from constitutional delay of puberty: partial growth hormone deficiency, early hypothyroidism, gonadal dysgenesis, and hypogonadotropic hypogonadism. Growth hormone deficiency and hypothyroidism are discussed in Chapters 3 and 5, respectively.

The treatment of choice is to reassure the girl that she is normal and that with time normal female sexual maturation will occur. These girls should be reevaluated at approximately 6-month intervals for assurance that the diagnosis continues to be that of constitutional delay of puberty.

There are no absolute data that indicate that effective substitutional estrogen therapy in a girl with constitutional delay of puberty does not compromise her adult height. In addition, administration of estrogen or estrogen-progesterone combination therapy will further retard maturation of the hypothalamic-pituitary-ovarian axis. It would seem wise to reserve therapy only for the adolescent girl who has marked psychological disability resulting from the delayed onset of puberty. In this rare instance, ethinyl estradiol, 5 μg/day orally, will induce growth acceleration and breast development.[8] Treatment is continued until stage 3 of breast development has occurred, which may take approximately 1 year.

HYPOGONADOTROPIC HYPOGONADISM

The secretion of gonadotropins may be decreased owing to abnormalities of either the hypothalamus or the pituitary. Hypogonadotropic hypogonadism may be familial or occur sporadically. Familial hypothalamic hypogonadotropic hypogonadism is probably transmitted as an autosomal dominant trait with variable expressivity. Inhibition of synthesis and release of GnRH may result from congenital anomalies, neoplasms, inflammatory disorders, or trauma to the hypothalamus. Familial hypogonadotropic hypogonadism may occur in association with several syndromes, such as Kallmann's syndrome, Laurence-Moon-Biedl syndrome (mental retardation, polydactylism, obesity, retinitis pigmentosa, nerve deafness, short stature, and diabetes insipidus), and the Prader-Willi syndrome.

Kallmann's syndrome consists of a triad of hyposmia or anosmia, hypogonadism, and color blindness. The histologic findings at autopsy have been olfactory bulb aplasia, normal pituitary glands, and hypoplasia of the hypothalamus. Evaluation of anterior pituitary function is normal except for the presence of low baseline gonadotropin levels. GnRH stimulation studies suggest there is a hypothalamic GnRH deficiency.[59] Females who have not previously received exogenous gonadotropins have immature ovaries. The only distinctive characteristic in Kallmann's syndrome may be some degree of anosmia. It has been suggested that the best compound to use to test for the sense of smell is phenylethylmethylcarbinol.

The major features of the Prader-Willi syndrome are neonatal hypotonia, mental retardation, short stature, hypogonadism, and marked obesity. Most of the studies of the hypogonadism in the Prader-Willi syndrome suggest that the basic defect is in the hypothalamus. However, recent studies suggest that the hypogonadism is due to combined hypothalamic and primary gonadal abnormalities.[22]

Isolated gonadotropin deficiency occurs as a heterogeneous syndrome. On the basis of the response to GnRH, three groups may be distinguished: (1) FSH and LH release after GnRH; (2) inconsistent release of LH only after GnRH; and (3) failure of release of FSH or LH after GnRH. In isolated gonadotropin deficiency there are no distinctive clues other than delay or absence of puberty. Only with the passage of time and the eventual normal appearance of all stages of pubertal development can constitutional delay in growth and puberty be definitely distinguished from isolated gonadotropin deficiency.

Hyperprolactinemia due to pituitary macro- or microadenomas may cause delayed puberty[20] and may or may not be associated with galactorrhea or any symptoms of pituitary dysfunction. It is therefore necessary to measure serum prolactin levels in females with delayed puberty. A pituitary lesion may not be detected in the patient with hyperprolactinemia. If a demonstrable pituitary lesion is not present, other causes of hyperprolactinemia must be ruled out. These include lesions in the hypothalamus or pituitary stalk, the empty sella syndrome, hypothyroidism, and drugs such as neuroleptics, antihypertensives, dopamine receptor antagonists, and antidepressants.[39] The mechanism by which hyperprolactinemia causes delayed puberty is most likely multifactorial. Elevated prolactin levels probably inhibit hypothalamic release of GnRH and cause decreased pituitary responsiveness to GnRH.

Females with anorexia nervosa have delayed onset of puberty and evidence of estrogen deficiency secondary to hypothalamic dysfunction.

There may be a significant delay in onset of puberty and menarche in girls with intensive premenarchal athletic training. In ballet dancers menarche was reported to occur at a mean age of 15.4 ± 1.9 years, which was significantly later than in age-matched controls (12.5 ± 1.2 years).[68] The combination of low percent body fat, high energy output, and stress are factors predisposing female athletes to menstrual dysfunction.

Females with hypogonadotropic hypogonadism have serum gonadotropins and E_2 levels which are prepubertal or inappropriately low for the stage of sexual development. Tests which may be used in the differential diagnosis are listed in Table 7–5. The pubertal increased secretion of LH with sleep and the clomiphene test after midpubertal development is reached are of aid when they are normal. If either test shows a normal response, hypogonadotropic hypogonadism is ruled out; if there is no response the possibility of hypogonadotropic hypogonadism still remains.

Therapy

Recent advances in transsphenoidal microsurgery have made the surgical removal of microadenomas causing hyperprolactinemia a procedure with low morbidity. Medical therapy with dopamine agonist drugs, which are potent inhibitors of prolactin secretion, effectively lower serum prolactin levels. Bromocriptine mesylate (Parlodel) and pergolide mesylate have been used to treat hyperprolactinemic syndromes. A multicenter study compared the effects of bromocriptine mesylate and pergolide mesylate in the suppression of prolactin secretion in patients with and without pituitary tumors

TABLE 7–6.

Gonadal Dysgenesis

Gonads	External Genitalia and Internal Duct System	Stature	Karyotype	Syndrome
Bilateral streaks	Female	Short	45,X and variants	Turner's
	Female	Normal or short	45,X/46,XX and variants	Turner's
	Clitoromegaly, female	Normal or tall	46,XY	Pure gonadal dysgenesis or Swyer's
	Female	Normal or tall	46,XX	Pure gonadal dysgenesis
Bilateral hypoplastic ovaries	Female	Short	45,X	Turner's
	Female	Normal or short	45,X/46,XX and variants	Turner's
Streak + ovary	Female	Normal or short	45,X/46,XX and variants	Turner's
	Female: vas deferens usually present with testis	Short	45,X/46,XY and variants	Mixed gonadal dysgenesis
Streak + testis	Ambiguous Male: rare			

and concluded that both dopamine agonists were effective and neither appeared to be superior to the other.[3]

In girls with functional gonadotropin deficiency, the primary disorder should be treated and female sex steroid therapy should not be prescribed unless absolutely necessary.

Girls with gonadotropin deficiency may be treated with oral ethinyl estradiol 0.02 to 0.1 mg/day for the first 21 days of each month. Medroxyprogesterone 10 mg/day is given from the 14th through the 21st day of each month.

HYPERGONADOTROPIC HYPOGONADISM

Syndrome of Gonadal Dysgenesis and Its Variants

In 1938 Turner described a syndrome in seven women consisting of sexual infantilism, short stature, webbed neck, and cubitus valgus.[66] The sexual infantilism was due to rudimentary streak gonads, and Grumbach et al.[14] used the term *gonadal dysgenesis* to describe the syndrome. It was subsequently determined that the typical patient with Turner's syndrome was missing one sex chromosome: 45,X.

Gonadal dysgenesis represents a wide spectrum of clinical phenotypes, gonadal structures that include the presence of at least one streak gonad and a variety of X chromosome abnormalities and mosaicism[64] (Table 7–6). Turner's syndrome is the best-known form of gonadal dysgenesis. The eponym should probably be restricted to those patients with the phenotype described by Turner: streak gonads or hypoplastic ovaries and an absent or abnormal X chromosome. Turner's syndrome occurs in 1 in 3,000 live female births.[64] Approximately 98% to 99% of pregnancies with Turner's syndrome abort spontaneously and approximately 10% of fetuses from pregnancies that have spontaneously aborted have Turner's syndrome.

The most common chromosomal anomaly in Turner's syndrome is a 45,X karyotype. The most common mosaic karyotype is 45,X/46,XX, which has been estimated to be present in 10% to 15% of patients while 2% to 5% of patients are estimated to be 45,X/46,XY mosaics.[64] Mosaicism may be demonstrated on culture of peripheral leukocytes alone in some patients. In others, cultures of skin or gonadal streak fibroblasts may be necessary, in addition to blood studies, to demonstrate mosaicism. The most important reason to determine if mosaicism is present is to identify those patients with a Y chromosome who are at risk for development of gonadoblastomas in their gonadal streak.[71] Gonadoblastomas develop in a high percentage of 45,X/46,XY patients in early childhood, thereby warranting removal of the streak gonads during preschool years. Dysgerminoma may occur in patients with 45,X karyotype and no Y chromosome, but occurs mainly in patients with 46,XY or mosaic karyotypes.[56]

Patients with a 45,X karyotype have been found to have normal or near-normal gonadal histology up to the fourth month of gestation. Thereafter, impaired maturation and accelerated degeneration of gonadocytes progress to a point at which the ovary consists of stromal connective tissue without any follicles. It has been postulated that regressive vascular changes occur causing atrophy and cicatrization of the gonad leading to the formation of a streak gonad. However, an occasional patient with a 45,X karyotype may have degenerated germ cells and atretic follicles present. It has also been suggested that the ovarian defect in Turner's syndrome results from the absence of genetic material on the X chromosome and is one of deficient maintenance of the endowment of primordial follicles and ova.

Short stature is almost a consistent finding in Turner syndrome, the cause of which is most likely multifactorial. The short stature of adults with Turner syndrome appears to be due to intrauterine growth retardation, to a gradual decline in height velocity in childhood, to the absence of a pubertal growth spurt, and to end organ resistance resulting from skeletal dysplasia.[37] Patients with Turner syndrome have abnormal body proportions characterized by markedly shortened lower extremities. The ultimate heights in published series range between 142.0 and 146.8 cm. Most clinicians have found no significant difference in the final heights between girls with 46,X karyotypes and those with other karyotypes. However, one group of investigators have repeatedly found greater adult heights in patients with 45,X karyotype compared with all other karyotypes. Familial height may play a role in determining the ultimate height in girls with Turner syndrome. Growth charts for Turner syndrome patients have been published.[34]

Girls with Turner syndrome may have the following physical findings: congenital lymphedema, low posterior hairline, webbed neck, prominent ears, high arched palate, micrognathia, broad chest, cubitus valgus, multiple pigmented nevi, abnormal fingernails, intestinal telangiectasia, and hypoplastic nipples. Cardiovascular anomalies are not unusual and the most frequent clinically recognized lesion is coarctation of the aorta. Coarctation of the aorta may be associated with aneurysmal dilatation of the aortic sinuses and ascending aorta, and with dissection of the aorta, and these combinations of lesions have occurred in Turner syndrome. Other abnormalities include hypertension, aortic valvular stenosis, partial anomalous pulmonary venous drainage, and mitral valve prolapse. Based on the echocardiographic study, isolated nonstenoic bicuspid aortic valve may be the most common cardiovascular lesion in Turner syndrome.

The webbed neck appears to result from in utero persistence of embryonic lymph sacs with resultant severe lymphedema. This usually resolves after birth, leaving redundant folds of skin. Patients who are mosaics for Turner syndrome appear to have fewer phenotypic stigmata, and patients with isochromosome of the short arm of the X chromosome often appear phenotypically normal. In general, the loss of the short arm (p) of the X chromosome appears to be most frequently associated with phenotypic findings of Turner syndrome.

Mosaic forms of gonadal dysgenesis are seen in female adolescents with primary amenorrhea and in young women with premature ovarian failure. It is estimated that 3% to 8% of 45,X karyotype patients and 12% to 21% of females with sex chromosome mosaicism may have normal pubertal development and spontaneous menstrual periods. Pregnancies have occurred in patients with 45,X and 45,X/46,XX karyotypes.

There is an increased frequency of chronic lymphocytic thyroiditis, and diabetes mellitus or carbohydrate intolerance. The impaired glucose tolerance may be due in part to decreased binding of insulin to specific erythrocyte receptors. Patients with Turner syndrome are prone to keloid formation. The prevalence of mental retardation appears to be no greater than that in the general population. However, many patients have a specific deficit in spatial ability and frequently exhibit both gross and fine motor dysfunction.

Laboratory Findings

The buccal smear is chromatin-negative and the sex chromosome karyotype is 45,X in the patient with classic Turner syndrome. Patients with mosaic sex chromosome karyotypes may have a chromatin-positive buccal smear. Culture of skin or other tissue fibroblasts may be necessary to demonstrate the presence of mosaicism.

Studies of serum growth hormone and insulin-like growth factor I (IGF-I) levels have yielded conflicting results. Patients with Turner syndrome are less likely to have a marked response to pharmacologic stimulation of growth hormone secretion. Serum IGF-I concentrations are usually at the lower end of the normal range, but increase with age. A study of 24-hour growth hormone secretion found very little difference in secretion in young patients when compared with normal controls.[50] However, in older girls with Turner syndrome, significantly less growth hormone was secreted when compared with normal controls.

Serum gonadotropin levels follow the diphasic curve of normal children but the concentrations in patients with Turner syndrome are elevated, with FSH levels being higher than LH levels.[6] Patients between birth and 4 years of age have gonadotropin concentrations that are four to ten times those of normal girls. Gonadotropin levels are usually low in all girls during midchildhood (4–9 years), even in patients with gonadal dysgenesis; therefore, serum gonadotropin levels may not be indicative of gonadal failure in this age group. At puberty the gonadotropins rise to markedly elevated levels characteristic of primary hypogonadism. The LH and FSH response to GnRH is elevated in the first 4 years and again after 9 years of age. However, between 4 and 9 years the response is closer to normal.

The bone age is retarded. Other radiographic manifestations of Turner's syndrome may be present. A positive metacarpal sign, consisting of shortening of the fourth metacarpal relative to the third and especially to the fifth, may be present. Characteristic changes in the knees consisting of enlargement and deformity of the medial tibial condyle have been reported. These are usually bilateral and symmetric. Osteoporosis may be seen and the pathologic findings are similar in several aspects to those found in primary or postmenopausal osteoporosis.

It has been suggested that renal anomalies occur in approximately one-third of girls with Turner syndrome, with monosomic patients at greatest risk.[32] The most common anomalies have been horseshoe kidney, embryologic malformation of the metanephros, and abnormalities in migration. The high frequency of renal abnormalities warrants the use of renal ultrasonography in all patients with Turner syndrome at the time of diagnosis.

Pelvic ultrasonography has been used to determine the presence of either streak or nonstreak gonads. The presence of nonstreak ovaries suggests that some ovarian function may be present with subsequent pubertal development to some degree. Laparoscopy can also be used to demonstrate the presence of streak ovaries and the absence of normal ovarian tissue.

Diagnosis

There should be no problem in diagnosing girls with the classic stigmata of Turner syndrome. Turner syndrome should be strongly suspected in any adolescent girl with short stature, primary amenorrhea, with no breast development but who has stage 3 pubic hair growth. Gonadal dysgenesis should be ruled out in all short girls, girls with unexpected primary or secondary amenorrhea, and girls with lymphedema. The most important and confusing entity in the differential diagnosis of Turner syndrome is Noonan syndrome, discussed next. Chromosome karyotyping and serum gonadotropin determinations are indicated in the workup of suspected patients with Turner syndrome. Cardiac and renal evaluation is indicated if the diagnosis is substantiated.

Therapy

Different groups of drugs have been used in Turner's syndrome in an attempt to increase linear growth and adult height. Low-dose estrogen therapy (ethinyl estradiol, 50–150 ng/kg/day) increases height velocity during the first year of therapy, but accelerated bone maturation and breast development may occur. Anabolic steroids also increase height velocity but serious side effects may occur and there is controversy regarding their use.

Several studies have shown that therapy with recombinant human growth hormone (rhGH) given three times a week alone or in combination with androgens or estrogens improves height velocity and probably ultimate height. There is a suggestion that administering rhGH daily improves the growth response.[12] These early results suggest that growth velocity can be stimulated without compromising final height and supports the use of rhGH in these patients.[12]

Most patients with Turner's syndrome will require substitution female hormone therapy for development of secondary sex characteristics and menstruation. It has previously been mentioned that a small percentage of nonmosaic and a slightly higher percentage of mosaic Turner syndrome patients will have spontaneous menarche and menstrual periods and may not require therapy initially. Serum LH and FSH determinations may be useful before starting therapy to determine whether the ovaries are functioning adequately. If the ovaries are functioning adequately, substitution therapy should probably not be started. At age 10 years, those patients with functional ovaries would be expected to have serum gonadotropin levels appropriate for their age, whereas those without sufficient ovarian function will have markedly elevated gonadotropin levels.

The time of initiation of therapy varies with each patient. We begin therapy when the patient expresses concern about the onset of puberty, with consideration for the familial timing of the age of onset of puberty. Early estrogen therapy (11 years of age) does not seem to compromise the final height when compared with late therapy (15 years of age).

Various estrogenic and progestational agents and schedules have been used. The response to hormone therapy varies from patient to patient. A suitable course of therapy consists of oral ethinyl estradiol 0.02 mg/day for 6 months or until menstruation occurs. Thereafter the estrogen can be given on the first 25 days of each calendar month. Withdrawal bleeding usually occurs 3 to 5 days after estrogen is stopped. Oral progestational agents such as medroxyprogesterone 5 to 10 mg/day should be given from the 15th to 25th day of each month to improve breast development, cause coiling of the glands of the endometrium, and increase the vascularity of the stroma. If the menstrual response is poor or breast development is inadequate, the dose of each hormone may be increased.

We prefer ethinyl estradiol, but an equivalent dose of any other estrogen can be used in replacement therapy, with the exception of diethylstilbestrol. Diethylstilbestrol is contraindicated because of reports of patients with Turner syndrome who developed endometrial carcinoma after its prolonged use. Estrogens should not be prescribed alone for prolonged lengths of time since they may provoke endometrial hyperplasia which might ultimately lead to malignant changes. Endometrial adenocarcinoma has been reported in patients with Turner syndrome. All patients on long-term exogenous female hormone therapy require periodic gynecologic examinations. Estradiol administered by a transdermal therapeutic system may soon be used in some patients in place of orally administered estradiol.

Patients with Turner syndrome have a high risk of developing neoplasms arising from the rudimentary streak gonads. This is another reason why these patients should be examined gynecologically at specific intervals. Periodic anteroposterior pelvic radiographs have been recommended, looking for calcification in the region of the rudimentary streaks. The gonadoblastoma, which characteristically undergoes calcification, is a common tumor which occurs in gonadal streaks. These neoplasms can be seen on the radiograph before they are palpable. The other common tumor is the dysgerminoma. If a mass is palpable or calcification is seen on x-ray film, surgical exploration is indicated and the streaks should be removed. Recently, laparoscopic gonadectomy has been used instead of exploratory laparotomy.

Noonan Syndrome

One aspect of Turner syndrome which has been difficult to explain has been the occurrence in males of features of the syndrome originally described in females. Also, normal female XX karyotypes have been described in some females with stigmata of Turner syndrome. It was appreciated that the clinical features in these cases differ from those found in patients with Turner syndrome and chromosomal abnormalities, and it is now accepted that they represent a separate entity, Noonan syndrome.[43]

The clinical findings in Noonan syndrome include hypertelorism, flat nasal bridge, ptosis of eyelids, low-set prominent ears, short or webbed neck, epicanthal folds, and cubitus valgus. The height is usually short. Males tend to have undescended or hypoplastic testes. Affected females usually have normal ovarian function although amenorrhea may occur. Congenital heart lesions are present in approximately 50% of patients. The most common cardiac lesion is pulmonary stenosis. Left ventricular disease may be present and echocardiography has been recommended for diagnosis since it is mostly unrecognized clinically. Moderate mental retardation may be present in contrast to Turner syndrome in which intelligence is generally normal.

The cause of Noonan syndrome is unknown and normal karyotypes have been reported in all cases.

XX AND XY GONADAL DYSGENESIS

Pure gonadal dysgenesis is a term applied to a heterogeneous group of disorders in phenotypic females with either XX or XY karyotypes, normal genitalia, normal müllerian duct development, bilateral streaked gonads, absent or poorly developed secondary sexual development, and primary amenorrhea.[55] In order to make an accurate diagnosis, the bilateral streak gonad must be verified histologically and karyotyping must be performed.

XX Gonadal Dysgenesis

These phenotypic females have a 46,XX karyotype, normal height, a eunuchoid habitus, absent or poorly developed secondary sexual characteristics, and primary or secondary amenorrhea.[1] The streak gonad is identical to that seen in Turner syndrome. The condition occurs either sporadically or in an autosomal recessive pattern. This syndrome is rarely recognized prepubertally. The patients are usually seen because of lack of secondary sexual development and primary amenorrhea. Clitoral enlargement is not present although hirsutism due to androgen production by the streak gonads has been reported. Serum FSH and LH levels are increased. Therapy is with the use of estrogen-progesterone preparations.

XX gonadal dysgenesis is distinguished from the testicular feminization syndrome and other forms of pure gonadal dysgenesis by the presence of a 46,XX karyotype. XX gonadal dysgenesis is further differentiated from isolated gonadotropin deficiency by the elevated FSH and LH levels and the presence of streak gonads. Karyotyping is essential to rule out X/XX mosaicism.

XY Gonadal Dysgenesis (Swyer Syndrome)

In 1955 Swyer described two phenotypic women with gonadal dysgenesis without stigmata of Turner syndrome.[63] The usual characteristics of this syndrome include bilateral streak gonads, normal or tall stature, sexual infantilism, female external and internal genitalia, a chromatin-negative buccal smear, and a 46,XY karyotype. Anomalies of ectodermal and mesodermal structures may be present. Clitoromegaly and postpubertal virilization may occur. Sexual infantilism usually persists without therapy but a patient has been reported with well-developed secondary sex characteristics. XY gonadal dysgenesis can be familial. Plasma LH and FSH levels are elevated.

The presence of a Y chromosome in these patients predisposes them to neoplastic changes in their streak gonads. The most common tumors are dysgerminoma and gonadoblastoma. The gonads should be removed as soon as possible as gonadal neoplasms have occurred in patients as young as 3 years of age.[35] Estrogen and progesterone therapy is given at the time of puberty.

Mixed Gonadal Dysgenesis

The term *mixed gonadal dysgenesis* has been proposed to describe patients with asymmetric gonadal differentiation consisting of a streaked gonad on one side and a dysgenetic testis on the contralateral side.[54] Normal müllerian structures are present. These patients may or may not have the somatic stigmata of Turner's syndrome, including short stature. The external genitalia are always masculinized to varying degrees and clitoral enlargement is a frequent finding. A chromatin-negative buccal smear has always been found in these patients, and XO/XY mosaicism is the most common cytogenetic abnormality.

Clitoroplasty or clitorectomy is indicated at an early age.[64] The presence of the Y chromosome predisposes the streaked gonad to neoplastic changes and surgical removal is indicated. The seminoma-dysgerminoma is the most common tumor in the streaked gonad. The dysgenetic testis is prone to neoplastic transformation and should also be removed. Estrogen and progesterone replacement should be started near the age of menarche.

OVARIAN DYSFUNCTION FOLLOWING TREATMENT OF MALIGNANCIES

Chemotherapy and radiotherapy as treatment for pediatric neoplastic diseases have significantly increased children's and adolescents' survival of various malignancies. Late endocrine sequelae of such therapies have increased as the patients live longer and, in girls, one of these is ovarian failure. The ovary may be damaged directly by irradiation or by certain cytotoxic drugs.[53] Cytotoxic chemotherapy causes inhibition of follicular maturation rather than depletion of primordial follicles and is therefore associated with reversible rather than permanent functional changes. Secondary ovarian failure may occur as a result of gonadotropin deficiency or hyperprolactinemia following cranial irradiation therapy.

AUTOIMMUNE OOPHORITIS

It is important to recognize autoimmune oophoritis because it may coexist with or precede other unsuspected autoimmune diseases. Evidence for an autoimmune cause includes histologic changes; presence of circulating antiovarian antibodies; association with other autoimmune disorders; and resumption of menstruation in some patients after therapy with glucocorticoids.[7,52] Ovarian biopsy in autoimmune oophoritis usually shows lymphocytic and plasma cell infiltration around developing cystic and atretic follicles.[52] Autoimmune oophoritis may be associated with either primary or secondary amenorrhea.

RESISTANT OVARY SYNDROME

A rare syndrome in which delayed pubertal development or primary amenorrhea, or both, are present is the resistant ovary syndrome.[23] Criteria for the diagnosis of this syndrome include (1) hypersecretion of gonadotropins; (2) presence of numerous primordial follicles on ovarian biopsy, a few of which progress to the antral stage, but almost none progressing further; and (3) hyporesponsiveness of the ovaries to exogenous stimulation with human menopausal or pituitary gonadotropin. The cause of this syndrome is not known. The most widely accepted hypothesis at the present time is that there is a defect in the FSH receptor protein.

17-HYDROXYLASE DEFICIENCY

Deficiency of 17-hydroxylase results in a decreased synthesis of all glucocorticoids and sex steroids and increased secretion of mineralocorticoids. Hypertension and hypokalemic alkalosis are present. Females have sexual infantilism and primary amenorrhea because 17-hydroxylase is necessary for synthesis of estrogen and androgen in the ovary and adrenal gland.

Laboratory studies show decreased production of glucocorticoids and sex steroids, elevated levels of corticosterone and deoxycorticosterone, and elevated levels of gonadotropins.

Therapy is with glucocorticoid and estrogen replacement. This will correct the hypertension and hypokalemia and induce feminization.

TOXIC SUBSTANCES

Hypergonadotropic hypogonadism may occur in females with galactosemia.[16] A high incidence of ovarian failure occurs most likely secondary to the toxic effects of galactose or its metabolites on the ovarian parenchyma.

MENSTRUAL DISORDERS

Menstrual irregularities in the adolescent are very common following menarche. The spectrum includes dysfunctional uterine bleeding, oligomenorrhea, and amenorrhea.

Dysfunctional Uterine Bleeding

Dysfunctional uterine bleeding (DUB) is defined here as abnormal bleeding not due to pathologic changes in the genital tract or to systemic disease and anovulatory. In anovulatory DUB, unopposed production of estrogen leads to excessive stimulation of the endometrium, with periodic breakdown and bleeding. Most pubertal episodes are self-limited. However, anemia may be severe. Iron therapy may be given and the patient reassured if anemia is not present.

The management of severe episodes of DUB requires (1) arrest of the bleeding and (2) the prevention of recurrence and restoration of cyclic menstruation. Uterine curettage is rarely indicated during adolescence as a method of stopping bleeding. Hormonal therapy is the treatment of choice in adolescents with anovulatory DUB. Several good reviews of DUB have recently been published.[40] Hormonal therapy in the form of an estrogen-progestin combination is the treatment of choice.

Adolescents with severe episodes of DUB should be followed indefinitely since a significant percentage of them will have recurrent problems. Those patients who have established normal menses before the dysfunctional episodes do better than those who have DUB from the onset. Decreased fertility is anticipated in those females with persistent problems.

Oligomenorrhea

Oligomenorrhea may be defined as the occurrence of one to six menstrual periods per year in a female at least 2 years post-menarche. Oligomenorrhea may occur at times of stress but may also be caused by endocrine abnormalities including polycystic ovary syndrome, adrenal hyperplasia, hypothyroidism, hyperprolactinemia, Cushing's disease, premature ovarian failure, and adrenocortical insufficiency. Each of these causes, except for the ovarian causes, is discussed elsewhere in this book.

Therapy of oligomenorrhea is treatment of the specific abnormality causing the oligomenorrhea. Infrequent menstrual periods occurring during the first 2 to 3 years following menarche should not be treated with estrogen-progestin preparations if at all possible. Since the usual cause of infrequent menstrual periods during these years is physiologic immaturity of the hypothalamic-pituitary-ovarian axis, administration of such therapy will only further suppress hypothalamic function, which may be irreversible. The preferred therapy is reassurance and reevaluation at specific intervals.

Primary Amenorrhea

Primary amenorrhea may be defined as the failure of menarche to occur by 16 years of age. Primary amenorrhea may be due to delayed onset of puberty, an endocrinopathy, or a congenital defect in the development of the genital tract. A careful gynecologic examination must be performed to exclude the last possibility.

Before proceeding on a complicated and expensive evaluation of a patient with primary amenorrhea, pregnancy must be ruled out. In the investigation of primary amenorrhea, it must be stressed that most of the conditions listed in Table 7–5 as causes of delayed onset of puberty can also cause primary amenorrhea. Therefore, many of the diagnostic steps used in evaluation of delayed onset of puberty are also used in the workup of girls with primary amenorrhea. I will not discuss again the specific diagnostic steps used. A clear indication of the probable lesion can often be obtained from the clinical features. It is helpful to divide patients into three categories:

those showing good secondary sexual development, those with poor or absent sexual development, and those showing heterosexual development. The more common possibilities are listed in Table 7–7.

Primary Amenorrhea With Good Secondary Sexual Development

In this category it is likely that an anatomic abnormality is present. Careful examination to determine the presence and patency of the vagina should be undertaken. If an imperforate hymen is present, there are likely to be associated symptoms of lower abdominal pain and urinary difficulty. A lower abdominal swelling may be present and on rectal examination a distended vagina may be felt.

If the vagina or uterus, or both, are presumably not present, a pelvic ultrasound study and buccal smear should be obtained. If the buccal smear is chromatin-negative, complete androgen insensitivity (testicular feminization) is the most likely diagnosis. These patients have a blind vagina without a cervix or uterus. This syndrome is discussed in Chapter 8.

If the buccal smear is positive, the most likely diagnosis is congenital absence of the vagina or uterus, or both. Pelvic examination and pelvic ultrasonography will reveal the anatomic defect. Congenital absence of the vagina is a müllerian system developmental abnormality which has also been called the Mayer-Rokitansky-Küster-Hauser syndrome (MRKH syndrome). The MRKH syndrome was defined by Hauser et al.[17] as consisting of (1) absence of the vagina; (2) primary amenorrhea; (3) normal female secondary sex characteristics; (4) normal ovaries; (5) a uterus that may be normal, be a streak, or be absent; (6) normal female karyotype; and (7) frequent association with other anomalies, most commonly renal and skeletal anomalies.

The incidence of congenital absence of the vagina varies from 1 in 4,000 to 1 in 5,000 female births. It ranks *second* to gonadal dysgenesis as the most common cause of primary amenorrhea. Treatment may be surgical or nonsurgical.[10]

If a normal vagina and uterus are found in the female with a chromatin-positive buccal smear, the clinical evaluation may suggest the presence of gonadal dysgenesis. Laboratory studies should include sex chromosome karyotyping, and serum gonadotropin and prolactin determinations. Primary amenorrhea associated with hyperprolactinemia due to prolactin-secreting pituitary tumors has been reported.

TABLE 7–7.

Causes of Primary Amenorrhea

Physiological	Gonadal
Delayed onset of puberty	Pure gonadal dysgenesis
Pregnancy	Prepubertal ovarian failure
Anatomic	Resistant ovaries failure
Abnormalities of vagina	Testicular feminization syndrome
Müllerian duct developmental abnormalities	Functioning ovarian tumors
Acquired abnormality of the endometrium	Polycystic ovarian disease
Hypothalamic-pituitary	Hyperthecosis syndrome
Hypogonadotropic hypogonadism	True hermaphroditism
Suprasellar and intrasellar tumors	
Psychogenic	

Heterosexual Development.—Primary amenorrhea in a girl showing signs of defeminization and virilization suggest the following causes: virilizing disorder of the ovary or adrenal gland; male pseudohermaphroditism in the form of incomplete androgen insensitivity; or true hermaphroditism. A buccal smear and chromosome analysis are the initial studies required. Further studies depend on these results (Fig 7–2).

Isolated clitoromegaly in neonates may be due to congenital adrenal hyperplasia (CAH), androgen-producing tumors in the mother, or administration of androgens to the mother in the second or third trimester of pregnancy. A rare cause of isolated clitoromegaly occurring after birth in preterm female infants is the presence of high serum levels of 3β-OH-5-ene steroids produced by the fetal adrenal zone.[38] The steroids are mainly dehydroepiandrosterone (DHEA) and its metabolites.

True Hermaphroditism.—True hermaphroditism is extremely rare. There are no characteristic features that distinguish these patients clinically. The differentiation of the genital tract and the development of secondary sexual characteristics are very variable. All patients have some müllerian duct development, with a variable degree of virilization of the external genitalia. Most have chromatin-positive buccal smears and an XX sex chromosomal karyotype. A few cases have exhibited a variety of other karyotypes, mostly mosaic karyotypes. The histologic presence of both ovarian and testicular tissue is essential for the diagnosis of true hermaphroditism.

Secondary Amenorrhea

Secondary amenorrhea may be defined as absence of menses for at least 6 months after menarche has occurred. Causes of secondary amenorrhea in adolescent girls are listed in Table 7–8.

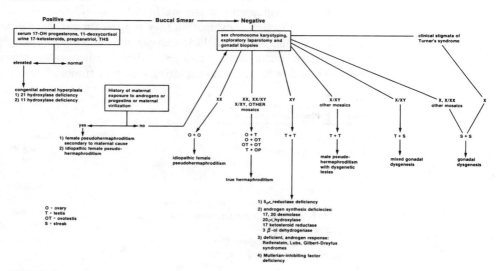

FIG 7–2.
A scheme for evaluation of abnormal sexual differentiation.

TABLE 7–8.

Causes of Secondary Amenorrhea in Adolescence

Hypothalamic-pituitary
Immaturity of hypothalamic-pituitary-ovarian axis
Hypothalamic oversuppression (post–oral contraceptive amenorrhea)
Psychological
Nutritional
Anorexia nervosa
Sudden massive weight gain
Organic diseases (trauma, tumors, toxic or infectious processes)
Ovarian
Tumors, estrogenic or androgenic
Gonadal dysgenesis
Premature ovarian failure
Uterine or vaginal defects (trauma or infections)
Systemic causes
Chronic illness
Metabolic or nonovarian endocrine disorders
Physiologic
Pregnancy

A thorough history and careful physical examination, including pelvic examination, should provide the diagnosis in many girls. In addition, obtaining a pregnancy test, radiographs of the sella turcica, thyroid function tests, and serum prolactin, FSH, and LH levels should allow the physician to make the diagnosis in the majority of patients.

The most common causes of secondary amenorrhea in adolescent girls are those thought to affect primarily hypothalamic-pituitary function. The diagnosis is frequently one of exclusion. The serum levels of FSH and LH in patients with hypothalamic types of amenorrhea are in the low-normal to low range, depending upon the severity of the process.

Galactorrhea-Amenorrhea

An unusual association in pediatrics is the occurrence of secondary amenorrhea and galactorrhea. The presence of this combination of findings should direct the physician's immediate attention to endocrinologic and neurologic evaluation of the pituitary gland. *Galactorrhea* may be defined as nonpuerperal or nonphysiologic lactation. Galactorrhea is not a disease entity in itself, but rather is a symptom of an underlying disorder. Amenorrhea is a frequent symptom of prolactin-producing microadenomas of the pituitary gland; therefore, determination of serum prolactin concentration is mandatory. Hyperprolactinemia associated with amenorrhea, with or without galactorrhea, represents a major disturbance of the hypothalamic pituitary system. Assessment of total anterior pituitary function is indicated.

The syndrome of nonpuerperal galactorrhea has eponymic designations that are often confusing (see Table 7–9). Both the Chiari-Frommel syndrome and del Castillo's syndrome imply that no organic lesion is present. When a pituitary lesion is demonstrated either initially or on follow-up, the eponym Forbes-Albright syndrome is used. Numerous reports emphasize that a lesion may become obvious only after

TABLE 7–9.

Syndromes of Amenorrhea and Nonpuerperal Galactorrhea

	Chiari-Frommel	del Castillo	Forbes-Albright
Onset	Post partum	Spontaneous	Post partum or spontaneous
Sella turcica	Normal	Normal	Enlarged
Duration	Usually transient	Usually permanent	Permanent

prolonged observation. These syndromes are seen mainly in adults, but cases have been reported in adolescent girls. Thyroid function studies should also be performed, as a syndrome of amenorrhea and galactorrhea due to hypothyroidism may be present.

Therapy for prolactin-secreting adenomas of the pituitary gland is discussed in Chapter 3.

Hypothalamic Oversuppression (Post–Oral Contraceptive Amenorrhea)

Many adolescent girls who have irregular menstrual periods have been placed on oral contraceptives to "regulate" them. Upon discontinuance of therapy, the result can be amenorrhea instead of regular cycles.[65] Endocrine studies have not revealed any consistent mechanism for the amenorrhea.

Psychogenic Causes

The menstrual irregularity and secondary amenorrhea that occurs in adolescent girls who have received emotional trauma is well known.

Nutritional Causes

Amenorrhea resulting from gross nutritional imbalance is similar in etiology to psychogenic amenorrhea. Anorexia nervosa is the condition which has been most frequently studied in this category and can be associated with delayed onset of puberty and either primary or secondary amenorrhea. Weight loss associated with injudicious dieting can result in hypothalamic dysfunction and secondary amenorrhea. Secondary amenorrhea may also occur in women who undertake chronic extensive exercise programs, particularly long-distance running. A high incidence of delayed puberty, and primary and secondary amenorrhea has been noted in young ballet dancers who restrict their food intake and are highly active. Simple weight loss is associated with primary or secondary amenorrhea when over 30% of body fat is lost.[69]

Low plasma FSH and LH levels are present but there is a normal release of FSH and LH after administration of GnRH. The 24-hour LH secretory pattern shows a regression to that found in prepubertal and pubertal children. Return of normal body weight causes a reversal to a LH secretory pattern seen in adult females and usually resumption of menses.

Organic Brain Disease

Intrasellar or suprasellar tumors of the pituitary gland may cause secondary amenorrhea.

Idiopathic hypogonadotropism has been discussed. It results mainly in primary amenorrhea, although an occasional patient may have secondary amenorrhea.

Ovarian Causes

Abnormalities of ovarian hormone production can produce menstrual abnormalities in several ways. Increasing amounts of estrogens can cause endometrial proliferation, and if the circulating level remains relatively constant, the endometrium may persist in a proliferative state for a long time. If the concentration of estrogen is decreased, then estrogen withdrawal bleeding occurs. If the concentration of estrogen remains unchanged, the persistent proliferative endometrium may partially slough, and breakthrough bleeding occurs.

Estrogen-secreting ovarian tumors such as granulosa cell tumors cause proliferation of the endometrium, and therefore amenorrhea, for months, as mentioned above. Estrogen-secreting tumors of the ovary are discussed later in this chapter.

Androgen-producing tumors of the ovary cause virilization. The differential diagnosis between an androgen-producing tumor, polycystic ovarian disease, and even late-onset adrenal hyperplasia may be extremely difficult at times and necessitate extensive laboratory evaluation. Androgen-producing tumors of the ovary are discussed later.

Uterine Defects

Severe infection of the endometrial cavity with its resultant obliteration, and the development of postcurettage synechiae (Asherman's syndrome) caused by overzealous curetting at the time of diagnostic studies can cause secondary amenorrhea. These are extremely uncommon causes of amenorrhea in the adolescent, but, nevertheless, they must be considered.

Nonovarian Endocrine Disorders

Thyroid disorders that can cause secondary amenorrhea include hypo- and hyperthyroidism. Clinical evaluation should provide the diagnosis. Appropriate laboratory studies include serum thyroxine (T_4) by radioimmunoassay (RIA), triiodothyronine (T_3) RIA, and TSH-RIA determinations.

Adrenal disorders include Addison's disease, Cushing's syndrome, and CAH. Again, careful clinical evaluation will provide the diagnosis in most patients. Laboratory studies which may be obtained to substantiate the clinical impression are discussed in Chapter 6.

CAH can cause secondary amenorrhea. Mild 21-hydroxylase deficiency can result in either primary or secondary amenorrhea.

Virilization occurs during childhood and typical plasma and urine steroid abnormalities are present, such as elevated urinary 17-ketosteroids and pregnanetriol and elevated serum 17-OH-progesterone levels (see Chapter 6).

The diagnostic features of the common causes of secondary amenorrhea have been enumerated but a brief outline of the general diagnostic approach seems warranted. The approach should be simple and clinical, progressing gradually to the more sophisticated procedures. The usual outline is presented below (not listed in order of importance):

1. Complete history and physical examination including pelvic examination
2. Pregnancy test if indicated
3. Serum FSH, LH, thyroid function studies, estrogens, progesterone, testosterone, 17-OH-progesterone, and 11-deoxycortisol determinations
4. Radiographs of the sella turcica
5. Twenty-four-hour urinary 17-ketosteroid, 17-hydroxycorticosterone, and THS determinations
6. Progesterone test
7. Estrogen-progesterone test

Progesterone Test.—A simple and easy test in the evaluation of secondary amenorrhea is the progesterone withdrawal test. Progesterone is given as a single 100-mg injection intramuscularly (IM), or medroxyprogesterone orally 10 mg twice a day is given for 4 days. If bleeding occurs following therapy (usually within 4–9 days), then one can conclude that the patient is not pregnant; that she has a functional endometrium; that she has an adequate amount of estrogen to "prime" the endometrium; that pituitary gonadotropins are present to stimulate the ovary; that GnRH is present; that the uterine cavity, cervix, and vagina are patent; and that her amenorrhea is probably due to a failure to ovulate (Fig 7–3).

If no withdrawal bleeding occurs, measurement of plasma FSH and LH is indicated. One must keep in mind that these values are subject to large variation and therefore a single value may not be significant.

Estrogen-Progesterone Test.—Patients who do not bleed after progesterone administration may be given estrogen with progesterone IM. Patients with a functional

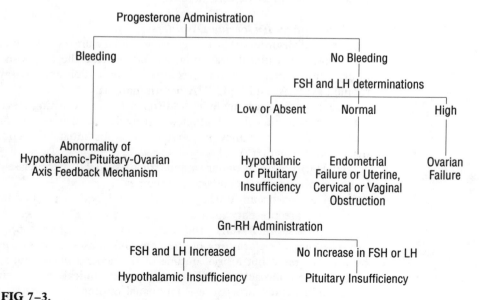

FIG 7–3.
Workup for secondary amenorrhea (pregnancy and ovarian tumors excluded). *FSH* = follicle-stimulating hormone; LH = luteinizing hormone; *Gn-RH* = gonadotropin-releasing hormone.

endometrium will bleed within 12 to 15 days after receiving the hormones. Failure to bleed after estrogen-progesterone therapy means endometrial failure (assuming the patient is not pregnant and cervical stenosis is not present).

Rarely, because of an ambiguity in test results, it is useful to test the potential normality of the hypothalamic-pituitary-ovarian axis. Clomiphene citrate can be administered, usually 100 mg/day for 5 to 10 days, with serum FSH and LH determined daily for 21 days. A rise in gonadotropins 2 or 3 days after the administration of clomiphene, and a subsequent fall followed by an ovulatory LH surge, is confirmation of a normal axis.

If no cause is found, the best therapy may be no therapy. The patient should be told that menses may be interrupted in normal girls under certain circumstances. However, she should be reevaluated at 9- to 12-month intervals for evidence of a previously occult disorder.

Polycystic Ovary Syndrome

In 1935 Stein and Leventhal[60] described a group of women with amenorrhea, infertility, obesity, hirsutism in most cases, and enlarged ovaries. This syndrome has been called the *Stein-Leventhal syndrome*. This syndrome has a wide spectrum since all, some, or only one of the originally described characteristics may be present in addition to the ovarian changes. There is, therefore, clinical and biochemical variability within this spectrum. During the past few years, the eponym Stein-Leventhal syndrome has been used infrequently and *polycystic ovary syndrome (PCOD)* has been adopted as the generic description for the broad spectrum of abnormalities in these females. PCOD may be familial. The cause(s) of PCOD has not been determined. Proposed mechanisms for the causation of PCOD include primary abnormalities of the hypothalamic-pituitary axis, the ovary, and the adrenal, and chronic hyperinsulinemia.

Most of the patients have a normal menarche and secondary sexual development but progressive hirsutism and obesity occur during the teenage years.[42] Virilization may rarely be present in premenarcheal girls. Occasionally, girls present with DUB at menarche. More often, anovulation, secondary amenorrhea, or oligomenorrhea occur. Frank virilization is rare during adolescence.

The ovaries may be enlarged and polycystic in the adolescent. It should be remembered that other hyperandrogenic states including androgen-producing tumors of the ovaries as well as some forms of CAH, may be associated with enlarged ovaries containing multiple subscapular follicles typical of PCOD.[42] Because of the difficulty in performing pelvic examination in obese adolescent girls, pelvic ultrasonography may be used to determine the presence or absence of enlarged polycystic ovaries. The adolescent with PCOD may have normal-sized ovaries. The tunica of polycystic ovaries is usually thickened and many small atretic follicles occupy the cortex. The follicles may be lined by a few layers of granulosa cells. The cells of the theca interna are swollen and the theca externa may be hyperplastic. Magnetic resonance imaging (MRI) has also been used in adolescents with PCOD and it has been suggested that it is more precise than sonography in defining the structure of lesions.

The serum hormonal profile usually demonstrates high pulsatile LH levels associated with normal or low levels of FSH, producing an elevated LH/FSH ratio. The 24-hour secretory pattern of LH has been studied in adolescent girls, 13 to 16 years of age, who had clinical and biochemical features of PCOD. The LH surge occurred in midday rather than nocturnally which is normal in the peripubertal period. It has been suggested that the primary defect in PCOD is at the level of the hypothalamus and that the repetitive positive feedback stimulating the ovarian theca to produce androgens in excess begins a cycle. The comparative deficiency of FSH has been attributed to either an inhibitory effect of the intraovarian androgens or to the high levels of inhibin produced by the ovarian follicles.

The formation of ovarian cysts, thecal hyperplasia, and other ovarian histologic changes are probably the effects of LH stimulation of ovarian follicular development. As a result of disordered follicular maturation, the ovary secretes abnormal levels of androgens.[36] Androgens of adrenal origin are also secreted in increased amounts. Increased ovarian secretion of androgens results in increased E_1 formation (by aromatization) which stimulates increased secretion of LH. The level of E_2 is usually low or normal.[36]

Twenty-four-hour profiles in adult females with PCOD of plasma LH, testosterone, and androstenedione concentrations have been found to be elevated, while concentrations of FSH, DHEA, androstenediol, and cortisol were similar to those seen in normal females. These studies demonstrate that the majority of Δ^5 androgens in PCOD are of adrenal origin while the preponderance of elevated testosterone and androstenedione is ovarian in origin. The cause of the increased levels of adrenal androgens has remained essentially unexplained. Serum ACTH levels in PCOD are normal. The increased serum levels of androgens are closely correlated with decreases in sex hormone–binding globulin and increases in free testosterone, androstenediol, and E_2. It has been suggested that the single most sensitive test for detecting PCOD is measurement of free testosterone before and after dexamethasone administration. The diagnosis is based on the presence of elevated serum free testosterone, which does not decrease after dexamethasone administration. The peripheral conversion of androstenedione to E_1 is correlated with body weight, especially adipose tissue. Elevated E_1 levels parallel androstenedione levels, reflecting peripheral estrogen synthesis.

Basal serum prolactin levels have been reported to be elevated in up to one-third of patients with PCOD. The hyperprolactinemia may be secondary to the elevated level of estrogens or androgens, or both, or may be the primary abnormality which gives rise to the abnormal gonadotropin release, chronic anovulation, and androgen excess. It has been suggested that patients with PCOD and hyperprolactinemia may have a relative deficiency of dopamine within hypothalamic nuclei.

Therapy

Ovarian wedge resection is infrequently used today because most patients respond to clomiphene citrate. Wedge resection of the ovaries in adolescent females is not recommended. Clomiphene citrate has been used for initiation of ovulation and has been recommended as therapy for adolescent girls. Other agents which have been used to induce ovulation include human chorionic gonadotropin (hCG)), human menopausal gonadotropin, and bromocriptine mesylate. Oral contraceptives and progestins have been used in the therapy of PCOD. These steroids interrupt the abnormal secretion of gonadotropins, thereby decreasing androgenic effects.

In PCOD, chronic stimulation of the endometrium by estrogen may produce endometrial hyperplasia, and adenocarcinoma of the endometrium has been reported in girls as young as 16 years of age. Consequently, an endometrial biopsy is advisable in adolescents with PCOD who have menometrorrhagia.

HYPERTHECOSIS OF THE OVARIES

The same clinical features described above for PCOD were later reported in women who had normal-sized ovaries with theca luteinization; this syndrome has been called the *hyperthecosis syndrome* or *hyperthecosis of the ovaries*. The characteristic histopathologic picture is clusters of luteinized cells scattered in hyperplastic ovarian stroma.[41] Patients with this syndrome may overlap both clinically and biochemically with PCOD but the patients with hyperthecosis of the ovaries may be virilized. Hyperthecosis of the ovaries can cause secondary amenorrhea and virilization in the adolescent. In contrast to PCOD in which a good response to clomiphene citrate therapy is expected, patients with hyperthecosis respond poorly, but patients occasionally respond to ovarian wedge resection.

PREMATURE OVARIAN FAILURE

The normal ovary has approximately 400,000 ova present at birth and this number declines gradually to virtually zero at the time of menopause. A decrease in the original number of follicles could result in premature menopause or premature ovarian failure (POF). POF is a syndrome consisting of the occurrence of menarche at a normal age followed by secondary amenorrhea, hypergonadotropinism, and hypoestrinism in females under 30 years of age. Two types of histopathologic pattern in POF have been described[25]: follicular and afollicular. The follicular type, the gonadotropin-resistant ovary syndrome, was discussed earlier. In the afollicular type of POF, there is premature attrition of follicles. The cause is unknown but it has been suggested that it may result from an autoimmune process. Studies have shown that 13% to 18% of patients with POF had an associated autoimmune disorder or detectable circulating autoimmune antibodies.[18] Circulating antibodies to human ovarian tissue have been demonstrated in some patients with POF using indirect immunofluorescence and by enzyme-linked immunosorbent assay (ELISA). Immunosuppressive therapy in some patients led to normalization of the menstrual cycle and pregnancy.

SEXUAL PRECOCITY

Isosexual Precocity

The onset of pubertal changes in a girl prior to 8 years of age is considered to constitute isosexual precocity. *True* isosexual precocity is due to mechanisms which cause premature activation of the hypothalamic-pituitary axis leading to increased circulating levels of gonadotropins. True isosexual precocity may be divided into cerebral and idiopathic causes. Pseudosexual precocity is due to nonpituitary gonadotropin causes of sexual precocity.

The differential diagnosis of isosexual precocity in girls is presented in Table 7–10. In the presence of well-defined central nervous system abnormalities, isosexual precocity is classified as the cerebral type. Tumors in or adjacent to the hypothalamus, pineal gland, or optic chiasm; hydrocephalus; congenital brain defects; postinfectious encephalitis; and craniopharyngioma have all been associated with the cerebral type of sexual precocity. In addition, neurofibromatosis and tuberous sclerosis have also been associated with sexual precocity.

The idiopathic type of isosexual precocity includes all patients in whom no central nervous system or gonadal abnormality is detected. The idiopathic group is the most common form of isosexual precocity. However a study utilizing cranial computed tomography (CT) in girls with "idiopathic" true sexual precocity suggest that the precocity is not idiopathic.[5] These investigators detected small hypothalamic masses in 33% of the girls. Most cases of isosexual precocity occur sporadically but there are familial cases. The incidence of idiopathic vs. cerebral types of true sexual precocity in girls is approximately 9:1. Serum concentrations of gonadotropin and E_2 have been studied during sleep in girls with idiopathic sexual precocity and nocturnal elevations of E_2 resulting from pituitary release of FSH and LH. The investigators suggest that there may be inappropriate timing of GnRH. Central isosexual precocity has followed

TABLE 7–10.

Differential Diagnosis of Isosexual Precocity in Girls

I. True sexual precocity
   A. Idiopathic
   B. Cerebral
      1. Tumors of central nervous system
      2. Congenital anomalies of central nervous system
      3. Trauma
      4. Postinfectious
      5. Specific syndromes
         a. Neurofibromatosis
         b. Tuberous sclerosis
         c. Silver's syndrome
         d. Hypothyroidism
         e. Congenital adrenal hyperplasia, belatedly or inadequately treated
II. Pseudosexual precocity
   A. Ovarian tumors
      1. Granulosa-theca cell tumors (Peutz-Jeghers syndrome)
      2. Granulosa-luteal and follicular cysts (McCune-Albright syndrome)
   B. Germ cell or gonadotropin-secreting tumors
   C. Feminizing adrenal tumors
   D. Iatrogenic
   E. Incomplete sexual precocity
      1. Premature thelarche
      2. Premature adrenarche
      3. Premature menarche

TABLE 7–11.

Laboratory Tests in Sexual Precocity in Girls*

	Serum				
	FSH	LH	Estrogens	Progesterone	Testosterone
True sexual precocity	4+	4+	2+ −4+	0−2+	1+
Gonadotropin-secreting tumor	0	4+	2+ −4+	0−1+	1+
Ovarian tumors					
Granulosa cell	0	0	1+ −4+	0	0
Granulosa-theca cell tumor, luteoma	0	0	1+ −4+	1+ −2+	0
Adrenal tumor	0	0	1+ −4+	0+ −1+	2+ −4+
Iatrogenic	0	0	0−1+	0	0

*FSH = follicle-stimulating hormone; LH = luteinizing hormone; 0 = normal for chronologic age.

cranial irradiation for therapy of brain tumors and after prophylactic cranial irradiation in acute lymphocytic leukemia.[30]

Sexual precocity may occur in girls with inadequately treated or late-treated CAH after proper glucocorticoid therapy is initiated and if the bone age has reached an approximate 13-year level (see Chapter 6).

Clinical Features

The most striking clinical feature of isosexual precocity is the presence of secondary sexual characteristics, but the sequence of their appearance may not, on occasion, follow the normal pattern. Sexual precocity is almost always associated with excessive linear growth and bone maturation which may result in short stature because of early epiphyseal fusion. However, in some girls normal linear growth continues with no reduction in predicted adult height. Menstruation can be the initial sign of sexual precocity. Ovulatory cycles can occur and fertility is usually normal. The patient may have psychological stress because of the sexual precocity (see Chapter 13).

Laboratory Findings

Plasma concentrations of FSH and LH are usually elevated (Table 7–11). However, the levels of LH and FSH may not be helpful in demonstrating idiopathic sexual precocity if they fall within the area of overlap. In fact, prepubertal levels of FSH and LH have been found in girls with sexual precocity. The determinations are useful although repeated serum levels may be necessary to document the presence of elevated values. Further, girls may demonstrate cyclic changes even before menarche and an initially low serum value may be higher if repeated shortly thereafter.[13]

Studies of the 24-hour LH, FSH, and E_2 concentrations and secretory patterns in patients with idiopathic sexual precocity have shown increased LH secretory activity that is synchronized with sleep similarly to that of normal pubertal girls but occurring earlier. GnRH stimulation causes marked LH release in girls with central sexual precocity in contrast to the minimal response in prepubertal girls.

Serum E_1 and E_2 and occasionally progesterone levels are elevated for the girl's chronologic age. There is also an increase in the mean free E_2 concentration. Urine 17-ketosteroid excretion is elevated for the patient's age. All laboratory values correlate better with the stage of sexual maturation and bone age than with chronologic age.

The bone age is advanced. Cranial CT or MRI should be performed in all girls suspected of having idiopathic sexual precocity. Pelvic ultrasonography can be of great help in differentiating the various forms of sexual precocity. Pubertal gonadotropin secretion characteristically results in a symmetric increase in ovarian volume, and the development of small follicular cysts in both ovaries causes a bilateral "multifollicular" pattern on ultrasonography. Ultrasonography is helpful in detecting an ovarian tumor or cyst as the cause of sexual precocity.

A vaginal smear or urocystogram may be helpful in confirming estrogenization and in following therapy.

Therapy of Idiopathic Central Isosexual Precocity

In the past, cyproterone acetate, medroxyprogesterone acetate, and danazol were used to treat central isosexual precocity. The treatment of choice at the present time is with long-acting synthetic agonist analogues of GnRH (GnRHa).[46] These agents stimulate release of LH and FSH and induce gonadotropin desensitization with continuous exposure to high concentrations in the pituitary. Desensitization depends on the potency of the GnRHa, and its bioavailability, frequency and method of administration, and rate of clearance. Some GnRHa given subcutaneously or intranasally is cleared very rapidly so that the pituitary is not completely suppressed. GnRHa suppresses release of LH and FSH, decreases E_2 levels to the prepubertal range, causes regression or lack of progression of breast development, and cessation of menstruation.[46] Daily subcutaneous injections of GnRHa can cause complete suppression of the pituitary-ovarian axis. Evidence of suppression can be obtained by demonstrating the failure of LH to increase when the pituitary is stimulated with GnRH or GnRHa. The assay used to measure LH should not measure alpha subunits, because alpha subunits continue to be released when LH and FSH are suppressed. Pelvic ultrasonography can be used to evaluate therapy since ovarian volume will decrease significantly with response to therapy.[51]

It has been suggested that not all girls with central sexual precocity require therapy. There is a group of girls that have slowly progressing sexual precocity and that can be identified when initially seen. These girls can be observed closely and therapy started if the sexual precocity accelerates. This group is characterized by having low plasma E_2 and somatomedin C levels and a normal or slightly advanced bone age, i.e., the bone age is less than 2 years advanced in comparison to the chronologic age.

Pseudosexual Precocity

Causes of pseudosexual precocity are listed in Table 7–10. The history has to exclude the possibility of exposure to oral estrogen preparations; geriatric multivitamins that contain estrogens; or to topical ointments, creams, or shampoos that contain estrogens. Breast development, pubarche, and menstruation may occur after prolonged exposure to these agents.

The incidence of ovarian tumors diagnosed before 16 years of age is approximately 1% to 2% of all ovarian tumors.[44] Ovarian tumors cause less than 10% of the cases of isosexual precocity in girls.[47] Granulosa cell tumors are the most common ovarian tumors causing isosexual precocity and less than 5% of them occur before the age of normal puberty. These tumors have distinctive microscopic and clinical features that differ from those of granulosa cell tumors in older women and have been termed *juvenile granulosa cell tumor*.[75] The precocity produced by these tumors may be rapid and striking. Vaginal bleeding without breast development or pubic hair growth may occur. The most frequent symptom is abdominal pain and the most frequent sign is a unilateral abdominal mass palpable on abdominal or rectal examination. Signs of puberty are due to excessive secretion by the tumor of estrogens or androgens, or both, and rarely progesterone or corticosteroids.

Laboratory Findings

The bone age is usually accelerated. Serum gonadotropins and progesterone are low while estrogens are moderately to markedly elevated[61] (see Table 7–11). Pelvic ultrasonography and MRI are valuable in detecting these tumors.

Therapy

Surgical removal of the tumor is the treatment of choice. The majority of tumors are benign but there is little correlation between the histologic picture and the degree of malignancy of any given granulosa cell tumor. Prognosis is good for localized tumors. Regression of sexual precocity occurs after removal of the tumor. These girls should be followed for a prolonged period of time because of the possibility of recurrence.

Ovarian growth and development have been studied fairly extensively by ultrasonography. Multiple small follicular cysts are not infrequently seen from birth through puberty[31] and surgical removal of these cysts is not indicated in every patient with cysts.

Ovarian follicular and luteal cysts may induce sexual precocity and the presence of an ovarian cyst is best confirmed initially by ultrasonography. Patients with central sexual precocity may have multiple small cysts (less than 10 mm) which are most likely gonadotropin-dependent. Ovarian follicular cysts are common in girls with sexual precocity. However, when a large ovarian cyst is detected, the possibility that pseudosexual precocity secondary to an autonomous functioning ovarian follicular cyst or a follicular cyst associated with McCune-Albright syndrome should be considered. Both of these entities are gonadotropin-independent. Clues as to whether the cysts are the cause or the result of sexual precocity may be found in the serum levels of FSH, LH, and estrogens.

If a cyst is considered to be the cause of pseudosexual precocity, a period of careful observation with repeat ultrasonographic examinations is reasonable, thereby reserving surgery as an option. Some of these cysts regress spontaneously with regression of signs of sexual precocity.[33] If the cysts continue to enlarge and signs of precocity progress, surgical removal is indicated. The suggestion has been made that ovarian IgG might cause development of these ovarian follicular cysts.[61] If the cyst is secondary to central sexual precocity, the use of a GnRHa might be appropriate.

The McCune-Albright syndrome was originally described as a triad of polyostotic fibrous dysplasia, café-au-lait pigmentation, and sexual precocity (Fig 7–4). Large

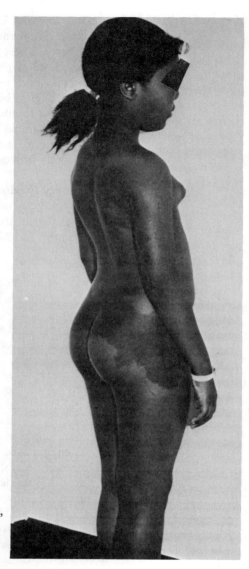

FIG 7–4.
An 8-year-old girl with McCune-Albright syndrome, showing sexual precocity and café-au-lait spots.

unilateral ovarian follicular cysts may be present and presumably are responsible for the sexual precocity. Recently other endocrine abnormalities have been described as part of the syndrome: autonomous endocrine hyperactivity including hyperthyroidism, Cushing's syndrome, hyperparathyroidism, and pituitary hypersecretion of growth hormone and prolactin. The sexual precocity is gonadotropin-independent. The skin hyperpigmentation may be absent or subtle in early childhood and the bony lesions may not be apparent on plain x-ray films early in life.[28]

The polyostotic fibrous dysplasia may involve any bone, but the femur and tibia are involved most frequently. Fractures are common. The skull may have hyperostotic lesions that produce frontal and occipital bulging (Fig 7–5). Obliteration of the sinuses, deafness, or blindness may arise as a consequence of the skull lesions.

Ovarian theca cell tumors may cause pseudosexual precocity. Peutz-Jeghers syndrome is a familial disorder consisting of isosexual precocity, mucocutaneous pigmentation, and intestinal polyposis (Fig 7–6). The secretion of estrogen is by a sex cord tumor which has a histologic appearance similar to that of granulosa–theca cell tumors.[74]

Feminizing adrenal tumors are rare causes of sexual precocity in girls and are discussed in Chapter 6.

Other rare causes of pseudosexual precocity are chorioepithelioma and hepatoma, which secrete gonadotropins, and detectable levels of the circulating beta subunit of hCG are present in the patient.

Incomplete Sexual Precocity

Premature thelarche is the appearance of breast development before the age of 8 years and is an isolated finding not accompanied by other signs of pubertal development (Fig 7–7). It may be present at birth.[21] The pathogenesis is controversial. The most

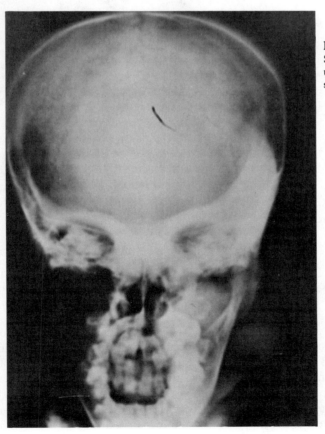

FIG 7–5.
Skull radiograph of patient in Figure 7–4, showing fibrous dysplasia.

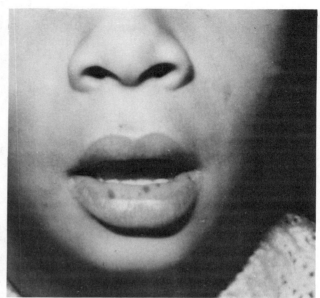

FIG 7–6.
A 7-year-old girl with Peutz-Jeghers syndrome with black-blue macules on lips and perioral area.

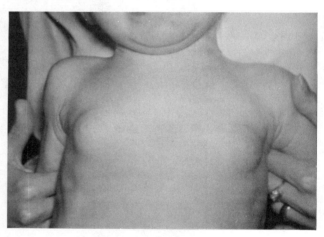

FIG 7–7.
An 18-month-old girl with premature thelarche.

widely accepted hypotheses include a defect in the maturation of the hypothalamic-pituitary-ovarian axis with higher-than-normal FSH secretion and increased peripheral sensitivity to the sex hormones.

The diagnosis of premature thelarche is made by exclusion of all causes of premature breast development, especially precocious puberty. Physical findings include increased height age and usually the presence of subareolar breast tissue of less than 4 to 5 cm diameter with no or little development of the areola or nipple. Breast development may be unilateral.

Most girls with premature thelarche have slightly elevated serum estradiol levels.[21] Basal levels of serum FSH and the response to GnRH are significantly higher than in normal controls. The serum LH response to GnRH is similar to that of prepubertal girls while the FSH response is similar to that of girls with isosexual precocity. Normal basal serum prolactin levels are present. The vaginal smear shows a slight but definite increase in estrinization as compared with normal controls. The bone age may be normal or slightly advanced.

The natural history of premature thelarche varies, but it is a benign condition. The breast tissue may disappear, persist without enlarging, or continue to enlarge. The changes may occur only on one side. Those girls in whom the breast tissue is present at birth and persists are more likely to have progressive enlargement. Premature thelarche does not appear to predispose to abnormalities in pubertal development, fertility, or breast neoplasia.[67]

Premature menarche is defined as transient isolated or cyclic vaginal bleeding in the absence of other signs of sexual development and with no evidence of an underlying genital disorder in a prepubertal girl.[4] Premature menarche may represent a similar response, as occurs in premature thelarche, to transient ovarian production of estrogens. Serum E_2 levels are significantly above the normal prepubertal range. The prepubertal girl may have menstruation lasting 1 to 5 days occurring once or in several monthly cycles. Other etiologies for vaginal bleeding must be excluded. The prognosis is good with normal pubertal development and normal menstruation occurring within the normal age range and fertility expected.

Premature adrenarche also is discussed in Chapter 6.

Heterosexual Precocity

Causes of heterosexual precocity in girls are listed in Table 7–12. A simplified flow sheet for workup is given in Figure 7–8. Heterosexual precocity is due to excessive exposure to androgens from any source. The precocity is manifested by virilization and the clinical findings may include the following: growth of pubic and facial hair; accelerated linear growth; deepening of the voice; acne; muscular development; and clitoral enlargement. If the girl is postmenarchal, secondary amenorrhea will occur,

TABLE 7–12.

Causes of Heterosexual Precocity in Girls

Ovarian
    Granulosa and granulosa-theca cell tumors
    Thecomas, fibrothecomas
    Sertoli-Leydig cell tumors (arrhenoblastoma)
    Adrenal rest tumors, including lipoid cell tumor
    Polycystic ovary disease/hyperthecosis syndrome
Adrenal
    Congenital adrenal hyperplasia
    Adenoma
    Carcinoma
    Cushing's syndrome
Intersex
    Gonadal dysgenesis
    True hermaphroditism
Iatrogenic
Tumors of the clitoris

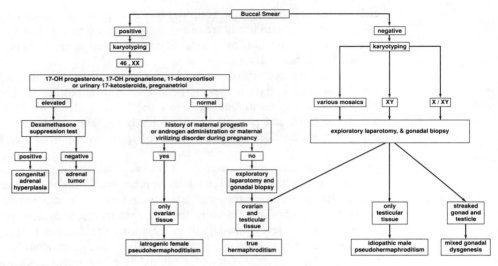

FIG 7–8.
A scheme for evaluation of amenorrhea with heterosexual development.

and atrophy of the breasts and enlargement of the clitoris may occur. The bone age is usually advanced.

Pubic hair growth is usually the initial physical finding, and may present difficulty in the differential diagnosis, because pubic hair growth may be the first sign of isosexual precocity or may represent premature adrenarche.

Androgen-producing tumors of the ovary and adrenal gland are extremely rare. An excellent review of androgen-producing tumors in children and adolescents has recently been published.[45]

Arrhenoblastoma of the ovary is an extremely rare tumor in the pediatric age range and approximately 25% are malignant.[27] Plasma testosterone and androstenedione levels are increased. Partial, rather than complete, suppression of urine 17-ketosteroid excretion during dexamethasone suppression studies suggests an ovarian rather than an adrenal source of the excessive androgens. The bone age is advanced. Pelvic MRI and ultrasonography may be helpful in localizing the tumor. Surgery is the treatment of choice.

Tumors of the clitoris consisting usually of situated tumors such as neufibromatosis can cause clitoromegaly.

Polycystic ovary syndrome and the hyperthecosis syndrome, as well as mixed gonadal dysgenesis, have been discussed earlier in this chapter. Diseases of the adrenal gland that may produce heterosexual precocity in girls are discussed in Chapter 6.

Hirsutism

The pediatrician is not infrequently asked to see a girl complaining of excessive hair growth. The clinician must first determine whether the hair growth represents true hirsutism, hypertrichosis, or a racial or ethnic variation in the distribution of hair follicle number. *Hirsutism* may be defined as the excessive growth of terminal hair (coarse and pigmented) in a male pattern. It must be differentiated from hypertrichosis in which there is a generalized increase in vellus hair (fine, soft, and unpigmented).

True hirsutism is due to androgen effect on the pilosebaceous units and other signs of virilization may be present. Ferriman and Gallwey[11] have proposed that hirsutism be classified according to terminal hair density in 11 zones of the body; hair density is graded 1 to 4 in each zone. A review of the pathophysiology of hirsutism has been published recently.[9]

Once true hirsutism is suspected, biochemical documentation of hyperandrogenemia is necessary. The differential diagnosis of hyperandrogenemia consists of defined disorders and those of unknown etiology. The defined disorders consist of CAH, particularly nonclassic or late-onset; Cushing's syndrome; hyperprolactinemia; and tumors of the ovary and adrenal glands. Each of these disorders has been discussed in this or other chapters in this book and will not be discussed further here. Exogenous agents such as androgens or anabolic drugs can cause hirsutism and must be excluded as causes. If defined causes of hirsutism have been excluded, the differential diagnosis is usually narrowed to idiopathic hirsutism (IH) or PCOD.

It has been suggested that the best method to screen for hyperandrogenemia is by measuring the serum levels of free testosterone, androstenedione, and DHEA-S.[9] A single normal determination of these hormones does not exclude the presence of hyperandrogenemia because of the episodic and cyclic secretion of androgens. Multiple blood sampling may be necessary. It has been suggested that measurement of serum 3α-androstenediol (3α-diol), which is produced exclusively in peripheral tissues, can serve as a marker of IH.[19]

Specific medical therapy or surgical therapies for the defined causes of hirsutism are discussed elsewhere. Mild hirsutism may be treated by local therapy such as bleaching or depilation. In patients with IH, glucocorticoids, combination estrogen-progestin therapy, and antiandrogens have been used.[9] Antiandrogens act primarily to inhibit binding of androgens to the androgen receptor. The most commonly used antiandrogen in the United States at the present time is spironolactone, in a dose of 50 to 100 mg twice daily. It is most effective when administered with cyclic estrogens. Side effects of spironolactone include headache, nausea, hypotension, and hyperkalemia.

MISCELLANEOUS USES OF FEMALE SEX STEROIDS

Constitutional Tall Stature

Estrogens have been prescribed to treat girls with constitutional tall stature who have psychosocial problems because of their tallness. Such therapy is controversial. High doses of ethinyl estradiol (0.3–0.5 mg/day) and low doses (0.05–0.1 mg/day)[15] have been used to hasten epiphyseal fusion in order to achieve a reduction in ultimate height. The clinician should remember that there are side effects, although rare, associated with this therapy. Thrombosis has been reported during high-dose ethinyl estradiol therapy in a tall girl.[70] It has been shown that ethinyl estradiol 0.1 mg/day is as effective as a higher dose in reducing final height.

Menstrual Suppression in Mentally or Physically Handicapped Girls

In certain girls with major physical handicaps or limited mental capacity, the total elimination of recurring menstruation by medical means may be advisable as an alternative to hysterectomy. One agent used for medical suppression of menstruation on a continuous basis is medroxyprogesterone acetate 150 to 250 mg by deep IM injection every 3 to 4 months. However, patient response is variable and breakthrough bleeding may occur. Another agent used is the oral progestin megestrol acetate 40 to 80 mg/day. Megestrol acetate is very expensive.

REFERENCES

1. Aleem FA: Familial 46, XX gonadal dysgenesis. *Fertil Steril* 1981; 35:317.
2. Apter D: Serum steroids and pituitary hormones in female puberty: A partly longitudinal study. *Clin Endocrinol* 1980; 12:107.
3. Blackwell RE, et al: Comparison of dopamine agonists in the treatment of hyperprolactinemic syndromes: A multicenter study. *Fertil Steril* 1983; 39:744.
4. Blanco-Garcia M, et al: Isolated menses in prepubertal girls. *Pediatrics* 1985; 76:43.
5. Cacciari E, et al: How many cases of true precocious puberty in girls are idiopathic? *J Pediatr* 1983; 102:357.
6. Conte FA, Grumbach MM, Kaplan SL: A diphasic pattern of gonadotropin secretion in patients with the syndrome of gonadal dysgenesis. *J Clin Endocrinol Metab* 1975; 40:670.
7. Coulam CB, Kempers RD, Randall RV: Premature ovarian failure: Evidence for the autoimmune mechanism. *Fertil Steril* 1981; 36:238.
8. Crowne EC, Shalet SM: Management of constitutional delay in growth and puberty. *Trends Endocrinol Metab* 1990; 1:239.
9. Ehrmann DA, Rosenfield RL: An endocrinologic approach to the patient with hirsutism. *J Clin Endocrinol Metab* 1990; 71:1.
10. Ellis CEG, Dewhurst J: A simplified approach to management of congenital absence of the vagina and uterus. *Pediatr Adolesc Gynecol* 1984; 2:25.
11. Ferriman D, Gallwey JD: Clinical assessment of body hair growth in women. *J Clin Endocrinol Metab* 1961; 21:1440.
12. Frasier SD, Lippe BM: The rational use of growth hormone during childhood. *J Clin Endocrinol Metab* 1990; 71:269.
13. Grumbach MM, Sizonenko PC, Aubert ML (eds): *Control of the Onset of Puberty*. Baltimore, Williams & Wilkins Co, 1990.
14. Grumbach MM, Van Wyk JJ, Wilkins L: Chromosomal sex in gonadal dysgenesis (ovarian agenesis): Relationship to male pseudohermaphroditism and theories of human sex differentiation. *J Clin Endocrinol Metab* 1955; 15:1161.
15. Gruters A, et al: Effect of different estrogen doses on final height reduction in girls with constitutional tall stature. *Eur J Pediatr* 1989; 149:11.
16. Hagenfeldt K, von Dobeln U, Hagenfeldt L: Gonadal failure in young women and galactose-1-phosphate uridyl transferase activity. *Fertil Steril* 1989; 51:177.
17. Hauser GA, et al: Das Rokitansky-Küster Syndrom: Uterus bipartitus solidus rudimentarius cum Vagina solida. *Gynaecologia* 1961; 151:111.
18. Ho PC, et al: Immunologic studies in patients with premature ovarian failure. *Obstet Gynecol* 1988; 71:622.

19. Horton R, Hawks D, Lobo R: 3α,17β-androstenediol glucuronide in plasma. *J Clin Invest* 1982; 69:1203.

20. Howlett TA, et al: Prolactinomas presenting as primary amenorrhea and delayed or arrested puberty: Response to medical therapy. *Clin Endocrinol* 1989; 30:131.

21. Ilicki A, et al: Premature thelarche—natural history and sex hormone secretion in 68 girls. *Acta Pediatr Scand* 1984; 73:756.

22. Jeffcoate WJ, et al: Endocrine function in the Prader-Willi syndrome. *Clin Endocrinol* 1980; 12:81.

23. Jones GS, Ruehsen MM: A new syndrome of amenorrhea in association with hypergonadotropins and apparently normal ovarian follicular apparatus. *Am J Obstet Gynecol* 1969; 104:597.

24. Jost A: Problems of fetal endocrinology: The gonadal and hypophyseal hormones. *Recent Prog Horm Res* 1953; 8:379.

25. Kinch RAH, et al: Primary ovarian failure. *Am J Obstet Gynecol* 1965; 91:630.

26. Lanes R, et al: The metoclopramide test: A useful tool with the luteinizing hormone-releasing hormone test in distinguishing between constitutional delay of puberty and hypogonadotropic hypogonadism. *Fertil Steril* 1989; 52:55.

27. Lauritzen C: Tumors of the ovary in childhood and adolescence. *Pediatr Adolesc Gynecol* 1984; 2:111.

28. Lee PA, Van Dop C, Migeon CJ: McCune-Albright syndrome: Long-term follow-up. *JAMA* 1986; 256:2980.

29. Lee PA, et al: Puberty in girls: Correlation of serum levels of gonadotropins, prolactin, androgens, estrogens, and progestins with physical changes. *J Clin Endocrinol Metab* 1976; 43:775.

30. Leiper AD, et al: Precocious and premature puberty associated with treatment of acute lymphoblastic leukemia. *Arch Dis Child* 1987; 62:1107.

31. Liapi C, Evain-Brion D: Diagnosis of ovarian follicular cysts from birth to puberty: A report of twenty cases. *Acta Pediatr Scand* 1987; 76:91.

32. Lippe B, et al: Renal malformations in patients with Turner syndrome: Imaging in 141 patients. *Pediatrics* 1988; 82:852.

33. Lyon AJ, De Bruyn R, Grant DB: Transient sexual precocity and ovarian cysts. *Arch Dis Child* 1985; 60:819.

34. Lyon AJ, Preece MA, Grant DB: Growth curve for girls with Turner syndrome. *Arch Dis Child* 1985; 60:932.

35. MacMahon RA, Cussen LJ, Walters WAW: Importance of early diagnosis and gonadectomy in 46, XY females. *J Pediatr Surg* 1980; 15:642.

36. Mahajan DK: Steroidogenesis in human polycystic ovary. *Endocrinol Metab Clin North Am* 1988; 17:751.

37. Massarano AA, et al: Growth hormone secretion in Turner's syndrome and influence of oxandrolone and ethinyl oestradiol. *Arch Dis Child* 1989; 64:587.

38. Midgley PC, et al: Virilization of female preterm infants. *Arch Dis Child* 1990; 65:701.

39. Molitch ME: Management of prolactinomas. *Annu Rev Med* 1989; 40:225.

40. Muram D: Vaginal bleeding in childhood and adolescence. *Obstet Gynecol Clin North Am* 1990; 17:389.

41. Nagamani M, et al: Clinical and hormonal studies in hyperthecosis of the ovaries. *Fertil Steril* 1981; 36:326.

42. New MI: Polycystic ovarian disease and congenital and late-onset adrenal hyperplasia. *Endocrinol Metab Clin North Am* 1988; 17:637.

43. Noonan JA, Ehmke DA: Associated noncardiac malformations in children with congenital heart disease. *J Pediatr* 1963; 63:468.

44. Norris HJ, Jensen RD: Relative frequency of ovarian neoplasms in children and adolescents. *Cancer* 1972; 30:713.
45. Padilla SL: Androgen-producing tumors in children and adolescents. *Adolesc Pediatr Gynecol* 1989; 2:135.
46. Pescovitz OH, et al: The NIH experience with precocious puberty: Diagnostic subgroups and response to short-term luteinizing hormone releasing hormone analogue therapy. *J Pediatr* 1986; 108:47.
47. Reiter EO, Kulin HE: Sexual precocity in the female: Normal development and precocious puberty. *Pediatr Clin North Am* 1972; 19:581.
48. Richards JS, et al: Ovarian follicular development in the rat: Hormone receptor regulation by estradiol, follicle stimulating hormone and luteinizing hormone. *Endocrinology* 1976; 99:1562.
49. Rosenfield RL: Diagnosis and management of delayed puberty. *J Clin Endocrinol Metab* 1990; 70:559.
50. Ross JL, et al: Growth hormone secretory dynamics in Turner syndrome. *J Pediatr* 1985; 106:202.
51. Schoenfeld A, et al: Ultrasonographic observations in girls with central precocious puberty before and during therapy with the GnRH analogue D-TRP-LHRH. *Adolesc Pediatr Gynecol* 1990; 3:31.
52. Sedmark DD, Hart WR, Tubbs RR: Autoimmune oophoritis: A histopathologic study of involved ovaries with immunologic characterization of the mononuclear cell infiltrate. *Int J Gynecol Pathol* 1987; 6:73.
53. Shalet SM: Endocrine consequences of treatment of malignant disease. *Arch Dis Child* 1989; 64:1635.
54. Shoval AR: Hermaphrodites with "atypical" or "mixed" gonadal dysgenesis. *Am J Med* 1964; 36:281.
55. Shoval AR: The syndrome of pure gonadal dysgenesis. *Am J Med* 1965; 38:615.
56. Sinisi AA, et al: Dysgerminoma in 45,X Turner syndrome: Report of a case. *Clin Endocrinol* 1988; 28:187.
57. Sippell WG, et al: Plasma levels of aldosterone, corticosterone, 11-deoxycorticosterone, progesterone, 17-hydroxyprogesterone, cortisol and cortisone during infancy and childhood. *Pediatr Res* 1980; 14:39.
58. Sizonenko PC, Aubert ML: Pituitary gonadotropins, prolactin, and sex steroids. Secretion in prepuberty and puberty, in Grumbach MM, Zizonenko PC, Aubert ML (eds): *Control of the Onset of Puberty*, Baltimore, Williams & Wilkins Co, 1990.
59. Soules MR, Hammond CB: Female Kallmann's syndrome: Evidence for a hypothalamic luteinizing hormone-releasing hormone deficiency. *Fertil Steril* 1980; 33:82.
60. Stein LF, Leventhal ML: Amenorrhea associated with bilateral polycystic ovaries. *Am J Obstet Gynecol* 1935; 29:181.
61. Stokvis-Brantsma WH, et al: Sexual precocity induced by ovarian follicular cysts. Is autoimmunity involved? *Clin Endocrinol* 1990; 32:603.
62. Swenson T, Havens B: Menarche and menstruation: A review of the literature. *J Commun Health Nurs* 1987; 4:199.
63. Swyer GIM: Male pseudohermaphroditism: A hitherto undescribed form. *Br Med J* 1955; 2:709.
64. Tho PT, McDonough PG: Gonadal dysgenesis and its variants. *Pediatr Clin North Am* 1981; 28:309.
65. Tolis G, et al: Prolonged amenorrhea and oral contraceptives. *Fertil Steril* 1979; 32:265.
66. Turner HH: A syndrome of infantilism, congenital webbed neck and cubitus valgus. *Endocrinology* 1938; 23:566.

67. Van Winter JT, et al: Natural history of premature thelarche in Olmsted county, Minnesota, 1940–1984. *J Pediatr* 1990; 116:278.
68. Warren MP: The effects of exercise on pubertal progression and reproductive function in girls. *J Clin Endocrinol Metab* 1980; 51:1150.
69. Wentz AC: Body weight and amenorrhea. *Obstet Gynecol* 1980; 56:482.
70. Werder EA, et al: Severe thrombosis during estrogen treatment for tall stature. *Eur J Pediatr* 1990; 149:389.
71. Wertelecki W, Fraumeni JF, Mulvihill JJ: Nongonadal neoplasia in Turner's syndrome. *Cancer* 1970; 26:485.
72. Winter JSD: Prepubertal and pubertal endocrinology, in Falkner F, Tanner JM (eds): *Human Growth*. New York, Plenum Press, 1979.
73. Winter JSD, et al: Pituitary-gonadal relations in infancy: 2. Patterns of serum gonadal steroid concentrations in man from birth to two years of age. *J Clin Endocrinol Metab* 1976; 42:679.
74. Young RH, Dickersin GR, Scully RE: A distinctive ovarian sex cord stromal tumor causing sexual precocity in the Peutz-Jeghers syndrome. *Am J Surg Pathol* 1983; 7:233.
75. Young RH, Dickersin GR, Scully RE: Juvenile granulosa cell tumor of the ovary. A clinicopathological analysis of 125 cases. *Am J Surg Pathol* 1984; 8:575.

Chapter 8

Testes and Variants of Male Sexual Development

Peter A. Lee
Louis St. L. O'Dea

Sexual differentiation of the developing male embryo, pubertal maturation, and the acquisition and maintenance of spermatogenesis depend on the normal functioning of the testis. Normal development of the testis during embryogenesis and the later acquisition of spermatogenesis in turn depend on the presence of a normal XY karyotype. However, the male phenotype may be present in the apparent absence of the Y chromosome, because many loci of male phenotypic expression are located on the X chromosome and on the autosomes. In addition, the male sex determining regulator gene(s) may be translocated within fragments of a Y chromosome onto an X. Function of the embryonic testis is initially stimulated by maternal chorionic gonadotropin and later comes under the control of the integrated functioning of the hypothalamic-pituitary unit. Failure to stimulate the differentiating testis, failure of the steroidogenic pathway, and failure of end organ response to the androgenic effects of gonadal steroids may all result in variable degrees of incomplete male genital differentiation. Subsequently, the process of sexual maturation during puberty depends on the presence of a functioning hypothalamic-pituitary-gonadal unit. The mature testis, through a system of hormonal messengers, has the capacity to modulate the influence of the hypothalamic-pituitary system.

This chapter outlines the mechanisms of male sexual differentiation during embryogenesis and of sexual maturation during puberty, and discusses the abnormalities that may disturb these critical phases of human development. The diagnosis and treatment of the clinical conditions that result are presented.

EARLY DEVELOPMENT OF MALE REPRODUCTIVE AXIS

Embryology

Development of the male reproductive system begins early in intrauterine life. Complete formation of the internal and external male genitalia depends on early and adequate development of testicular function.

The process of testicular differentiation is directed by testes-determining gene(s) or sex-determining region (SRy) located on the Y chromosome.[52,54,55] Small deletions or translocations of genetic material may result in marked differences in sexual differentiation. Males with 46,XX karyotypes who have male external genital differentiation but who are infertile have been found to have Y chromosomal material in their DNA,[48] and phenotypic females with true gonadal dysgenesis with 46,XY karyotypes have small deletions of Y chromosomal material.[53]

The earliest recognizable precursors of the testis can be identified in the yolk sac ectoderm by 2 to 2½ weeks. These primordial germ cells are the precursors of the spermatogonia and migrate along the mesonephric ridge, drawing in epithelial cells and nesting in the mesenchyme to form the primordial gonad at 5 to 6 weeks.[24] The first morphologic evidence of testicular differentiation is the development of Sertoli cells, which secrete two substances, müllerian inhibiting hormone (MIH) and serologically detectible H-Y antigen.[7,34] In the differentiating gonad, seminiferous cords become discernible at 7 to 8 weeks. These germ cells, along with other primitive cells, form testicular cords; mesenchymal cells fill in the interstitial space, and Leydig cells and Sertoli cells can be distinguished.

Prior to the differentiation of the embryonic gonad into a testis or ovary, a dual ductal system has developed: first the wolffian or mesonephric ducts, then the müllerian ducts. Under the influence of testosterone from the Leydig cells, the cells of the proximal wolffian ducts invaginate into the developing gonad to form the collecting system and epididymsis as the mesonephric kidney regresses. At about 7 weeks, concomitant with gonadal differentiation, the müllerian ducts develop lateral and adjacent to the wolffian ducts whose proximity appears essential for the development of the müllerian system. The müllerian ducts then fuse distally with the wolffian system to form the urogenital sinus.

In the absence of testicular controls, the constitutive program of female differentiation occurs with female internal and external genital development, and with ovarian differentiation occurring late in the first trimester. For male external genital development not only is testosterone from the fetal gonad necessary but also intracellular conversion of testosterone to dihydrotestosterone by the enzyme 5α-reductase. Dihydrotestosterone mediates the development of the undifferentiated genital tubercle, genital swellings, and the genital folds bordering the urogenital sinus into the penis, scrotum, and the penile urethra with the overlying perineal raphe. The perineal opening of the sinus is surrounded by the genital swellings or labioscrotal folds, which fuse to become the scrotum, and by the more medial genital or labiourethral folds, which fuse to form the penile urethra and surrounding corpus spongiosum. The sinus is bordered anteriorly by the genital eminence or tubercle, which will later, under hormonal stimulation, form the main corpora of the penis. The prostate and seminal vesicles arise from the endodermal floor of the genital sinus.[17]

Endocrinology

Testosterone is produced by the fetal Leydig cells (Fig 8–1) by 8 weeks of gestation and stimulates further differentiation of the primordial gonad, thereby providing the androgen necessary for the development of the penis and scrotum from the undifferentiated primordial external genitalia. The formation of the external genitalia requires dihydrotestosterone (DHT) synthesized by reduction from testosterone within the androgen-sensitive cells of the genital anlage which are richly supplied with the 5α-reductase enzyme. Testosterone from the fetal Leydig cells, rather than DHT, stimulates the development of the primordial wolffian ducts into the epididymis, vas deferens, and seminal vesicles, with the prostate gland developing from outgrowths of the urogenital sinus. The fetal Sertoli cells secrete MIH which inhibits the further development of the müllerian female genital structures and may initiate the formation of spermatic cords. Regression of the müllerian system begins as the Sertoli cells start functioning at 9 weeks. In the absence of MIH, these ducts progress to form the fallopian tubes, uterus, and, together with the urogenital sinus, the vagina. Unless stimulated with testosterone, the wolffian ducts will not develop further into the internal male ducts and glands. MIH has primarily a local effect so müllerian structures may develop to varying degrees on the side of defective testicular MIH secretion and regress normally if testicular function is adequate on the contralateral side.[35]

Thus it appears that male sexual differentiation requires testosterone for pro-

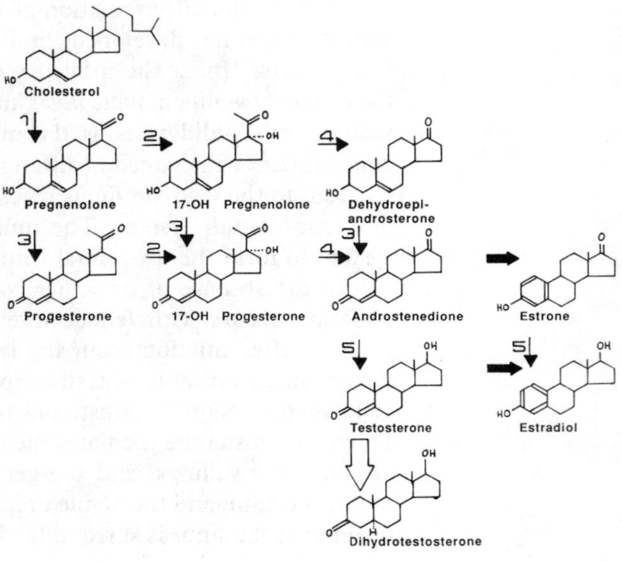

FIG 8–1.
Sex steroid biosynthetic pathway. Numbers 1–5 represent intratesticular enzymes: (1) 20, 22-desmolase, P-450$_{scc}$; (2) 17-hydroxylase, P-450$_{c17}$; (3) 3-β-ol-dehydrogenase; (4) 17-20 lase, desmolase; also P-450$_{c17}$; (5) 17-ketosteroid reductase, 17-β-hydroxysteroid dehydrogenase, or 17-β-oxidoreductase. Conversion of testosterone to dehydrostestosterone by 5α-reductase occurs within androgen-sensitive tissues. The testis also does not contain aromatase for conversion from androgen to estrogen.

motion of wolffian development, MIH for regression of müllerian structures, and DHT for development of the male external genitalia.

Sexual Differentiation

The differentiation of the male external genitalia from the bipotential undifferentiated anlage begins at around 9 weeks and is complete within 4 weeks. The midline genital tubercle, under DHT stimulation, forms the bulk of the shaft of the penis, the corpora cavernosa. The genital folds fuse ventrally from posteriorly to anteriorly enclosing the urethral groove to form the penile urethra, creating a common conduit for the urinary and reproductive system openings. When fusion is complete, this meatus is at the tip of the glans penis. The paired genital swellings likewise fuse from posteriorly to anteriorly forming the scrotum. Fusion extends to enclose the shaft of the penis, continuing distally to envelope the glans within the prepuce. The line of fusion is evident in the raphe which extends at midline from the anus onto the surface of the scrotum and up the ventral side of the penis onto the foreskin.

Male external genital differentiation is complete by 13 weeks of fetal life. Normally, differentiated male genitalia indicate that adequate androgen was present during this critical period, and conversely, if differentiation is incomplete, that androgen stimulation was inadequate or not properly synchronized. Androgen stimulation beyond this gestational age can cause no further differentiation but is necessary for normal genital growth. Increase of penis size occurs primarily during the third trimester and is dependent upon testosterone secretion from the fetal testes.

Therefore, inadequate differentiation (virilization) of genitalia in a male is evidence of defective stimulation prior to 13 weeks; normally differentiated genitalia but an abnormally small penis suggest defective androgen stimulation later in fetal life. Ambiguous or underdeveloped male genitalia may be consistent with inadequate androgen exposure in the genetic male or of excessive or inappropriate androgen exposure in the genetic female. If genitalia in a developing female are exposed to androgen during this period of fetal life, 9 to 13 weeks, variable degrees of fusion of the perineum may similarly occur. Differentiation may range from minimal posterior fusion of the genital folds and swellings to fully differentiated male genitalia with absent testes. Excessive androgen exposure later in intrauterine life results in variable degrees of clitoral enlargement, but fusion does not occur. Thus, perineal fusion and clitoromegaly may occur in the setting of continuous intrauterine androgen exposure, whereas perineal fusion alone or clitoromegaly alone suggests more limited early or late exposure, respectively.

PROBLEMS OF GENITAL DEVELOPMENT

Failure of complete sexual differentiation in the male may generally be classified as resulting from abnormalities of genetic control of sexual differentiation, from abnormalities of gonadal differentiation, or from abnormalities of the endocrine modulators of genital development. Other factors, such as medications, may interfere with normal intrauterine sexual development, but frequently the cause cannot be clearly identified.

The spectrum of abnormalities of phenotypic sex in the male may range from complete feminization through hypospadias, to failure of complete testicular descent. The same range of ambiguity may be present in excessive virilized genetic females, with the exception that testes are always absent.

Ambiguous Genitalia

Classification

Abnormalities of sexual differentiation may be classified on the basis of the genetic, gonadal, or phenotypic sex. However, such classification fails to account for the degree of variability found in any one disorder, for the common phenotypic manifestations of divergent etiologies, or for the exceptions to these rules of classification. For example, individuals with ambiguous genitalia and a 46,XY karyotype may, depending on other findings, fit a classification as male pseudohermaphroditism, mixed gonadal dysgenesis, or true hermaphroditism.

A clinical classification of ambiguous genitalia in the newborn may be made on the basis of chromosomal status and on the presence of symmetric or asymmetric gonads. Asymmetry of the gonads refers to the presence of an "unmatched" pair of gonads (Fig 8–2) and may be found in true hermaphrodites, either 46,XX, 46,XY, or mosaics, and in mixed gonadal dysgenesis, possibly the commonest nonadrenal cause of ambiguous genitalia in the neonate. Mixed gonadal dysgenesis is also important in that one gonad is usually a streak gonad and therefore associated with persistence of ipsilateral müllerian structures. The other gonad is usually a dysgenetic testis and at increased risk for malignancy.

When all possible karyotypes are considered, ambiguous development of the external genitalia can be classified into four categories: (1) female pseudohermaph-

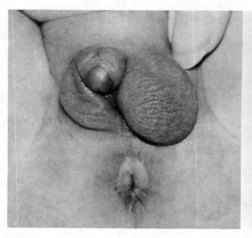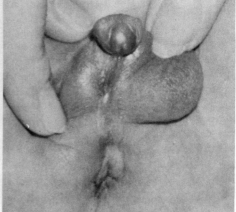

FIG 8–2.
Asymmetric genital development in a newborn infant, suggestive of asymmetric gonadal differentiation. This patient had mixed gonadal dysgenesis with a palpable testes on the left and a streak gonad on the right.

roditism, characterized by a 46,XX karyotype, ovaries, and female internal reproductive organs; (2) male pseudohermaphroditism, with 46,XY karyotype, testes which may be defective, and varying degrees of development of internal wolffian- and müllerian-derived structures; (3) mixed gonadal dysgenesis, characterized by a streak gonad and a dysgenetic testis; and (4) true hermaphroditism in which the karyotype varies, both ovarian and testicular tissue is present, and internal development depends upon ipsilateral testicular function.

Female Pseudohermaphroditism

Female pseudohermaphroditism occurs when the external genitalia are excessively virilized for a female in a patient with a 46,XX karyotype. These patients have ovaries; the source of excessive androgen is not gonadal. The most common etiology of female pseudohermaphroditism is excess adrenal androgen secretion as a consequence of congenital virilizing adrenal hyperplasia (CVAH). The most common CVAH is 21-hydroxylase (cytochrome $P-450_{c21}$) deficiency, which accounts for 80% to 90% of female pseudohermaphroditism. Much rarer is 11-hydroxylase deficiency ($P-450_{c11}$), and far rarer as a cause of neonatal genital ambiguity is 3β-ol-dehydrogenase. Also, rarely, excessive transplacental passage of androgen, from either an exogenous source or from pathologic maternal production, causes masculinization of the genitalia of a female in utero. The external genitalia of females may also appear to be virilized in instances in which there are other congenital anomalies.

Male Pseudohermaphroditism

In association with sexual ambiguity, the presence of symmetric gonads in an XY individual with testes is classified as male pseudohermaphroditism, and in the XX individual with ovaries as female pseudohermaphroditism (Fig 8–3). Male pseudohermaphroditism may be associated with varying degrees of incomplete external and internal virilization.

Dysgenetic Testes.—Male pseudohermaphroditism may result from developmental abnormalities of the testis, abnormalities of androgen production, or disorders of androgen effect. It is characterized by the XY karyotype, by the presence of testes with varying degrees of functional adequacy, and generally by regressed or partially developed müllerian duct derivatives. Developmental abnormalities of the testis other than severe Leydig cell dysgenesis rarely result in male pseudohermaphroditism because of the apparently adequate early function of the organ. In these entities, MIH-induced müllerian regression is complete and androgen-stimulated fusion of perineal structures is also adequate and complete. Thus, the vanishing testis syndrome, XY gonadal dysgenesis, and Klinefelter's syndrome are not associated with pseudohermaphroditism. However, Leydig cell dysgenesis or hypoplasia may result in some androgen secretion, albeit inadequate, and therefore may present with ambiguous genitalia. If the dysgenetic testis fails to produce sufficient MIH, müllerian structures may be present. A specific example of dysgenetic testes associated with partial persistence of müllerian structures is the Drash syndrome, also associated with renal malformations.[51]

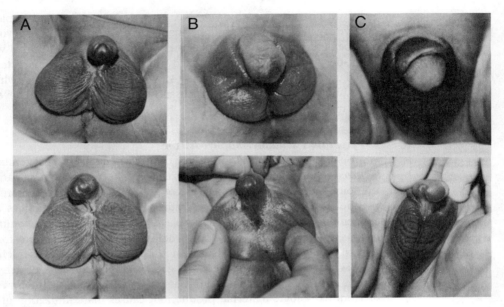

FIG 8–3.
Male pseudohermaphroditism. Genital development in three newborn 46,XY male infants. The *upper* and *lower* photos show different views of the same genitalia in each instance. Testes were palpable in each infant, in the scrotum (**A**), in the upper scrotum (**B**), and in the inguinal canal (**C**). Phallus size varies. Perineoscrotal hypospadias was present in each case, with varying degrees of chordee. The unfused urethrolabial folds are visible ventrally.

Biosynthetic Defects.—Disorders of androgen biosynthesis (see Fig 8–1) affect the virilization of the internal and external genitalia of the male embryo but do not interfere with regression of the müllerian system. These defects may be of variable severity, partial or complete, and may present at puberty as well as in the newborn period. Variable degrees of ambiguity of the genitalia, from complete feminization to mild hypospadias, may be apparent at birth. All but one of the enzymes involved in these defects are present in both the gonad and the adrenal and may present as congenital adrenal hyperplasia. In both 17α-hydroxylase/17,20-lyase and cholesterol desmolase deficiencies, male infants are undervirilized while female infants have normal female external genitalia. In 3β-hydroxysteroid dehydrogenase deficiency, male infants are undervirilized while female infants are virilized. Defects of 17-ketosteroid reductase, an enzyme present in the gonad but not in the adrenal cortex, result in deficient male genital development and present with ambiguous genitalia, although virilization may occur at puberty.

The most proximal block in the pathway from cholesterol to testosterone is that of the 20,22-desmolase enzyme, a $P-450_{scc}$ (side chain cleavage) enzyme which is ACTH-responsive and which facilitates the conversion of cholesterol to pregnenolone. Therefore, in addition to absent or minimal virilization of the affected male fetus owing to the deficiency of testicular androgen steroidogenesis, this enzyme deficiency causes a profound pandeficiency of adrenal steroidogenesis and results in severe salt-losing hypoadrenalism and neonatal mortality.

The 3β-hydroxysteroid dehydrogenase enzyme catalyzes the next step—the conversion of pregnenolone to progesterone, 17-hydroxypregnenolone to 17-hydroxyprogesterone, and dehydroepiandrosterone (DHA) to androstenedione. Decreased activity compromises the production of all adrenal and gonadal steroids. Therefore, in the severely affected male fetus, testosterone production is markedly diminished, while DHA levels are increased. This then results in partial male external genital differentiation (male pseudohermaphroditism). In the severely affected female fetus, the increased androgen effect from elevated DHA levels causes excessive virilization (female pseudohermaphroditism). The neonatal presentation is usually that of severe salt-losing hypoadrenalism with a high mortality.

Although 17-hydroxylase[13,33,36] and 17,20-desmolase[72] deficiencies have been described as two different syndromes, both enzymatic conversions are accomplished by a single enzyme, P-450$_{c17}$. The 17-hydroxylase step converts progesterone to 17-OH-progesterone and pregnenolone to 17-hydroxypregenolone. Blockage at this point results in shunting of progesterone to 11-deoxycorticosterone (DOC) and corticosterone in the adrenal gland. The increased mineralocorticoid potency of these steroids results in a hypokalemic alkalosis and suppression of aldosterone. Cortisol levels are low. In the testis, deficiency of the 17-hydroxylated precursors results in absent or low levels of androgens and poor virilization of wolffian and genital structures. In the male, defective 17,20-desmolase activity results in decreased conversion of 17-hydroxypregnenolone and 17-hydroxyprogesterone, substrates which are already low if there is impaired 17-hydroxylase activity, to dehydroepiandrosterone (DHEA) and androstenedione, respectively. The degree of male pseudohermaphroditism associated depends upon the severity of the compromised enzyme activity and the resulting diminished androgen synthesis.

17-Ketosteroid reductase (17-β-hydroxysteroid dehydrogenase) is present in the testis but not in the adrenal cortex. Deficiency impairs the conversion of androstenedione to testosterone. This uncommon deficiency is characterized by elevated serum androstenedione and low serum testosterone. The increased androstenedione secretion of puberty may result in both increased androgenic and estrogenic manifestations with both virilization and breast enlargement occurring.

Defect in Androgen Action.—Abnormalities of androgen effect can be characterized as those due to defects of the androgen receptor, both partial and complete, (complete or partial androgen insensitivity syndromes, CAIS, PAIS) and to abnormalities of the 5α-reductase enzyme converting testosterone to dihydrotestosterone. With the exception of CAIS, these defects present with ambiguous genitalia in the newborn.

Complete Androgen Insensitivity Syndrome.—CAIS is characterized by the development of female external genitalia (Fig 8–4) and failure of masculinization of the wolffian system, but regression of the müllerian system. Inguinal or labial testes may be palpable in the neonate or older patient although they may not be detected or the diagnosis suspected until they are discovered during exploration of an inguinal hernia. A vagina is present, but because the upper portion is derived from the fused distal müllerian ducts, it may be short. If testes remain functional, the increased

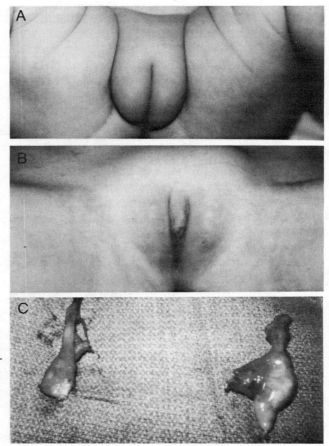

FIG 8–4.
Complete androgen insensitivity syndrome. **A,** genitalia of a newborn infant with palpable labial-inguinal testes. **B,** genitalia at 8 years of age. **C,** resected testes, removed at age 8 years.

testicular stimulation by elevated gonadotropins at puberty results not only in high-normal or elevated testosterone levels to which the patient is nonresponsive but also in high or high-normal estrogen levels which promote normal female breast development. Adult height is relatively tall when compared with the female population. Sexual and body hair is scant. If the diagnosis is not made before puberty, primary amenorrhea or infertility may be the presenting complaint.

The diagnosis of CAIS is made based on clinical findings including a female phenotype with a short vagina, absent uterus, and inguinal hernias with palpable gonads in a patient with a 46,XY karyotype. During the neonatal and pubertal years and thereafter, elevated testosterone, luteinizing hormone (LH), follicle-stimulating hormone (FSH), and estradiol levels may be found. Additional studies may include androgen-binding studies and human chorionic gonadotropin (hCG) or testosterone stimulation. The abnormalities may be found to be receptor-mediated or post-receptor depending on the presence or absence of androgen binding, respectively. Lack of virilization is expected in response to testosterone or hCG stimulation, although circulating levels of testosterone rise.

There is an increased incidence of testicular tumors in CAIS and therefore orchidectomy should be performed by the end of the second decade of life, following completion of puberty. However, if there is a possibility that the patient has a partial form of androgen insensitivity with the risk of masculinization during puberty, the testes should be removed prior to that time.

Partial Androgen Insensitivity Syndrome. — The less common PAIS presents with variable degrees of virilization, the phenotype varying from slightly virilized female genitalia, through the perineoscrotal hypospadias of Reifenstein's syndrome, to penile hypospadias, undescended testis and adolescent gynecomastia, micropenis, or perhaps only as decreased spermatogenesis.[19] Patients who present with ambiguous genitalia or micropenis in the neonatal period may or may not have detectable defects in androgen binding, but they have characteristic hormonal profiles. In the neonatal period, elevated testosterone, LH, and FSH are indicative of androgen insensitivity. Further diagnostic testing involves in vivo androgen stimulation. The lack of detectable or adequate penile growth in response is consistent with the diagnosis of androgen insensitivity. Marked ambiguity and biochemical evidence of severe androgen insensitivity dictate a female sex of rearing. In addition, a partial defect may result in further masculinization at puberty and gonadectomy should therefore be performed before puberty in contrast to the recommendation for the complete defect.

5α-Reductase Deficiency. — Male pseudohermaphroditism may also result from defective function of the 5α-reductase enzyme with inadequate conversion of testosterone to dihydrotestosterone. This enzyme acts within androgen-responsive cells of the perineum. Defective conversion of testosterone to dihydrotestosterone at the genital tubercle and labioscrotal folds gives rise to only partial masculinization of the external genitalia. From 7 to 12 weeks of fetal life, when masculinization of the male genitalia should be completed, 5α-reductase activity in the fetal genital area peaks. Later androgen exposure fails to correct the defect. This form of male pseudohermaphroditism is also known as *pseudovaginal perineoscrotal* hypospadias because of the specific sexual ambiguity most commonly encountered with it. Testicular testosterone and MIH production is normal so that müllerian regression occurs and internal wolffian structures are developed to varying degrees. However, as is true of most patients with male pseudohermaphroditism, the sperm-carrying ducts end blindly before the prostate gland, so even if spermatogenesis occurs, the ejaculate is azoospermic. Inheritance is X-linked recessive and is more common in certain ethnic groups. A number of specific defects of the 5α-reductase enzyme have been described including impaired binding of testosterone, heat lability, and a combination of the two. In the undiagnosed patient or in the patient in whom orchidectomy is not accomplished by the age of puberty, there is further virilization of the ambiguous genitalia with phallic growth, development of a muscular male habitus, and male body hair patterns.

Hormonal profiles include normal or elevated testosterone levels with low DHT levels in relation to testosterone levels, an elevated ratio of testosterone to DHT, and a high ratio of 5-β- to 5-α-reduced urinary steroid metabolites. Stimulation with hCG further accentuates this altered ratio. Decreased conversion of testosterone to DHT can also be demonstrated in cultured fibroblasts from androgen-sensitive tissues.[19]

The virilization which occurs at puberty can be very disconcerting to patients raised as females. The switch from a female to male gender role reported from the Dominican Republic provides interesting insights into factors influencing gender identity. While initial reports suggest an easy switch to a male gender role in a male-dominated culture, subsequently, with a greater awareness of the situation, there may be greater problems for those children growing up with recognized genital ambiguity.

Unidentified In Utero Defects.—Patients with male pseudohermaphroditism may have no identifiable defect of androgen secretion or action. While the etiology remains unknown, the incomplete differentiation may result from lack of synchronization of androgen secretion and effect during the critical period of sexual differentiation. Ineffective or abnormal hCG stimulation of Leydig cell steroidogenesis at this critical time is also a potential cause of abnormal differentiation. While such abnormalities have not been identified, patients with 46,XY karyotypes born with genital ambiguity have had significant virilization at puberty without evidence of Leydig cell dysgenesis, androgen insensitivity, 5α-reductase or other enzyme deficiency.

Because fetal pituitary gonadotropin stimulation of testicular function is predated and preempted by placental hCG stimulation, gonadotropin deficiency does not contribute significantly to sexual differentiation, although subjects with hypogonadotropic hypogonadism may have undescended testes or micropenis, evidence of androgen deficiency, later in fetal life.

While exogenous hormones may also interfere in the normal differentiation of male genitalia, the etiology of male sexual ambiguity is frequently indeterminate.

Mixed Gonadal Dysgenesis

The term *mixed gonadal dysgenesis* has been defined in two ways. The anatomic definition is based on a unilateral streak gonad on one side and testicular tissue, usually within a dysgenetic testis, on the other side. The chromosomal definition involves chromosomal mosaicism that includes at least one Y chromosome, most commonly 45,X/46,XY. Most patients qualify by both criteria but among some patients, the degree of gonadal dysgenesis may vary in each of the gonads and the karyotype may be 46,XY. Conversely, the influence of the Y chromosome upon gonadal differentiation may have been lost so that the external genitalia are female and the presentation may be with features comparable to Turner's syndrome.

The physical findings in patients with mixed gonadal dysgenesis reflect the level of function of the fetal dysgenetic testis. The degree of virilization of the external genitalia and size of the penis depends on relative androgen stimulation present at 9 to 13 weeks and during the second and third trimester of gestation, respectively. Scrotal development may be asymmetric, greater on the side occupied by a testis, and related to relative testicular descent (Figs 8–2 and 8–5). Internal development may also be asymmetric. The side of the streak gonad commonly has some development of müllerian-derived structures while the contralateral side has varying development of the vas deferens and wolffian structures commensurate with the degree of androgen production by the testis. Patients raised as girls should have gonadectomy

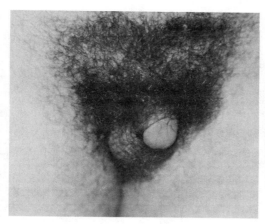

FIG 8–5.
Mixed gonadal dysgenesis. Genitalia of teenaged youth with karyotype 45,X/46,XY. A gonadal streak and müllerian remnants on the *left* were removed during childhood. The testis on the *right* is intrascrotal, and grew during spontaneous puberty. The hypospadias has been repaired so that urination and erections are normal.

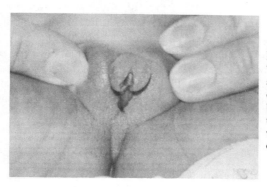

FIG 8–6.
True hermaphroditism. Ambiguous genitalia of a newborn infant found to have differentiated ovarian and testicular tissue. The patient is being raised as a girl because of phallus size. A unilateral ovary with ipsilateral fallopian tube was developed, and a uterus was present. The ovotestis was removed.

to avoid the risk of tumor development. Those raised as males may have adequate androgen secretion for pubertal virilization. Furthermore, if the single testis is left intact, a scrotal location should be ensured to facilitate examination.

True Hermaphroditism

The diagnosis of true hermaphroditism is based on the presence of both differentiated testicular tissue and ovarian tissue containing oocytes within the same individual. The testicular and ovarian tissue may be combined within an ovotestis, on one or both sides, or in distinct opposite gonads. External genitalia are usually but not always ambiguous (Fig 8–6) and a wide variety of ambiguity of internal and external genitalia may exist. The testis or ovotestis may be descended to varying levels and may present as an inguinal hernia. Scrotal development may be asymmetric. Internal duct development varies depending on the hormonal milieu determined by the presence and function of an ipsilateral testis, and by the amount of testosterone and MIH produced. A uterus is often at least partially developed. True hermaphroditism is most commonly associated with 46,XX karyotype, but 46,XY, 46,XX/46,XY, and other mosaic patterns may also occur. Spontaneous puberty and menses may occur in the 46,XX form and occasionally in mosaics. Fertility has been documented.[65] In some patients, the phallus is relatively well developed as a result of some testicular function, although it is usually hypospadic. Such patients may therefore be reared as male.[5]

Evaluation of Ambiguous Genitalia

Disorders of genital differentiation often present with ambiguous external genitalia at birth. Ambiguous genitalia in the newborn should be considered a potential neonatal emergency. The determination of life-threatening hypoadrenalism, the detection of associated congenital anomalies, and the alleviation of parental concerns justify this approach. The appearance of the genitalia does not reflect the chromosomal sex, but the prenatal hormonal millieu. Appropriate sex of rearing must be determined as soon as possible. Parents should be told that there is a problem in the development of the genitalia and that they should delay announcing the birth of their child for a few hours or days until an evaluation indicates whether the sex should be male or female.

Evaluation should begin with a careful physical examination to determine the degree of sexual ambiguity and to detect any other developmental anomalies. The symmetry of gonadal development is a critical feature of this evaluation. The size and position of the phallus, the extent of fusion of the labioscrotal and urethrolabial folds, the position of the urethral meatus, and the presence of a vagina, vaginal pouch, or urogenital sinus should be noted. The scrotum or labioscrotal folds and the inguinal region should be carefully palpated for gonadal tissue and hernias. A rectal examination may detect a midline uterine cervix. Incomplete genital development, such as epispadias, which does not represent incomplete virilization and does not result from a hormonal defect, may occur.

The initial diagnostic tests for genital ambiguity include establishment of a karyotype, determination of levels of serum gonadotropins, testosterone, and 17-hydroxyprogesterone (to detect the most common enzyme defect causing genital ambiguity), pelvic ultrasound, and a genitogram with retrograde injection of contrast media to outline the lumina of the urethra and vagina, if present. The karyotype is helpful in deciding subsequent diagnostic tests and sex assignment. Although the karyotype may indicate that the chromosomes are 46,XX or 46,XY, that alone is insufficient to determine the sex of rearing but does provide information to more reasonably assess the appropriateness of sex assignment. The karyotype is also insufficient to categorize ambiguous genitalia since, for example, both female pseudohermaphroditism and true hermaphroditism may occur with a 46,XX karyotype. If chromosome tests are inconclusive, a gonadal biopsy may be indicated.

Serum gonadotropins and testosterone will provide information concerning primary gonadal failure or feedback defects as in PAIS. 17-Hydroxyprogesterone will be markedly elevated in the most common causes of female pseudohermaphroditism, 21-hydroxylase and 11-hydroxylase congenital adrenal hyperplasia (CAH). The pelvic ultrasound and bimanual rectal examination may establish the presence of a complete vagina, a uterus and ovaries, or a partly descended testis.

Gender Assignment

It may be difficult to recommend a sex of rearing before a definitive diagnosis is made. However, if lack of phallic development precludes a male gender assignment, a female sex of rearing may be made even before the karyotype is known. Gender and sexual orientation is not dependent on chromosomal, gonadal, or in utero hormonal factors and may be learned in the rearing environment. However, a male sex of rearing should not be assigned until the karyotype is known, even if genital development is adequate for the male sexual role, with or without surgical intervention. This approach prevents the inappropriate sex assignment of a genetic female with normal ovaries and internal female organs.

Three basic considerations for a recommendation of sex of rearing are (1) the potential for sexual intercourse, (2) the potential for gonadal hormone production adequate to induce puberty and maintain sexual maturity in the adult, and (3) the potential for fertility. The sex of the child should be that for which the potential for these three is greatest. A child with ovaries, internal female structures, and a 46,XX karyotype, but with severely virilized external genitalia, has the potential for normal pubertal development and may, after appropriate genital surgery, assume a satisfactory female sexual role and have normal fertility. An infant with a 46,XY karyotype with adequate penis development to anticipate normal size and erectile function may appropriately be raised as a male even though testicular hormone production and fertility are unlikely.

Sex of rearing for a child with female pseudohermaphroditism should always be female, if the choice is made in infancy. Most patients with female pseudohermaphroditism have virilizing adrenal hyperplasia, a condition in which the ovaries, fallopian tubes, and uterus can be expected to be adequately developed at birth. With appropriate treatment of the adrenal hyperplasia, normal pubertal development and fertility can be expected. If raised as a male, even though the child may have a phallus adequate for penetration, the absence of a testicle would require continued hormonal supplementation before and after puberty and fertility would be precluded.

Conversely, in no instance should a child be raised a male, even if the karyotype is 46,XY, if the potential of a functional penis of adequate size for penile-vaginal intercourse is not present. The decision of gender assignment among patients with male pseudohermaphroditism is primarily based on potential penile adequacy since the other two considerations, pubertal hormonal secretion and fertility, are both unlikely. The causes of inadequate male genital development are usually associated with significant disruption of gonadal function and internal genital development such as to preclude adequate maturation and delivery of spermatozoa, and therefore the probability of normal fertility is remote. Because penis size is the major consideration in the assignment of male sex of rearing, and since the partial androgen insensitivity syndrome is a cause of male pseudohermaphroditism, a trial of androgen stimulation of penile growth may be indicated and, if positive, may provide reassurance that the appropriate assignment is being made.

The sex assignment of patients with mixed gonadal dysgenesis is more commonly female because genital development is only mildly or moderately virilized. The male gender should only be assigned to those with adequate phallic development and preferably with hormonal or physical evidence of a functional testis.

The diagnosis of true hermaphroditism, a condition associated with several karyotypes, is seldom made before gender is decided. However, the assignment of sex can still be made appropriately since patients with masculinized genitalia will usually be raised as females, and should be. If the fallopian tube is developed on the side of a functional ovary, even though uterine development is asymmetric, puberty and fertility are possible. A male sex of assignment should be made only if penile development is potentially adequate and a testis is partially or completely descended.

Diagnostic Criteria and Management

Female Pseudohermaphroditism.—A 46,XX karyotype allows tentative classification of patients into the category of female pseudohermaphroditism. As mentioned above, this disorder is classified on the basis of a normal female karyotype, the presence of ovaries and internal female structures, and usually results from the virilizing effect of excess of adrenal androgens.

Since the CAHs—primarily 21-hydroxylase deficiency—are the most common causes of female pseudohermaphroditism, metabolites of adrenal steroid synthesis in blood and urine need to be assayed. For example, significant elevation of 17-hydroprogesterone is indicative of defective 21-hydroxylase action. A careful history is needed to determine the causes resulting from androgen excess of transplacental origin, either maternal or exogenous. Both history and physical findings suggest the etiologies associated with in utero insults and other congenital defects. A pelvic ultrasound and genitogram may help to determine internal genital development and to plan surgical repair. If the etiology is not determined, exploration at the time of genitoplasty may be desirable to verify internal development. Exploratory surgery may be required at a later date to verify the correct classification from those possible given a 46,XX karyotype: female pseudohermaphroditism, true hermaphroditism, or mixed gonadal dysgenesis.

Male Pseudohermaphroditism.—The diagnosis of male pseudohermaphroditism is based on the presence of a male 46,XY karyotype in the presence of incompletely virilized or variably feminized external genitalia (see Fig 8–3). The failure of virilization may reflect the inadequate production of androgen or the failure of androgen effect at the cellular level in androgen-responsive tissues. Abnormalities of androgen production are reflected by low serum testosterone and high LH and FSH levels. If Leydig cells are dysgenetic, all precursor hormone levels will be low, while among the enzyme deficiencies, whether or not the defect involves the adrenal as well as the gonad, levels proximal to the defect are generally elevated while those distal are low. High-level blocks in the androgen pathway, such as 20,22-desmolase and 3β-hydroxysteroid dehydrogenase defects, present with evidence of adrenal insufficiency. All adrenocortical steroids are low in the former while pregnenolone, 17-hydroxypregnenolone, and DHEA can be expected to be elevated in the latter. Defects of 17-hydroxylase/17,20-desmolase action result in diminished amounts of steroids from the glucocorticoid pathway in the adrenal gland, and decreased steroid levels from the sex steroid pathways of both the adrenal and gonad while DOC and corticosterone levels are elevated. Deficiency of 17-ketosteroid reductase affects only the sex steroid pathway, and therefore is not associated with abnormal levels of steroids from mineralocorticoid or glucocorticoid production. Serum testosterone and androstenedione levels are low and LH is elevated. Estrone levels may also be increased. Stimulation with hCG to accentuate the abnormal steroid levels may be helpful in diagnosing these testosterone synthetic defects.

The diagnosis of 5α-reductase deficiency may be made based upon an elevated testosterone-DHT ratio in early infancy following hCG or testosterone stimulation, or after puberty. Because urinary C-19 and C-21 steroid 5α-metabolites are also reduced in 5α-reductase deficiency, low ratios of 5α– and 5β–urinary metabolites or urinary tetrahydrocortisol (THF) to 5α-THF provide a basis for the diagnosis as does decreased 5α-reductase activity (decreased conversion of testosterone to DHT) in cultured fibroblasts from genital skin.[28,29] Gonadotropins, particularly LH, may be elevated in early infancy and after puberty.

Patients with PAIS have elevated male levels of serum LH, FSH, and testosterone, a lack of penile growth in response to testosterone administration, and may or may not have reduced androgen binding in cells from the usual androgen-sensitive sites. In male pseudohermaphroditism, failure to make a diagnosis would indicate surgical exploration and gonadal biopsy. Concomitantly, surgical repair involving genital reconstruction and scrotal replacement or removal of the testes may be indicated.

Mixed Gonadal Dysgenesis.—The diagnosis of mixed gonadal dysgenesis can usually be made based on the presence of variably ambiguous genitalia, asymmetry of gonadal location and development, a mosaic karyotype (usually 45X/46XY, but also 46,XY), and elevated serum gonadotropin levels. A dysgenetic testis is present, descended to varying degrees, with a streak gonad on the opposite side. Exploratory surgery is indicated to document gonadal development. Histology shows Leydig cells and varying seminiferous tubule defects which may be as severe as the tubule profile of Sertoli cell–only syndrome.

The streak gonad should be removed. In the case of the formed gonad, removal or placement in the scrotum is recommended (see Fig 8–5). In the subject raised as female, removal is additionally indicated to prevent masculinization at puberty.

True Hermaphroditism.—True hermaphroditism (see Fig 8–6) can only be established by gonadal biopsy which documents true ovarian and testicular elements existing in the same subject. Clinical evaluation of the external and internal genitalia will not establish the diagnosis and the phenotypic manifestations may vary greatly. Müllerian structures will usually be absent or rudimentary on the side of the testis or ovotestis. The testis or ovotestis may produce a serum testosterone level in infancy, after hCG stimulation, and after puberty, which exceeds age-appropriate female levels. Normal or elevated gonadotropin levels are present in the neonate and in the postpubertal patient. Karyotype is usually 46,XX and therefore a 46,XX female with ambiguous genitalia, asymmetric gonads, and an elevated serum testosterone without an etiologic diagnosis warrants a gonadal biopsy. A 46,XX/46,XY karyotype suggests this diagnosis. Any patient with either of these karyotypes or a 46,XY karyotype without an etiologic diagnosis should also have gonadal biopsies to rule out true hermaphroditism.

Hypospadias

Hypospadias is defined as failure of complete development and incorporation of the penile urethra within the shaft of the penis (Fig 8–7). The urethral opening may

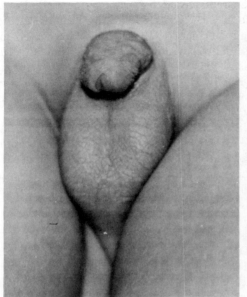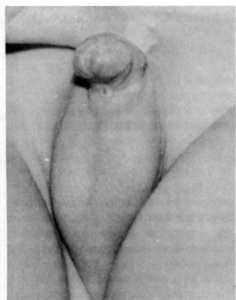

FIG 8–7.
A, 46,XY male with hypospadias accompanied by chordee. **B,** urethral meatus at the penoscrotal junction can be seen.

therefore be at any point from the perineum to the glans and its position forms the basis of classification. Hypospadias may be classified as glanular, coronal, distal, or midshaft, penoscrotal or perineoscrotal. More proximal defects of urethral development are associated with failure of development of the corpus spongiosum and shortening of the ventral shaft of the penis, or chordee. There may also be underdevelopment of the penis, but the term *micropenis* should not be used in this context.

Because hypospadias is failure of androgen-stimulated midline fusion, hypospadias represents a form of ambiguous genitalia. It is estimated to occur in 8 in 1,000 males. The milder forms with the urethral meatus close to the tip of the penis are more common. The more severe forms may be characterized by such severe underdevelopment of the urethrolabial folds that there is simply inadequate tissue to fuse and form the urethra. The control of the midline fusion is by testosterone via DHT, but defects in androgen synthesis are seldom identified among patients with hypospadias without additional manifestations of ambiguous genitalia. Potential etiologies include failure of testosterone secretion, failure of testosterone effect, genetic causes, and idiopathic cases, which constitute the majority.

Mixed gonadal dysgenesis, true hermaphroditism, and occasionally cryptorchidism (10%) are associated with hypospadias, the former two with severe hypospadias and ambiguous genitalia. Failure of testosterone effect, as in Reifenstein syndrome, incomplete androgen insensitivity, or 5α-reductase deficiency, may also be associated with hypospadias. More distal and therefore milder forms are usually idiopathic, not associated with testicular or endocrine dysfunction, and may frequently be familial. In families with idiopathic hypospadias, there is a 12% recurrence rate in subsequent males. This figure increases to 26% if the father is also affected. Idiopathic hypospadias is also generally the most distal type when associated with other congenital anomalies.[1,37,67]

Hypospadias may be found frequently in the presence of major congenital abnormalities of the lower half of the trunk such as myelomeningocele and imperforate anus. Renal abnormalities may occur in 5% of patients with idiopathic hypospadias. However, associated abnormalities need not be confined to the local area or to the genitourinary system.[3,16,38]

The ventral portion of the foreskin, formed as part of the same fusion process, may be deficient. Because surgical correction may be required, circumcision should be delayed so that the foreskin can be available for surgical repair.

Hypogenitalism (Micropenis)

Micropenis or *hypogenitalism* (Fig 8–8) refers to the presence of a fully formed but small penis in the absence of other abnormalities of sexual differentiation.[43] The definition is therefore statistical and refers to a penis which is 2.5 SD below the normal

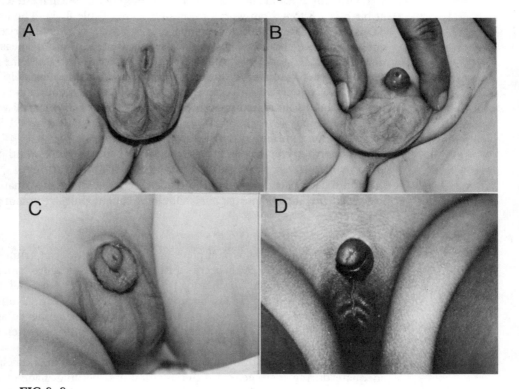

FIG 8–8.
Genital development in two patients referred for evaluation of inadequate penile development. Genitalia before androgen therapy (**A and B**) and after (**C**). This is an example of the buried penis syndrome in which corpora development within the penile shaft is adequate, and the skin does not cover the shaft but is continuous with suprapubic skin from just below the corona. **D**, micropenis; an adequately formed, but underdeveloped scrotum; and palpable testes.

TABLE 8–1.

Mean Stretched Penile Length (cm)

Age	Mean ± 1 SD	− 2.5 SD
Birth		
30 weeks' gestation	2.7 ± 0.5	1.5
34 weeks' gestation	3.0 ± 0.4	2.0
Full term	3.5 ± 0.4	2.5
0–5 mo	3.8 ± 0.8	1.8
6–12 mo	4.1 ± 0.8	2.1
1–2 yr	4.6 ± 0.8	2.6
2–3 yr	5.0 ± 0.8	3.0
3–4 yr	5.4 ± 1.0	2.9
4–5 yr	5.6 ± 0.7	3.4
5–7 yr	6.0 ± 0.9	3.8
7–9 yr	6.3 ± 1.0	3.8
9–11 yr	6.3 ± 1.0	3.8

standards for age and stage of pubertal development. Normal stretched penile length at birth is 2.8 to 4.2 cm with a mean of 3.5 cm (Table 8–1). The lower limit for 2.5 SD is 1.9 cm. The question of hypogenitalism most commonly arises during infancy and during late childhood just before pubertal onset. Careful measurement, particularly in the infant with a thick suprapubic fat pad, will limit the overdiagnosis of this problem. Observation of a spontaneous erection may be helpful. Little penile growth occurs relative to increasing body length during childhood and therefore the presentation of this question is frequently just before the pubertal years, particularly in the obese boy. At whatever age the question arises, stretched length should be compared with published norms (see Table 8–1).

The term *micropenis* should not be used in the presence of other developmental abnormalities of the penis, such as simple hypospadias or forms of genital ambiguity, including male pseudohermaphroditism. Once it is established that a penis is significantly small, an etiologic diagnosis should be sought and a treatment plan formulated.

Etiology

Penile development is complete at the end of the first trimester, but further growth in length and breadth occurs during the second and third trimesters in response to continuing androgen stimulation. Therefore, abnormalities of hypothalamic-pituitary function resulting in low androgen production, including Kallmann syndrome, may be associated with micropenis.[63] In addition, abnormalities of androgen production in the presence of appropriate stimulation, as in Klinefelter syndrome, or of androgen effect (partial androgen insensitivity syndrome) may be associated with micropenis. In both of these instances, androgen stimulation and responsiveness were adequate during male genital differentiation and became inadequate subsequently. Abnormalities of growth hormone (GH deficiency) or GH effect (Laron-type dwarfism) may also be associated with micropenis, suggesting a supportive role for GH in genital development. Finally, idiopathic micropenis may be the most common form of the defect seen in clinical practice.[44] The etiology of idiopathic micropenis is unclear, and the diagnosis is by exclusion. There may be evidence of attenuated scrotal development, and cryptorchidism may be associated.

Conditions associated with both primary hypogonadism and micropenis include the following: Klinefelter, Robinow, Laurence-Moon-Biedl, and multiple X syndromes. Micropenis and secondary hypogonadism are associated with Kallmann syndrome, hypopituitarism, Laron-type dwarfism, septo-optic dysplasia, and the syndromes of Laurence-Moon-Biedl, Prader-Willi, and Rud. Associated with unexplained (idiopathic) micropenis are the following syndromes: Carpenter, Cornelia de Lange, Down, Fanconi pancytopenia, Hallerman-Streiff, long-arm 18 deletion, Noonan, Smith-Lemli-Opitz, triploidy, and Williams.

Examination

Measurement of the fully stretched length of a penis is the most accurate measurement. Flaccid penile length varies considerably, and is not useful. A stretched length measurement requires that the glans be grasped between the thumb and finger of the examiner and the penis pulled to the point of slight discomfort. With the other hand, the examiner holds a nonflexible ruler along the dorsal surface while depressing the suprapubic fat pad so that the measurement begins at the base of the penis and extends to the tip of the glans. This length should be compared with published normal values for age (see Table 8–1). An estimation of the relative corporal volume should be made. The location of the urethral meatus, scrotal development, and testicular descent and size should be verified.

Hormonal Assessment

Measurement of gonadotropins, testosterone and, if indicated, GH profiles may be helpful in determining the etiology of micropenis in the newborn. Elevated levels of gonadotropins indicate primary hypogonadism. Mildly elevated levels in the presence of high or high-normal testosterone levels suggests partial androgen insensitivity since the insensitivity is also expressed at the hypothalamic-pituitary level. Normal or low levels associated with low serum testosterone may be indicative of hypothalamic-pituitary dysfunction and secondary hypogonadism. Normal testosterone and gonadotropins, with no evidence of GH deficiency, suggest idiopathic micropenis. Determination of the cause by hormone determinations after 6 months of age and before the pubertal years may be difficult, although hCG administration can be used to assess testicular steroidogenesis during this time. If partial androgen insensitivity is suspected, androgen-binding studies in cells from androgen-responsive tissues may be done to assess receptor level or function.

Androgen or hCG administration may stimulate further penile development during infancy or childhood. This can be a practical test to exclude androgen insensitivity. Significant penile growth rules out androgen insensitivity and predicts further growth potential. A single injection of testosterone in oil, 25 or 50 mg, may be sufficient, but this dose may be repeated once or twice at monthly intervals, if necessary.

Therapy and Counseling

Concern about penile size is a common anxiety. For infant males and young boys, the concern is parental. Later, the parent and child may share the concern. These concerns are probably related to societal views that greater size means greater masculinity, potency, and appeal. Adult erect penis size varies in a normal distribution, as do all body organs, and reassurance of normalcy may be all that is required.

Most often, micropenis is not present when this concern is raised by patients or parents (Fig 8–9). The common ages of questioning are infancy and between 9 and 12 years, just prior to puberty. Frequently, the concern among the older group is an overweight boy with a thick suprapubic fat pad with the penis appearing small relative to body size. In almost all such boys, normal penile size can be demonstrated by careful penile measurement while depressing the suprapubic subcutaneous tissue. The stretched length can be demonstrated to the parents and patient, with reference to normal ranges for age, and with the explanation that the root of the penis is obscured in the suprapubic fat pad and that little penile growth occurs from age 5 years until the onset of puberty (see Table 8–1). Because the body grows continuously, penile size appears progressively smaller relative to body size over the prepubertal years. This explanation usually suffices to convince the patient and his parents of adequate and normal size.

When a micropenis is present and a search has been made to identify the underlying cause, an age-appropriate treatment plan should be made. Assignment to the female sex is rarely indicated even in severe cases, and should be considered only if the patient is younger than 18 months of age. Marked degrees of hypogenitalism,

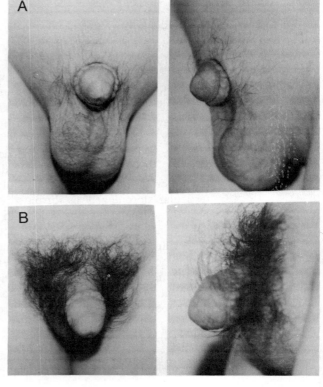

FIG 8–9.
A, Genitalia in a 14-year-old boy with the complaint of a small penis. Pubertal development had begun, evidenced by testicular size and pubic hair. A daytime testosterone level did not indicate that progression of pubertal development would proceed rapidly, so the patient was given exogenous testosterone for 4 months. **B,** subsequent penis development was occurring normally and appropriately.

particularly if associated with other features of ambiguous genitalia or with minimal development of erectile tissue, can occasionally justify sex assignment to the female sex. Such situations may arise with partial androgen insensitivity or in cases of severe maldevelopment of the erectile apparatus. Failure of penile growth in response to androgen stimulation must be demonstrated before sex assignment is contemplated.

The decision of sex assignment to female should always be carefully considered and discussed in detail with the parents. The decision can only be justified in the absence of a reasonable expectation of further penile growth. After appropriate counseling and discussions, parents can understand that rearing their child as a female is the only reasonable course for their child. The same principles of counseling apply to these cases as for parents of children with ambiguous genitalia. The bipotential onset of physical sexual differentiation, the learned rather than genetic nature of gender identity, and the fact that female gender assignment can be successful should be stressed. When female gender assignment is indicated and occurs, appropriate plans for surgical and medical treatment should be made and discussed with the parents, and continued support and counseling for the parents and child should be planned for the future.

While consideration of sexual identity is not usually part of the therapy for the patient with micropenis, appropriate therapy throughout childhood and adolescence is indicated. The most important aspect of this therapy is counseling. It is not clear that penile growth missed during the final third of in utero development is lost forever. Some patients may achieve normal adult penile length after full pubertal androgen stimulation, although a small relative size is more likely. The emphasis of counseling should be that size is unimportant for sexual satisfaction and adjustment and that the development of the usual male sexual roles and orientation can be expected to develop.[59] Parents need to hear repeatedly that parental attitude provides the strongest influence, that parents who are supportive, who explain the problems, and who encourage and expect a male gender identity can expect their son to reflect their attitudes.

Androgen administration, 25 or 50 mg of testosterone enanthate intramuscularly (IM), may be indicated not only as a diagnostic test but to stimulate penile growth at key times during childhood to avert or address psychological concerns. Since normal penile growth is greater during the first rather than the second 5 years of childhood, response to therapy may be greater if it is administered early. The age at which such treatment may be helpful is from 2 to 3 years when comparisons are first being made, and again when starting school when bathroom exposure may be more frequent. When psychological concerns are evident, therapy may be considered at any age. Treatment should be carefully monitored to avoid excessive stimulation of general growth and skeletal maturation by androgen. If more than two injections are given, radiologic bone age should be assessed.

Persistent Müllerian Structures

The discovery of a uterus and fallopian tubes in males without ambiguous genitalia is usually an unexpected finding during surgery for inguinal hernias (hernia uteri inguinale) or cryptorchidism. The etiology is presumed to be defective MIH secretion in utero but may be a receptor defect. Until diagnosed, genital development is presumed to be normal although the testes may be dysgenetic and prone to germ cell malignant degeneration. The disorder may be familial. Surgical removal of the müllerian structures is recommended.

46,XY Pure Gonadal Dysgenesis

Gonadal agenesis or gonadal dysgenesis with absent steroidogenesis, whether the karyotype be 46,XX or 46,XY, results in female genital differentiation. Patients with 46,XY pure gonadal dysgenesis have normal stature, lack pubertal development, have hormonal evidence of primary hypogonadism, and frequently have eunuchoid proportions. Because of the risk of malignant degeneration, gonadectomy is indicated. The etiology of the failure of testicular differentiation is unclear, is not explained by H-Y antigen alone, and is likely due to small deletions of the Y chromosome which contain the testis-determining gene or genes. Rarely, patients have features of Turner syndrome and may fit the syndrome complex that is associated with 45,X and with 45,X/46,XY or 45/46,XY mosaic combinations. Hormonal replacement is by estrogen and progesterone after puberty.

Phenotypic males with small testes, possibly associated with cryptorchidism or a degree of hypospadias, may have a 46,XX or 45,X karyotype. Presentation may be at or after puberty with pubertal delay or hypogonadism due to deficient testicular steroidogenesis or later with azoospermic infertility. Mental retardation may be associated with the 45,X form. In utero male differentiation suggests effective early androgen production and the absence of the Y chromosome may be explained by translocation of the critical portion of the Y chromosome to an autosome or to the X chromosome.[2] Occurrence of 46,XX males may be familial and may be in association with 46,XX true hermaphroditism.[61]

Males with 46,XX gonadal dysgenesis share some features of Klinefelter syndrome such as testicular volume and histology, hypergonadotropic hypogonadism, and gynecomastia, but not eunuchoid proportions and psychological problems. Intellectual deficits, not a characteristic of XXY Klinefelter syndrome, but more commonly a problem in the multiple X forms, do not seem to be a characteristic of 46,XX males. Again, counseling and appropriate explanations are essential and treatment is by androgen replacement therapy.

MALE PUBERTAL DEVELOPMENT

Puberty is the period during which the final maturation of growth and development occurs, resulting in a physically adult, sexually mature individual. The physiologic hormonal changes which stimulate puberty are actually a resurgence of secretory mechanisms which were already functional during in utero life and infancy but which became quiescent during childhood. The central focus of the increased hormonal secretion is the augmentation of both the frequency and magnitude of gonadotropin pulsatile secretion. There is an escalation of hypothalamic gonadotropin-releasing hormone (GnRH) episodic secretion initiating this process. This increased secretion of GnRH may result from removal of inhibition or from increased stimulation of higher central nervous system (CNS) centers. Increased gonadotropin secretion ensues; urinary, blood, and model studies indicate that elevation of FSH secretion precedes LH in puberty. The gonadotropins, particularly FSH, together with androgen stimulate spermatogenesis. LH stimulates secretion of testosterone by the Leydig cells of the testis and thereby induces the anabolic androgen effects characteristic of puberty, including sexual hair growth, genital maturation, and somatic growth with increased muscle and bone mass. The process results in a sexually mature individual capable of reproduction.[41,42]

In Utero

The initial development of the hypothalamic-pituitary-testicular axis occurs during fetal life and plays a role in male sexual differentiation, as discussed above. GnRH can be detected by 6 weeks after conception and pituitary LH and FSH by 10 weeks. Within a few days, integrated function of the hypothalamic-pituitary unit is present with gonadotropin release in response to GnRH. Gonadotropin levels rise progressively until midgestation, after which they decline until birth. This pattern is consistent with an increasing androgen secretion from the testes, which in turn is subsequently suppressed by the adjusting negative feedback mechanism. The decline in gonadotropin secretion during the second half of gestation probably represents further suppression by the high levels of maternal estrogen which persist until birth. Concomitantly, an increase in neuroendocrine inhibition of GnRh secretion develops which, except for a readjustment during the neonatal period, persists until puberty.

Newborn and Childhood

At birth there is a resurgence of gonadotropin secretion consistent with a reduction of the negative effect of maternal sex steroid on hypothalamic-pituitary-gonadal activity. Mean serum LH, FSH, and testosterone levels rise after birth to a peak at 6 to 12 weeks of age, an interval of temporary reactivation of the hypothalamic-pituitary-gonadal unit. During this time, gonadotropins are released in the same episodic fashion as during puberty and in the sexually mature individual. After 3 months of age there is a gradual fall of serum gonadotropin levels to the low levels characteristic of childhood. During these years there is a persistence of periodic release of gonadotropins at a diminished frequency and amplitude, more apparent during sleep.

Puberty

Puberty is initiated by the resurgence of episodic gonadotropin secretion, first occurring during sleep. Mean circulating levels of gonadotropins rise, the elevation of FSH levels preceding those of LH. Gradually the diurnal variation in gonadotropin secretion is lost as puberty is established.[64]

Before the hormonal elevations characteristic of testicular reactivation (gonadarche) are apparent, an increase in adrenal androgen secretion (adrenarche) occurs.

Adrenarche is the result of the progressive development of the adrenocortical zona reticularis and occurs before pubarche. The control of steroidogenic shift and the cause of the resulting adrenache is unknown but is unrelated to gonadarche. Adrenarche can be verified by determining DHEA sulfate (DHEA-S) serum levels. The DHEA-S concentration, because of its long half-life, increases before other adrenal androgens. This hormonal evidence of adrenarche can usually be detected 2 or more years before hormonal evidence of gonadarche can be detected.

The principal adrenal androgens are DHEA and androstenedione. Both are relatively weak androgens but may stimulate increased sebaceous gland secretion and the development of acne and body odor, clinical markers of adrenarche. Rarely, adrenal androgens may be responsible for pubic hair development in males, as in the absence of testicular steroids, e.g., Kallmann syndrome.

The earliest sign of puberty on physical examination is testicular enlargement. Testicular volume greater than 4 mL or a longitudinal axis length more than 2.5 cm is evidence of the onset of puberty resulting from FSH stimulation. Subsequent physical development of puberty can be usefully documented using the Tanner staging of genital and pubic hair development (see Chapter 2), with serial testicular volume measurements. The rate of pubertal progression may vary, but the sequence of progression is consistent. The mean age of onset of puberty is between 11.5 and 12.5 years, with a wide normal range extending from 9.5 to about 14 years. Onset of puberty at an age younger than 9.5 is precocious and after age 14 in males is delayed. Pubertal development correlates more closely with biologic development as indicated by skeletal age than by chronologic age. The first signs of puberty are therefore expected to be present by the time a bone age of 12.5 years is achieved.

Growth of the penis is the next physical change of puberty after testicular growth. However, because neither the initial growth of the testes nor the penis is likely to be recognized without one or more careful examinations, the onset of the first coarse, pigmented pubic hairs is often the earliest evidence of puberty noted. Both genital and pubic hair growth progresses over the next 3 to 4 years. These stages of development, as classified by Tanner, proceed similarly but may not necessarily be correlated. Pubic hair and genital staging should therefore be recorded separately. The development of axillary and facial hair, acne, and voice change occur in the latter half of puberty. The maximum growth rate, both in height and weight gain, also occur during this time. Mature sperm is present with attainment of midsized testicular volume (10–12 mL) at midpuberty.[63] Sperm may also be detected in the morning urine sample.[40] The sperm count gradually increases throughout puberty to adult levels.[30,31] Pubertal and sexual maturation are usually complete by age 16 years.

Problems of Pubertal Development

Pubertal Delay

Delayed pubertal development may be defined as the failure to mature sexually in an age-appropriate fashion. Failure to complete pubertal development over the normal 3- to 4-year period despite normal age of onset, as well as delayed onset, is considered pubertal delay. Causes of pubertal delay may be grouped into those related to failure of the testis to respond to appropriate pubertal stimulation (primary hypogonadism); failure of the appropriate signal to appear at the expected time of puberty (hypogonadotropism or secondary hypogonadism); or, most commonly, delayed initiation of the activation of a normal hypothalamic-pituitary-testicular axis including both the entity of constitutional delay of puberty and delay in relation to chronic disease and malnutrition.[45]

Primary Hypogonadism.—Primary hypogonadism may involve partial or complete testicular failure (Table 8–2). Congenital abnormalities of testicular function presenting at this time are, among others, Klinefelter syndrome, gonadal dysgenesis, and congenital anorchia as well as those associated with congenital syndromes such as Prader-Willi and Laurence-Moon-Biedl. Acquired forms of testicular failure presenting at puberty are those associated with orchiectomy, viral or autoimmune orchitis, and testicular damage as a consequence of chemo- or radiotherapy. Frequently, primary testicular failure is associated with incomplete masculinization, i.e., failure to complete pubertal development rather than failure to enter puberty.

If the failure involves inadequate Leydig cell production of testosterone, the presentation may be pubertal delay. At pubertal age, normal reactivation of the hypothalamic-pituitary unit occurs. Failure of the testicular steroidogenetic response results in the absence of the appropriate negative feedback modulation of gonadotropin secretion. Therefore LH and FSH levels are in the castrate range. This elevation may be apparent even before the usual age of puberty, first manifest by elevated circulating FSH levels.[11]

The types of testicular failure that present with failure of pubertal development can often be suspected before the age of puberty. The clinical finding of absent testes or abnormally small or firm testes during infancy and childhood suggests primary hypogonadism. The diagnosis can be made before the age of pubertal development by the lack of response to hCG stimulation testing or, during early infancy, by pathologically elevated gonadotropin levels with concomitantly low testosterone levels.

Types of primary hypogonadism that do not necessarily present with pubertal delay are most commonly diagnosed during adulthood because of infertility, inadequate virilization, or gynecomastia, or occasionally in infancy because of absent or small testes. Seminiferous tubule dysfunction may be present with only partial Leydig cell insufficiency. These may include the Klinefelter[58] and Sertoli cell–only syndromes, and may also occur following chemo- and radiotherapy since spermatogenic elements are much more sensitive to damage than the Leydig cells.

Secondary Hypogonadism.—*Secondary hypogonadism* is defined as failure of testicular function on the basis of failure of the hypothalamic-pituitary unit. The term *hypogonadotropic hypogonadism* is usually reserved for permanent forms of hypothalamic-pituitary dysfunction causing testicular failure rather than the transient forms characterizing pubertal delay. The problem more commonly resides at the hypothalamic level causing GnRH deficiency, but may be associated with pituitary dysfunction. Hypothalamic dysfunction should be suspected in the presence of multiple hormone defects. Commonly, the hypopituitarism which results from intracranial space-occupying lesions or their treatment with surgery, irradiation, or chemotherapy is a reflection of, or is associated with, hypothalamic dysfunction as well. Clues to hypogonadotropic hypogonadism during childhood include the presence of additional

TABLE 8–2.

Categories of Pubertal Delay

Primary hypogonadism
  Androgen enzymatic synthesis defects
  Androgen insensitivity syndrome, partial
  Anorchia
  Autoimmunity
  Chemotherapy
  Cryptorchidism
  Galactosemia
  Gonadal dysgenesis
    Pure 46,XY
    Mixed 45,X/46,XY
  Infections
    Coxsackie
    Mumps
    Sexually transmitted diseases
  Irradiation
  Klinefelter syndrome (47,XXY, multiple X-Y syndrome)
  Luteinizing hormone–resistant testes
  Müllerian inhibiting hormone defect
  Myotonic dystrophy
  Noonan (Ullrich-Noonan) syndrome
  Partial androgen insensitivity
  5α-reductase deficiency
  Sertoli-cell-only syndrome
  Sickle cell disease
  Spinal cord neurologic disorders
  Surgical consequence
  Syndromes
    Laurence-Moon-Biedl
    Prader-Willi
    Robinow
  Testicular torsion
  Toxic orchitis
  Traumatic testicular destruction
  Vanishing testis syndrome
  XX males
  XYY syndrome and multiple Y syndrome
Secondary (hypogonadotropic) hypogonadism
  Autoimmune disease (also cause of pituitary defects)
  Craniopharyngioma
  Fertile eunuch syndrome
  Granulomatous disease
  Hemosiderosis, thalassemia
  Hypothalamic tumors
  Idiopathic hypopituitarism
  Irradiation
  Isolated follicle-stimulating hormone deficiency
  Isolated gonadotropin deficiency
  Kallmann syndrome

TABLE 8–2.
Categories of Pubertal Delay—cont'd

    Laron-type dwarfism
    Pituitary tumors
        Adrenocorticotropin-secreting tumors
        Growth hormone–secreting tumors
        Prolactinoma
    Septo-optic dysplasia (DeMorsier syndrome)
    Sickle cell disease (also delayed and primary failure)
    Steroid sulfatase deficiency
    Suprasellar tumors
    Surgery
    Syndromes
        Borgeson-Forssman-Lehman
        CHARGE
        Laurence-Moon-Biedl
        Leopard (multiple lentigenes)
        Lowe
        Martsoff
        Prader-Willi (also primary)
        Rothmund-Thomson
        Rud
        Steroid sulfatase deficiency
Delay of pubertal onset
    Anorexia nervosa
    Chronic systemic illness or treatment effects
        Cardiac
        Gastrointestinal (e.g., Crohn's disease)
        Hematologic (e.g., sickle cell)
        Malignancy
        Malnutrition
        Pulmonary
        Renal, chronic
    Constitutional delay of puberty
    Emotional stress
    Endocrinopathies (untreated)
        Cushing's disease
        Cushing's syndrome (e.g., iatrogenic)
        Diabetes mellitus
        Growth hormone deficiency
        Hyperprolactinemia
        Hypothyroidism
Excessive exercise
    Physical stress or overexertion
    Psychosocial dwarfism

---

hypothalamic-pituitary dysfunction, hypogenitalism with small testes or micropenis, cryptorchidism, cleft lip or palate, and anosmia or hyposmia (Kallmann syndrome) since the olfactory lobe is the site of origin of GnRH-secreting cells.[69] In cases of hypopituitarism, the risk of GnRH deficiency is proportional to the number of other hypothalamic-pituitary deficits.

The diagnosis of secondary hypogonadism may be verified only after enough years have passed without gonadotropin secretion since there is no consistent procedure to differentiate delayed maturation from a permanent defect.[6] Serum gonadotropins and testosterone are low and bone age may be retarded as in physiologic delay. Stimulation tests as well fail to distinguish secondary hypogonadism and constitutional delay of puberty.

Hypogonadotropism or secondary hypogonadism may be associated with the conditions and syndromes listed in Table 8–2 including congenital midline fusion defects, congenital and acquired hypothalamic tumors, infiltrations, and multiple complex syndromes. However, most cases presenting at puberty are idiopathic; the reason for the inability to secrete GnRH is unknown. Defects may involve either inadequate development of GnRH-secreting neurons or lack of stimulation of secretion. Inadequate development of the GnRH-secreting cells may result from defects of the primordial cells in the olfactory lobe as seen in patients with anosmia.

Physiologic Delay of Puberty (Including Constitutional Delay).—Constitutionally delayed puberty is essentially a diagnosis of exclusion and can be suspected in the absence of the above physical findings, significant health disorders, and in the presence of a normal physical examination. In addition, a family history, short stature, and delayed bone age may be supportive. However, there is no objective, definitive physical or laboratory confirmation of the diagnosis.

Puberty may also be delayed in individuals with the normal potential for sexual maturity as the result of any disorder which interferes with factors essential for progressive biologic maturity (see Table 8–2).

Evaluation of Pubertal Delay.—The initial assessment of pubertal delay involves a careful history and physical examination; basic hormonal testing, i.e., measurements of LH, FSH, and testosterone; and a bone age radiograph.[45] The medical history should include heights and weights throughout childhood to determine the pattern of growth and development up to puberty. Consistent delay of growth is more indicative of delay of growth and development. A normal pattern until the age of puberty suggests gonadal or pituitary deficiency. A history of cryptorchidism, small testes, and small penis is compatible with either primary or secondary deficiency. CNS tumors and their treatment, thyroid and pituitary dysfunction, or a history of hernia or genital surgery as well as the general medical history may be pertinent.

The physical examination should begin with a careful measurement of height, weight, upper-lower segment ratio, and arm span. A complete examination should be performed. Detailed evaluation of pubertal and genital development, particularly testicular size, should be performed, and evidence of hypogonadism, such as gynecomastia, recorded.

Serum testosterone, if elevated to the pubertal range, is supportive of initiation of puberty. Because there is diurnal variation of gonadotropin and testosterone secretion, particularly evident in early and midpuberty, morning venous sampling may be necessary to detect evidence of increased testosterone secretion. Serum LH and FSH levels should be measured to detect primary testicular failure. The wide range of normal and the overlap of gonadotropin levels before and across puberty limit the value of these tests except to exclude hypergonadotropic states. Neither gonadotropin, testosterone, or other hormone levels will differentiate between hypogonadotropism and delayed maturation. If bone age is greater than 12.5 years, the hypothalamic-pituitary axis should be active with normal pubertal gonadotropin and testosterone levels.

Further gonadotropin or gonadal hormone testing is seldom helpful. GnRH stimulation testing yields similar responses in physiologically delayed puberty and hypogonadotropic hypogonadism, and the hyperresponse of primary hypogonadism can be predicted by elevated basal hormone levels.[15] hCG testing, useful during childhood to test testicular function, will provoke a response in both the delayed and hypogonadotropic subject.[14] Gonadotropins will already be elevated in the pubertal-age male with primary hypogonadism. Frequent sampling of gonadotropin levels may reveal pulsatile patterns suggestive of puberty, but these may occur in hypogonadotropism.[63] Such testing is too expensive to be practical.

Treatment of Pubertal Delay and Hypogonadism.—Therapy for lack of pubertal development, regardless of the cause, is testosterone. Androgen therapy will stimulate somatic growth and pubertal maturation. The usual treatment utilizes the long-acting testosterone esters in oil (e.g., testosterone enanthate or cyprionate). This form will maintain reasonable levels for up to 2 weeks or may be administered less frequently if the goal is to initiate pubertal development. Small dosages will initiate pubertal changes so a regimen of 25 to 75 mg (commonly 50 mg) given every 4 weeks is adequate to gradually stimulate changes even though circulating values are not maintained above prepubertal values. Adult replacement therapy is 100 mg/wk, and since levels peak in 4 to 6 days and decline gradually thereafter, a regimen of 200 mg every 2 weeks will provide replacement therapy. Larger dosages given less frequently result in higher supraphysiologic levels during the first week with a decrement to subnormal levels during the third week and later.[62]

To stimulate pubertal development, dosages may be begun using a low, less frequent regimen (e.g., 50 mg every 4 weeks) and then gradually increasing dosage and frequency over 2 to 4 years to full adult therapy of 200 mg every 2 weeks.

Androgen therapy should be begun at the usual age of puberty or as soon thereafter as the diagnosis is made in patients with primary hypogonadism. Age of onset of therapy in patients with secondary hypogonadism depends upon other defects, the status of other therapy, and overall development and maturation. Androgen therapy could dramatically shorten adult height if given too soon in a hypopituitary patient before optional therapy with GH. The skeletal age and height standard deviation (z) score should be carefully evaluated to be sure that androgen therapy is not premature and will not prevent attainment of the boy's height potential. If constitutional delay of puberty is the tentative diagnosis, temporary androgen therapy may be given for several months to provide pubertal development for psychosocial reasons[60] without detrimental effect upon subsequent development.[47,71] If such patients are treated, subsequent evaluation is needed to verify whether pubertal hormonal secretion has begun.

Synthetic androgens available in oral or sublingual forms do not stimulate full pubertal development and are inadequate therapy. Transdermal applications and injections of depot forms of testosterone may become available in the future.

While GnRH or gonadotropin therapy could be used to stimulate testicular androgen synthesis in patients with hypogonadotropism,[23] such therapy is expensive and impractical for long-term therapy and should be reserved for stimulation of spermatogenesis in adult men when impregnation is being attempted.

Precocious Puberty

The onset of physical pubertal development before the age of 9.5 years in males is precocious. Early pubertal development may result from the early activation of pubertal gonadotropin secretion, or be the result of increased episodic secretion of GnRH from the hypothalamus (true or central precocious puberty, CPP) or of any other process that results in increased androgen stimulation causing physical maturation (precocious peripheral or pseudopuberty, PPP). CPP is characterized by a mature response to GnRH testing, while in PPP, the response to GnRH is comparable to the childhood pattern. Early onset of sexual hair, with acne and body odor, may not represent the onset of puberty but only adrenarche (Fig 8–10).

True (Central) Precocious Puberty.—If true puberty occurs early, the physiologic alteration is at the level of the hypothalamus. The prepubertal testes and pituitary are both capable of a mature pattern of response if appropriately stimulated. The down-regulation of the hypothalamic-pituitary-gonadal axis during childhood and its subsequent increased activity at puberty is not primarily due to a shift in the sensitivity of the feedback mechanism but is the result of less influence from higher CNS centers upon pulsatile GnRH release.

True isosexual precocious puberty may or may not have an identifiable cause (Table 8–3). However, the cause should always be sought in detail because of the frequent occurrence of CNS dysfunction as a cause and because of the possibility of successful treatment once the cause is identified. CPP occurs less frequently in males than females but is more commonly associated with the identification of a CNS lesion in the male. About 50% of male CPP is idiopathic whereas about 90% of female CPP is.

CPP may be the presenting sign of an intracranial space-occupying lesion, may

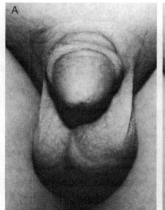 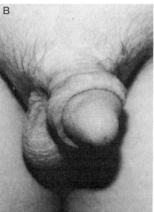

FIG 8–10.
A, early pubertal growth of genitalia in a boy after gonadarche with increased testicular size. **B,** prepubertal genitalia and Tanner stage 2 pubic hair in a boy with premature pubarche secondary to premature adrenarche.

TABLE 8–3.
Etiology of Precocious Puberty

Central (true)
  Idiopathic, sporadic, familial
  CNS abnormalities
    Arachnoid cysts
    Astrocytomas
    Brain abscess
    Congenital anomalies
    Craniopharyngioma
    Dysgerminomas
    Ependymomas
    Ganglioneuromas
    Granulomas
    Hydrocephalus
    Hypothalamic hamartoma
    Inflammatory (meningitis, encephalitis)
    Irradiation
    Neurofibromatoses
    Optic gliomas
    Prader-Willi syndrome
    Russell-Silver syndrome
    Septo-optic dysplasia
    Suprasellar cysts
    Surgery
    Tay-Sachs disease
    Trauma
    Tuberous sclerosis
Secondary to pseudoprecocious puberty
  Congenital adrenal hyperplasia
  Gonadotropin-independent precocious puberty
  Virilizing tumors (adrenal or Leydig cells)
Peripheral (pseudo)
  Adrenal tumors, adenomas, carcinomas
  Congenital virilizing adrenal hyperplasia
  Exogenous gonadotropin
  Gonadotropin-independent precocious puberty (testotoxicosis)
  Luteinizing hormone–secreting pituitary adenoma
  McCune-Albright syndrome
  Nonpituitary or ectopic gonadotropin-producing tumors (chorioepithelioma, choriocarcinoma, germinoma, hepatoblastoma, teratoma)

---

follow surgical intervention or radiotherapy, and need not be associated with additional endocrine abnormalities. CNS tumors associated with CPP are craniopharyngiomas, hamartomas, astrocytomas, gliomas, and others. CPP may also be associated with meningitis, encephalitis, and abscess formation as well as with inflammatory or granulomatous conditions such as histiocytosis. Neurocutaneous syndromes such as tuberous sclerosis and neurofibromatosis may also be associated with CPP, as may increased intracranial pressure of whatever etiology. Hypothyroidism is associated with both delayed and advanced pubertal development. The mechanism of precocious puberty associated with chronic primary hypothyroidism is related to excessive TSH and alpha-subunit secretion and may be the result of direct gonadal stimulation rather than central activation of the hypothalamic-pituitary axis. It is not true CPP with episodic gonadotropin secretion.

Patients with precocious puberty present with a history of growth acceleration and early onset of pubertal changes. On physical examination, the growth of pubic hair, penis, and testes is usually evident in central precocious puberty (Fig 8–11).

The natural history of precocious puberty is the early completion of physical growth and sexual maturation. Bone age is relatively more accelerated than height age, resulting in reduced final height despite the early acceleration ahead of peers. In addition to early physical maturation, gonadotropin stimulation of the testes may induce spermatogenesis in CPP. Major psychosocial and psychosexual consequences are entailed in precocious puberty. Educational, parental, and peer relationships may be disrupted and some aspects of "adolescent" behavior may be exhibited although such children do not immediately acquire a teenage psychosexual mind-set. These manifestations of precocious puberty may be found equally in central and peripheral causes of the disorder. Sexual behavior, such as increased fondling and masturbation, may be found in both, but often it is not noticeably present and only infrequently presents a problem. Sexual interest, if greater than prepubertal, is usually self-directed and does not pose a threat to other children. On the contrary, the advanced sexual maturity may place these children at increased risk of being abused. Adults tend to relate to such children in response to their size and physical development rather than age, and peer relationships may be hampered.

Pseudo (Peripheral) Precocious Puberty.—PPP can be defined as any form of PP not normally mediated through activation of the hypothalamic-pituitary-gonadal axis. History and physical findings may contain clues to etiology. Age of onset, rapidity of progression, and associated changes may be helpful. Lack of unilateral or bilateral testicular enlargement suggests difficult etiologies.

The most common form of PPP in males is CAH, specifically the simple virilizing form of 21-hydroxylase deficiency. Failure of earlier recognition, in the presence of compensated cortisol secretion, or inadequate treatment may result in precocious

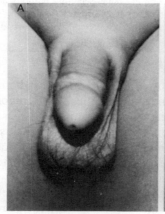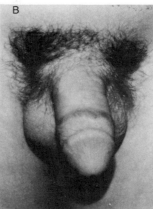

FIG 8–11.
A, genital development in a 3-year-old boy with male gonadotropin-independent precocious puberty (testotoxicosis). Testes growth is apparent. **B,** genital development in a 7-year-old boy with idiopathic central precocious puberty. Penile, testicular, and pubic hair growth are obvious.

onset of pubertal development. Rarely, androgen-secreting tumors of the testicle or adrenal may initiate pubertal change. Gonadotropin-independent autonomous testicular function (gonadotropin-independent precocity [GIP] or testotoxicosis) is a poorly understood cause of PPP, presenting at a very young age and occurring in both sporadic and autosomal dominant forms. In GIP, pubertal development is complete, with spermatogenesis occurring as well as physical development, as if all of the mechanisms which are normally stimulated by gonadotropins are operative.

Forms of gonadotropins or subunits may be secreted ectopically by hepatoblastomas, teratomas, embryomas, or chorioepitheliomas and activate testicular androgen production. Hypothyroidism may stimulate PPP through TSH or the alpha subunit.

Prolonged androgen exposure resulting from PPP can result in activation of the hypothalamic-pituitary-gonadal axis and the addition of CPP to the clinical situation. This may require combined treatment of both entities.

The early development of one or more characteristics of precocious puberty does not necessarily mean precocious puberty, and careful assessment and observation may be necessary to make the correct diagnosis. Persistence of elevated androgen secretion will result in onset and progression of the combined sexual and somatic manifestations of puberty: genital development, growth of pubic, facial, and axillary hair; mature body odor; acceleration in linear growth; and increase in musculature and bone mass.

Evaluation. — Evaluation of precocious puberty includes a careful history, family history, and physical examination with detailed documentation of secondary sexual characteristics and testicular volume. Height, weight, growth curves, and bone age determinations are essential to an accurate diagnosis. Biochemical separation of CPP from PPP can be made through gonadotropin determination with or without GnRH stimulation. Adrenal origins should be apparent by urine collections for 17-ketosteroids and 17-hydroxysteroids and determination of serum cortisol, 11-deoxycortisol, DHEA-S, testosterone, androstenedione, and 17-OH-progesterone. CNS lesions can be assessed by CT or MRI scanning. Thyroid function studies and testicular tumor markers, hCG, and α-fetoprotein should also be measured. Failure to delineate the cause of precocious puberty by these means will point to a diagnosis of idiopathic CPP.

Treatment. — Because pubertal changes in a prepubertal boy have an impact on his psychosocial relationships and psychosexual development, counseling is important to allow him to understand that his body has begun changing from a boy's to a man's too soon, that testing needs to be done to find out why, that treatment may be given to slow or stop development, and that essentially his body will be like that of any other man. Sex education geared to his level of understanding is crucial. The counseling process must also include the parents, since they too may carry many misconceptions about the implications of early pubertal development.

The therapy for the types of pseudoprecocious puberty is directed toward each specific etiology. Androgen-producing tumor should be removed. Excessive androgen production in adrenal hyperplasia should be appropriately suppressed. Adequate treatment of primary hypothyroidism results in cessation of pubertal change. Treatment of gonadotropin-independent puberty involves interference with androgen production (e.g., ketoconazole) plus in some instances inhibition of aromatase activity (e.g., testolactone) and androgen action (e.g., spironolactone or flutamide).

Treatment of central precocious puberty, which may also occur as a consequence of longstanding peripheral precocious puberty, is with GnRH analogue therapy.[10,46,50,56,66] Therapeutic agents previously used to suppress gonadotropins or to interfere with hormone action were at best only partially effective.

GnRH analogue treatment of children with central sexual precocity is efficacious and the treatment of choice. Therapy suppresses gonadotropin secretion resulting in cessation or regression of physical pubertal development and a slowing of the accelerated growth rate and skeletal maturation. Growth rate and bone maturation during treatment slows, depending on skeletal maturation at the onset of treatment. Adult height can be expected to be achieved or reclaimed with such therapy if begun early enough.

During therapy, not only does physical pubertal development cease or regress, and growth and skeletal maturity rates slow, but behavioral characteristics also return to those typical of childhood. Resumption of normal gonadal functions occurs after therapy is stopped.[49]

TESTES

Development

The fetal gonad is bipotential; testicular determining factors regulate development into testes. The posterior portion of the mesonephros develops into the genital ridge; on its medial side a thickening of mesenchymal cells form the gonadal ridge. Cells of the germinal epithelium proliferate inward to form the undifferentiated gonad. This development is accomplished by 6 weeks when primordial germ cells first become established in the undifferentiated gonad. These cells, the precursors of spermatogonia, can be recognized in the yolk sac ectoderm by 2.0 to 2.5 weeks. They migrate along the mesonephric ridge, which becomes the genital ridge, to form the primitive gonad.

The differentiation of this gonad into a testis begins at about 7 weeks. Within the cortical portion of the indifferent gonad, germ cells, with other primitive cells, form testicular cords, mesenchymal cells fill in interstitial space, and Sertoli and Leydig cells can be seen. The wolffian or mesonephric duct develops by about 4 weeks prior to the fetal age when the gonad becomes a testis. The rete testis, the ductal network of the medullary portion of the undifferentiated gonad, develops from portions of the mesonephros; the mesonephric tubules form the efferent ducts, and the wolffian duct, under the influence of testosterone, develops into the male genital tract.

The testicular cords become transformed into convoluted seminiferous tubules. Their peripheral ends anastomose and open through the rete tetes into the mesonephric tubules (which become the efferent ducts) and on into the portion of the wolffian duct that becomes the vas deferens. The cords are made up of two cell types, the gonocyte, which undergoes mitosis, and the Sertoli cell, which proliferates during fetal life and into the neonatal period. Differentiation occurs slowly and it is not until puberty that a hollow lumen develops and the maturation process from spermatogonium to spermatozoa becomes complete.

At about 7 weeks, the embryonic Sertoli cells in the differentiating testis begin to secrete MIH and nurture the proliferation of the spermatogonia. FSH stimulates the differentiation of the seminiferous cords and the development of seminiferous tubules, at least in part via stimulation of the Sertoli cells. Spermatogonia can be seen by 14 weeks.

MIH and testosterone are the major controls of testicular descent. Abnormalities of the abdominal wall, its tone, and intraabdominal pressure may interfere in the expression of the normal modulation of testicular descent. Early control of testicular descent appears to be a combination of MIH and testosterone, while later testicular descent is under the influence of testosterone alone.[26] Therefore, the failure of testicular descent may be related to abnormalities of hypothalamic control of testosterone secretion such as Kallman syndrome[63] or hypopituitarism, or to primary testicular dysfunction such as Klinefelter syndrome. Failure of testicular descent is also reported to be a consequence of diethylstilbestrol (DES) exposure and has been reproduced in animals exposed to high intrauterine estrogen levels.[21] The mechanism is reported to be estrogen-induced atrophy of the gubernaculum.[25] Testicular dysfunction and primary testicular failure is associated with increased testicular estrogen production in the adult. It can be hypothesized that a similar increase in local estrogen is responsible for maldescent in dysfunctional testes and for the association of maldescent with dysgenetic testes. It is also reported that innervation of the testes may also play a role in the process of descent since maldescent is more common in spinal cord lesions, and section of the genitofemoral nerve may result in failure of descent in animals.[4]

Testicular growth during infancy, childhood, and puberty results from gonadotropin stimulation and is reflected by changes in testicular volume (Table 8–4).[8,12,70] A size increase is noted at 2 and 3 months of age, the time of the peak neonatal gonadotropin secretion and again with pubertal growth, particularly by midpuberty. A somewhat larger volume of the right testis is apparent at puberty. Testicular growth

TABLE 8–4.

Testicular Size

Age (yr)	Length (cm) (Mean ± SD)	Corresponding Volume (mL) (Approximate)
<2	1.4 ± 0.4	
2–4	1.2 ± 0.4	
4–6	1.5 ± 0.6	1
6–8	1.8 ± 0.3	
8–10	2.0 ± 0.5	2
10–12	2.7 ± 0.7	5
12–14	3.4 ± 0.8	10
14–16	4.1 ± 1.0	20
16–18	5.0 ± 0.5	29
18–20	5.0 ± 0.3	29

is the earliest sign of puberty. Testicular volume of greater than 4 ml or a long axis greater than 2.5 cm is evidence that pubertal testicular growth has begun.

Problems of Testicular Development

Cryptorchidism

Cryptorchidism, the undescended or hidden testis, is the condition in which one or both testes do not reside in the normal location well within the scrotal sac. Cryptorchidism may occur unilaterally or bilaterally. The testis may be palpable and located along its line of descent at the external ring of the inguinal canal, within the canal, at the internal ring, just within the abdomen, or not palpable (truly hidden). If neither testis is palpable, an intersex problem may exist or the testis may be absent. Anorchia occurs in 4% of cases of nonpalpable testis.

The palpable testis may be somewhat mobile, particularly in the young boy with a very active cremasteric reflex, so a cryptorchid testis must be differentiated from a retractile testis. A retractile testis remains in the correct scrotal position most of the time but may readily recede into the inguinal canal as high as the internal ring. On examination, a retractile testis can be pulled into the scrotal sac and remains in that position after release. A cryptorchid testis cannot be drawn fully to the base of the scrotum and when released will immediately withdraw into its original position.

Cryptorchidism is one of the most frequent developmental abnormalities of the human male. Lack of descent occurs in 2% to 5% of newborns, being more common among premature infants. Lack of testicular descent has an incidence three to four times greater among those born before the seventh month of intrauterine life, since these males are born before the age when the normal process of testicular descent is completed. As a result of spontaneous descent after birth, the incidence decreases to 0.7% to 1.6% at 1 year of age.[32,39]

Complications of maldescent are inguinal hernia, infertility, malignant transformation, and hypogonadism. Herniorraphies can be accomplished at the time of orchidopexy. Correction of cryptorchidism is indicated because spermatogenesis is impaired and the incidence of testicular cancer is increased in its undescended situation.[18] Infertility is a common consequence of cryptorchidism.[9]

Infertility has also been reported in as many as 50% of cases with unilateral descent, evidence to support the hypothesis that cryptorchidism is frequently a manifestation of a bilateral testicular defect. Cryptorchid testes are histologically normal at birth, but beyond infancy progressively acquire a more abnormal microscopic appearance. Morphologic abnormalities have been consistently documented by 2 years of age with more severe abnormalities occurring progressively thereafter with increasing age.[20,22] However, it is not clear that repositioning alters the potential for fertility in either bilaterally or unilaterally cryptorchid males.[9] Nevertheless, until the efficacy of treatment concerning fertility is verified, the current recommendation for treatment of cryptorchidism between 1 and 2 years of age, before the age of detectable anatomic abnormality, is appropriate and should be followed.

Malignant transformation is more common in undescended testes, up to ten times the normal incidence, and occurs in the third and fourth decades of life.[18] Seminoma accounts for 60% of cases. Because of this incidence of malignant change, it is recommended that any testis not reaching a scrotal position by the end of the second year of life should undergo orchidopexy. While there is no conclusive evidence that such repositioning alters the incidence of malignant transformation, it clearly makes earlier detection possible. If maldescent is a marker of primary testicular dysfunction, surgical correction does not remove the need for vigilance.

Etiology.—Since the control of testicular descent is not understood, and since lack of descent may be due to various etiologies which are not well delineated, patients with cryptorchidism usually cannot be classified so that an accurate prognosis of potential testicular function can be given.

It is clear that fetal testicular testosterone secretion in response to gonadotropin secretion during the final trimester of pregnancy plays a critical role in the final phase of descent. Therefore, while maldescent may be associated with primary or secondary hypogonadism and with impaired androgen effect as is found in the androgen insensitivity syndromes and 5α-reductase deficiency, there may be many other causes of maldescent. Potential causes include early maldevelopment resulting in dysgenetic testes; inadequate hormone stimulation, including insufficient gonadotropin, testosterone, or thyroid hormone production; and anatomic hindrance with associated defects, either because of obstruction or lack of development of the usual pathway of descent or because of lack of abdominal wall integrity and low intraabdominal pressure, as in the prune-belly syndrome.

Determination of the cause of the failure of descent in the newborn is facilitated by measurement of serum FSH, LH, and testosterone and by the presence of other stigmata of syndromes which may be associated with cryptorchidism. Primary testicular failure, GnRH deficiency, and panhypopituitarism can be determined at this age.

Defects of gonadotropin secretion cannot be identified during childhood but can be at any time after pubertal age by characteristic low LH, FSH, and testosterone levels. Conversely, if the testis is dysgenetic or damaged by its cryptorchid state, elevated levels of LH and FSH and a low testosterone level indicative of testicular failure are present during puberty and adulthood, but not during childhood. During the childhood years testosterone responsiveness to hCG can be used to assess testicular function.

Evaluation.—Evaluation of the boy with possible cryptorchidism includes a careful antenatal and perinatal history, family history, and physical examination, with particular attention to whether the abnormality is unilateral or bilateral and to distinguish cryptorchidism from retractile testis. A history of drug use in pregnancy and a family history of cryptorchidism, hypogonadism, hypogenitalism, and anosmia should be sought. Associated abnormalities may suggest congenital hypothyroidism. Micropenis and hypospadias associated with maldescent may suggest primary or secondary disorders of androgen secretion or altered androgen responsivity.

Careful clinical examination will avoid unnecessary surgery and unnecessary parental concern. When examining a boy for testicular location, it is important to provide a private, quiet setting where the room temperature is comfortable. The examiner's hands should be warm. There are several positions that may be helpful. The position with the patient lying prone with his legs slightly spread allows a sheet or gown to be draped over the patient, minimizing exposure. A useful approach is to palpate one side of the scrotum at one time while gently placing the fingers of the other hand over the inguinal canal to obstruct retraction of the testis by a vigorous cremasteric reflex. While pressing over the internal ring with one hand, the testis located distal to it can be grasped between the thumb and fingers of the other hand and gently pulled into the scrotal sac. If the testis cannot be definitely palpated within the inguinal canal, it is often helpful to stroke the area gently and slowly with a small amount of soap on the fingers. Using this technique, the testis will often slip or pop noticeably under the examining fingers as they pass over it. The cross-legged Indian-style sitting position seems to inhibit the cremasteric reflex. Whenever the testes are palpated, they should be measured, and either testicular volume or the length of the long axis should be recorded.

Before a definite diagnosis of cryptorchidism is made, the patient should be examined on at least two occasions, and by more than one examiner if possible. A testis which is apparently cryptorchid or even nonpalpable on one examination may clearly be a retractile testis when examined at another time.

Laboratory evaluation is particularly important in the presence of bilateral cryptorchidism or of associated hypospadias or micropenis. It is essential to establish the presence of appropriate testosterone levels and to distinguish primary from secondary hypogonadism. If the child is less than 2 years old or older than 10 years, determination of serum testosterone, LH, and FSH levels may be helpful. If LH and FSH are elevated, this is indicative of testicular failure. Elevation of FSH suggests seminiferous tubule failure. During childhood, levels are low and not discernibly different from normal. At any age during childhood, an hCG stimulation can be done as a diagnostic test to verify Leydig cell response by measuring testosterone levels after three or more injections. If there is an absence of detectable androgen in bilateral cryptorchidism, a karyotype and surgical search for identifiable testicular tissue and biopsy are indicated. Ultrasonography is seldom helpful in localizing testicular tissue.

Treatment.—A testis that is undescended should be brought into the scrotum. Treatment may include hormonal stimulation, surgery, or both. Hormonal treatment has included testosterone, GnRH, or hCG. Gonadotropin stimulation, which stimulates an androgen response, is more frequently used than testosterone. GnRH stimulation provides no advantage over hCG. The reported success of both hormonal and surgical therapy varies considerably; patient series are generally small, probably not representative of the general population, and do not consider pretreatment testicular location. Hormone treatment is most likely to be successful in the more distally placed testes.[27,57,68] If surgical therapy is chosen, it should be done as soon after the first year of life as possible to obtain the maximum benefit.

Because adequate data are not available to judge the efficacy of one treatment vs. another, it is reasonable to use general guidelines. If an inguinal hernia is present, herniorrhaphy is indicated, and a concomitant orchiopexy is logical. If no testes are palpable bilaterally, an hCG test is a reasonable initial treatment, both to document testosterone response and to stimulate descent. If hCG stimulation causes partial descent, orchiopexy can promptly follow while the hormonal benefit of partial descent and stimulation of the vascular supply to the testis and supporting structure is still present. Hormonal stimulation may be beneficial when the testes are at the external inguinal ring or in the scrotal neck, a position which may be difficult to improve surgically but which may be readily responsive to hormonal stimulation. While hCG stimulation may be efficacious in some instances of bilateral cryptorchidism, its usefulness in unilateral cryptorchidism is unclear. If there is a mechanical or anatomic reason for lack of descent, hCG stimulation is contraindicated.

Adequate stimulation of hCG is obtained by using 3,000 U/m^2 body surface per injection with injections given two or three times a week IM for 4 to 6 weeks. Descent, if it occurs, may be apparent within the first 2 weeks. If so, it is reasonable to complete the prescribed course in an attempt to enhance the persistence of descent. Although hCG has been widely used without clear evidence of significant long-term side effects, a maximum total dosage of 20,000 U is reasonable.

Parents of cryptorchid boys and the patient himself, at an appropriate age, should be told of the increased risk of infertility and malignancy and, after puberty, semen analyses should be done and self-examination of the testes taught.

Small Testes

Prepubertal boys may be referred for evaluation of small testes. In adults, since about 90% of testicular volume is made up of the spermatogenic apparatus, low testicular volume reflects either failure of central activation of testicular function or an intrinsic abnormality of testicular function. Because the normal prepubertal testis may be very small, small testes in a boy may not indicate a pathologic condition. Small testes may be present in the situations listed in Table 8–5. Pathologically small testes generally fall into one of two categories: hypogonadotropic hypogonadism or primary hypogonadism. In both categories, if the problem existed before birth, the testes may be undescended as well as small. Idiopathic hypogonadotropic hypogonadism, Kallmann syndrome, and hypopituitarism involving GH with or without gonadotropin secretion may all present with small testicular volume in infancy or childhood although size often overlaps the normal range. Primary hypogonadism, particularly Klinefelter syndrome and variants, but also the rudimentary testis syndrome or testicular regression syndrome, may present with decreased testicular volume in childhood. The decreased volume is due to lack, or loss of development of seminiferous tubules and germ cells. Primary hypogonadism may also be acquired and may affect one or both testes. If only one testis is small, the cause is likely local or acquired. Damage to the prepubertal testes may result from cryptorchidism, orchitis, irradiation, chemotherapy, an autoimmune process, and trauma with or without compromise of the vascular supply. Patients with the Sertoli cell–only syndrome have somewhat small testes during adulthood but have not been identified in childhood.

It is most likely that, even if a child presents with a complaint of small testes, that the testis is within normal limits for a prepubertal male. The mean length of a prepubertal testis is 1.5 to 2.0 cm and the volume is between 1 and 2 ml. However, the distribution around the prepubertal size indicates that normal prepubertal males may have testicular volume of less than 1 ml or length as short as 1 cm.

A useful examination technique is to isolate the testis from other scrotal contents laterally and anteriorly within the scrotal sac. The testis can be held in one hand, with the fingers palpating the ends of the long axis, being careful to exclude the

TABLE 8–5.

Variations in Testicular Size

	Unilateral	Bilateral
Small testes		
Hypothalamic-pituitary dysfunction		
Gonadotropin deficiency, idiopathic or organic		X
Growth hormone deficiency		X
Normal variant		X
Primary hypogonadism		
Autoimmune destruction		X
Chemotherapy		X
Cryptorchidism	X	X
Irradiation		X
Klinefelter syndrome		X
Orchiditis	X	X
Rudimentary testes syndrome		X
Surgery	X	X
Testicular regression syndrome		X
Torsion	X	X
Trauma	X	X
Large testes		
Adrenal rest tissue	X	X
Compensatory	X	
Fragile X syndrome		X
Growth hormone excess		X
Hypothyroidism		X
Idiopathic	X	X
Tumor	X	X

epididymis, and any blood vessels or hydrocele. The other hand can hold a centimeter ruler to measure the long axis, or an orchidometer to compare testicular volume. In addition, a complete genital and general physical examination should be done.

If testicular volume is less than mean prepubertal size or if consistency is particularly firm or soft, laboratory testing to be considered includes determination of LH, FSH, and testosterone levels and karyotype. If no abnormality is found, patients with small testes should be monitored until puberty is established.

Large Testes

Both prepubertal and pubertal boys may present with a complaint of unilateral or bilateral testicular enlargement (see Table 8–5). Bilateral enlargement may or may not be symmetric and unilateral enlargement may be uniform. The initial assessment should exclude extratesticular scrotal contents including hydrocele, varicocele, hernial sac, or adrenal rest tissue.

Bilateral enlargement for stage of pubertal development may frequently be idiopathic, but also occurs with congenital or chronic primary hypothyroidism, the fragile X syndrome, or GH excess. Hyperplasia of adrenal rest tissue in the testes of patients with inadequately treated CAH may be unilateral or bilateral.

Unilateral enlargement or asymmetry of size may occur in testicular tumors, as a variant of normal puberty, or as simple compensatory hypertrophy in the contralateral testis following damage of the opposite testis for whatever reason. When compensatory hypertrophy occurs, the opposite testis may be absent, obviously atrophic, or simply smaller with normal consistency. Compensatory hypertrophy may occur secondary to torsion, cryptorchidism, orchidopexy, herniorrrhaphy, or other trauma on the opposite side, or for no apparent reason.

Enlargement of one or both testes may represent a benign physiologic response but also may represent an underlying pathologic condition. If the etiology is explained by such an expected physiologic response, treatment may not be indicated. If the cause is unknown, ultrasound studies and biopsy may be indicated.

REFERENCES

1. Allen TD, Griffin JE: Endocrine studies in patients with advanced hypospadias. *J Urol* 1984; 131:310–314.
2. Anderson M, Page DC, laChapelli AD: Chromosome Y-specific DNA is transferred to the short arm of X chromosome in human XX males. *Science* 1986; 233:786–788.
3. Bauer SB, Retik AB, Colodny AH: Genetic aspects of hypospadias. *Urol Clin North Am* 1981; 8:559–564.
4. Beasley SW, Hutson JM: Effect of division of the genitofemoral nerve on testicular descent in the rat. *Aust NZ J Surg* 1987; 57:49–51.
5. Benirschke K, Naftolin F, Gittes R, et al: True hermaphroditism and chimerism. *Am J Obstet Gynecol* 1972; 113:449–458.
6. Bourguignon JP, Vanderschueren-Lodeweyckx M, Wolter R, et al: Hypopituitarism and idiopathic delayed puberty: A longitudinal study in an attempt to diagnosis gonadotropin deficiency before puberty. *J Clin Endocrinol Metab* 1982; 54:733–744.
7. Brunner M, Moreira-Filho CA, Wachtel G, et al: On the secretion of H-Y antigen. *Cell* 1984; 37:615–619.
8. Cassorla FG, Golden SM, Johnsonbaugh RE, et al: Testicular volume during early infancy. *J Pediatr* 1981; 99:742–743.
9. Chilvers C, Dudley NE, Gough MH, et al: Undescended testes: The effect of treatment on subsequent risk of subfertility and malignancy. *J Pediatr Surg* 1986; 21:691–696.
10. Comite F, Pescovitz OH, Rieth KG, et al: Luteinizing hormone–releasing hormone analog treatment of boys with hypothalamic hamartoma and true precocious puberty. *J Clin Endocrinol Metab* 1984; 59:888–892.
11. Conte FA, Grumbach MM, Kaplan SL: A diphasic pattern of gonadotropin secretion in patients with the syndrome of gonadal dysgenesis. *J Clin Endocrinol Metab* 1975; 40:670–674.
12. Daniel WA Jr, Feinstein RA, Howard-Peebles P, et al: Testicular volumes of adolescents. *J Pediatr* 1982; 101:1010–1012.
13. Dean HJ, Shackleton CHL, Winter JSD: Diagnosis and natural history of 17-hydroxylase deficiency in a newborn male. *J Clin Endocrinol Metab* 1984; 59:513–520.
14. Dunkel L, Perheentupa J, Sorva R: Single versus repeated dose human chorionic gonadotropin stimulation in the differential diagnosis of hypogonadotropic hypogonadism. *J Clin Endocrinol Metab* 1985; 60:333–337.
15. Dunkel L, Perheentupa J, Virtanen M, et al: Gonadotropin-releasing hormone test and human chronic gonadotropin test in the diagnosis of gonadotropin deficiency in prepubertal boys. *J Pediatr* 1985; 107:388–392.
16. Fallon B, Devine CJ Jr, Horton CE: Congenital anomalies associated with hypospadias. *J Urol* 1976; 116:585–586.

17. George FW, Wilson JD: Embryology of the genital tract, in Walsh PC, Gittes RF, Perlmutter AD, et al (eds): *Campbell's Urology*, ed 5. WB Saunders Co, 1986.

18. Giwercman A, et al: Testicular cancer risk in boys with maldescended testes: A cohort study. *J Urol* 1987; 138:1214–1216.

19. Griffin JE, Wilson JD: The syndrome of androgen resistance. *N Engl J Med* 1980; 302:198–209.

20. Hadziselimovic F, Herzog B, Buser M: Development of cryptorchid testes. *Eur J Pediatr* 1987; 146(suppl 2):S8–S12.

21. Hadziselimovic F, Herzog B, Kruslin E: Estrogen-induced cryptorchidism in animals. *Clin Androl* 1980; 3:166–174.

22. Hedinger C: Histological data in cryptorchidism, in Job, J-C (ed): *Cryptorchidism, Diagnosis and Treatment. Pediatric and Adolescent Endocrinology*, vol 6. New York, Karger, 1979, pp 3–13.

23. Hoffman AR, Crowley WF Jr: Induction of puberty in men by long-term pulsatile administration of low-dose gonadotropin-releasing hormone. *N Engl J Med* 1982; 307:1237–1241.

24. Hughes IA, Pinsky L: Sexual differentiation, in Collu R, Ducharme JR, Guyda HJ (eds): *Pediatric Endocrinologoy*, ed 2. New York, Raven Press, 1989, pp 251–293.

25. Hutson JM: Testicular feminization: A model for testicular descent in mice and men. *J Pediatr Surg* 1986; 21:1985–1998.

26. Hutson JM, Donahoe PK: The hormonal control of testicular descent. *Endocr Rev* 1987; 7:270–283.

27. Illig R, Bucher H, Prader A: Success, relapse and failure of intranasal LH-RH treatment of cryptorchidism. *Eur J Pediatr* 1980; 133:147–150.

28. Imperato-McGinley J, Gantier T, Pichardo M, et al: The diagnosis of 5-alpha-reductase deficiency in infancy. *J Clin Endocrinol Metab* 1986; 63:1313–1318.

29. Imperato-McGinley J, Petersen RE, Gautier T, et al: Decreased C19 and C21 steroids, 5 alpha-metabolites in parents of male pseudohermaphrodites with 5 alpha-reductase deficiency: Detection of carriers. *J Clin Endocrinol Metab* 1985; 60:553–558.

30. Janczewski Z, Bablok L: Semen characteristics in pubertal boys. I. Semen quality after first ejaculation. *Arch Androl* 1985; 15:199–205.

31. Janczewski Z, Bablok L: Semen characteristics in pubertal boys. IV. Semen quality and hormone profile. *Arch Androl* 1985; 15:219–223.

32. John Radcliffe Hospital Cryptorchid Study Group: Cryptorchidism—an apparent substantial increase since 1960. *Br Med J* 1986; 293:1401–1404.

33. Jones HW, Lee PA, Archer DF, et al: A genetic male patient with 17α-hydroxylase deficiency. *Obstet Gynecol* 1982; 59:254–259.

34. Jost A, Magre S, Agelopaulou R: Early stages of testicular differentiation in the rat. *Hum Genet* 1981; 58:59–63.

35. Jost A, Vigier B, Prepin B, et al: Studies on sex differentiation in mammals. *Recent Prog Horm Res* 1973; 29:1–41.

36. Kater CE, Biglieri EG, Brust N, et al: The unique patterns of plasma aldosterone and 18-hydroxycorticosterone concentrations in the 17α-hydroxylase deficiency syndrome. *J Clin Endocrinol Metab* 1982; 55:295–302.

37. Kenawi MM: Sexual function in hypospadias. *Br J Urol* 1975; 47:883–890.

38. Khuri FJ, Hardy BE, Churchill BM: Urologic anomalies associated with hypospadias. *Urol Clin North Am* 1981; 8:565–571.

39. Koyle MA, Rajfer J, Ehrlich RM: The undescended testis. *Pediatr Ann* 1988; 17:39, 42–46.

40. Kulin HE, Frontera MA, Demers LM, et al: The onset of sperm production in pubertal boys. *Am J Dis Child* 1989; 143:190–193.

41. Lee PA: Neuroendocrinology of puberty. *Semin Reprod Endocrinol* 1988; 6:13–20.
42. Lee PA: Pubertal neuroendocrine maturation: Early differentiation and stages of development. *Adolesc Pediatr Gynecol* 1988; 1:3–12.
43. Lee PA: Micropenis, in Forest MG (ed): *Androgens in Childhood. Pediatric Adolesc Endocrinol*, vol 19. Basel, Karger, 1989, pp 149–154.
44. Lee PA, Mazur T, Danish R, et al: Micropenis. I. Criteria, etiologies and classification. *Johns Hopkins Med J* 1980; 146:156–163.
45. Lee PA, O'Dea L St L: Primary and Secondary testicular insufficiency. *Pediatr Clin North Am* 1990; 37:1359–1387.
46. Lee PA, Page JG, Leuprolide Study Group: Effects of leuprolide in the treatment of central precocious puberty. *J Pediatr* 1989; 114:321–324.
47. Ley SB, Leonard JM: Male hypogonadotopic hypogonadism: Factors influencing response to human chorionic gonadotropin and human menopausal gonadotropin, including prior exogeneous androgens. *J Clin Endocrinol Metab* 1985; 61:746–752.
48. Magenis RE, Webb MJ, McKean RS, et al: Translocation (X;Y) (p22.3;p11.2) in XX males: Etiology of male phenotype. *Hum Genet* 1982; 62:271–276.
49. Manasco PK, Pescovitz OH, Feuillan PP, et al: Resumption of puberty after long term luteinizing hormone-releasing hormone agonist treatment of central precocious puberty. *J Clin Endocrinol Metab* 1988; 67:368–372.
50. Manasco PK, Pescovitz OH, Hill SC, et al: Six-year results of luteinizing hormone releasing hormone (LHRN) agonist treatment in children with LHRH-dependent precocious puberty. *J Pediatr* 1989; 115:105–108.
51. Manieul JC, Sibley RK, Dehner LP: Complete and incomplete Drash syndrome: A clinicopathologic study of five cases of a dysontogenetic-neoplastic complex. *Hum Pathol* 1987; 18:80–89.
52. Müller U: Molecular genetic approaches to testis differentiation, in Collu R, Ducharme JR, Guyda HR (eds): *Pediatric Endocrinology*, ed 2. New York, Raven Press, 1989, pp 295–305.
53. Müller U, Donlon T, Schmid M, et al: Deletion mapping of the testis determining locus with DNA probes in 46,XX males and in 46,XY and 46,X,dic(Y) females. *Nucleic Acids Res* 1986,14:6489–6505.
54. Page DC, Mosler R, Simpson ER, et al: The sex determining region of the human Y chromosome encodes a finger protein. *Cell* 1987; 51:1091–1104.
55. Palmer MS, Sinclair AH, Berta P, et al: Genetic evidence that 2FY is not the testes-determining factor. *Nature* 1989; 342:937–939.
56. Pescovitz OH, Comite F, Hench K, et al: The NIH experience with precocious puberty: diagnostic subgroups and response to short-term luteinizing hormone releasing hormone analogue therapy. *J Pediatr* 1986; 108:47–54.
57. Rajfer J, Handelsman DJ, Swerdloff RS, et al: Hormonal therapy of cryptorchidism: A randomized, double-blind study comparing human chorionic gonadotropin and gonadotropin-releasing hormone. *N Engl J Med* 1986; 314:466–470.
58. Ratcliffe SG, et al: Klinefelter's syndrome in adolescence. *Arch Dis Child* 1982; 57: 6–12.
59. Reilly JM, Woodhouse CRJ: Small penis and the male sexual role. *J Urol* 1989; 142:569–571.
60. Rosenfeld RG, Northcraft GB, Hintz RL: A prospective, randomized study of testosterone treatment of constitutional delay of growth and development in male adolescents. *Pediatrics* 1982; 69:681–687.
61. Skordis NA, Stetka DG, MacGillivray MH, et al: Familial 46,XX males coexisting with familial 46,XX true hermaphroditism in the same pedigree. *J Pediatr* 1987; 110:244–248.

62. Snyder PJ, Lawrence DA: Treatment of male hypogonadism with testosterone enanthate. *J Clin Endocrinol Metab* 1980; 51:1335–1339.

63. Spratt DI, Carr DB, Merriam GR, et al: The spectrum of abnormal patterns of gonadotropin-releasing hormone secretion in men with idiopathic hypogonadotropic hypogonadism: Clinical and laboratory correlations. *J Clin Endocrinol Metab* 1987; 64:283–291.

64. Spratt DI, O'Dea L St L, Schoenfeld D, et al: Neuroendocrine-gonadal axis in men: Frequent sampling of LH, FSH, and testosterone. *Am J Physiol* 1988; 254; E658–666.

65. Starceski PJ, Sieber WK, Lee PA: Fertility in true hermaphroditism. *Adolesc Pediatr Gynecol* 1988; 1:55–56.

66. Styne DM, Harris DA, Egli CA, et al: Treatment of true precocious puberty with a potent luteinizing hormone–releasing factor agonist: Effect on growth, sexual maturation, pelvic sonography, and the hypothalamic-pituitary-gonadal axis. *J Clin Endocrinol Metab* 1985; 61:142–151.

67. Sweet RA, Schrott HG, Kurland R, et al: Study of the incidence of hypospadias in Rochester, Minnesota 1940–70, and a case control comparison of possible etiologic factors. *Mayo Clin Proc* 1974; 49:52–58.

68. Urban MD, Lee PA, Lanes R, et al: hCG stimulation in children with cryptorchidism. *Clin Pediatr* 1987; 26:512–514.

69. Wray S, Nieburgs A, Elkabes S: Spatiotemporal cell expression of luteinizing hormone-releasing hormone in the prenatal mouse: Evidence for an embryonic origin in the olfactory placade. *Dev Brain Res* 1989, 46:309–318.

70. Zachmann M, Prader A, Kind HP, et al: Testicular volume during adolescence: Cross-sectional and longitudinal studies. *Helv Paediatr Acta* 1974; 29:61–72.

71. Zachmann M, Studer S, Prader A: Short-term testosterone treatment at bone age of 12 to 13 years does not reduce adult height in boys with constitutional delay of growth and adolescence. *Helv Paediatr Acta* 1987; 42:21–28.

72. Zachmann M, Werder EA, Prader A: Two types of male pseudohermaphroditism due to 17,20-desmolase deficiency. *J Clin Endocrinol* 1982; 55:487–490.

Chapter 9

Diabetes Mellitus

Allen M. Glasgow

Type I diabetes mellitus is a chronic disorder caused by deficiency of insulin.

INSULIN AND INSULIN SECRETION

Insulin is the primary hormonal regulator of glucose metabolism. The insulin gene has been isolated, cloned, and sequenced.[78] The gene has three exons and two introns, is located on the short arm of chromosome 11, and is active only in beta cells. The mechanism by which regulatory proteins interact with the insulin gene to regulate transcription is an area of active investigation. In the past few decades, significant progress has been made in understanding the synthesis, secretion, and mechanism of insulin action.

Proinsulin,[78] the immediate precursor of insulin, is a single-chain protein produced from preproinsulin, which is formed on the rough endoplasmic reticulum of the beta cell.[15,84] Proinsulin is thought to produce a configuration that favors the formation of appropriate disulfide bridges for insulin. A connecting (C) peptide is then cleaved out by protolytic enzymes. The resulting insulin contains an α chain with 21 amino acid residues and a β chain with 30 amino acid residues, linked by two disulfide bridges. In addition, there is a disulfide bridge between amino acid residue 6 and 11 of the α chain (Fig 9–1). The normal pancreas contains a 4- to 6-day supply of insulin stored in granules. Insulin is released by the fusion of the granule with the plasma membrane (exocytosis). Although the concentration of serum glucose is the principal regulator of insulin secretion, a number of other factors also modulate

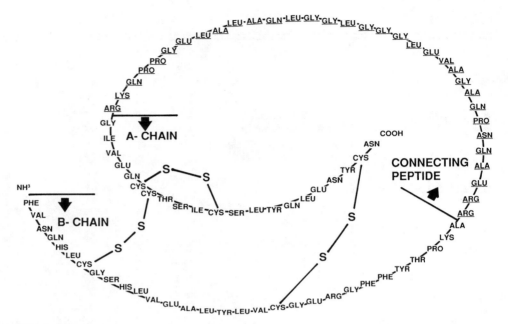

FIG 9–1.
Proinsulin. C peptide is underlined; insulin is not.

insulin secretion.[69] For example, increases in the serum concentration of several amino acids stimulate insulin secretion, as do gastrointestinal hormones, such as secretin, pancreozymin, gastrin, and galanin. These hormones are important in the initial rise of insulin after a meal and may account for the greater rise in insulin after oral (as compared to intravenous [IV] glucose. Other hormones, such as glucagon, growth hormone, and cortisol, stimulate insulin secretion under certain conditions, whereas catecholamines and somatostatin inhibit insulin release.

The existence of gap junctions (areas of intracellular communication between the cells of the islets) suggests that insulin secretion may be coordinated with the secretion of glucagon and other pancreatic hormones.[64,65] Somatostatin, an inhibitor of glucagon and insulin secretion, has been found in high concentrations in the islets of the pancreas. Finally, insulin secretion may be regulated by the autonomic nervous system.

Insulin release is regulated by intercellular concentrations of Ca^{2+}, cyclic adenosine monophosate (cAMP), and inositol triphosphate.[21,68] These messengers activate protein kinases that phosphorylate the proteins that move secretory granules to the cell membrane. Glucose metabolites increase potassium efflux through adenosine triphosphate (ATP)–sensitive channels. The resulting depolarization of the beta cell membrane increases Ca^{2+} influx into the cell. Calcium influx increases insulin secretion. Insulin secretion resulting from a relatively constant stimulus occurs in two phases: an initial peak of insulin release lasting a few minutes is followed by a gradual sustained rise in secretion.[67]

The first step in insulin degradation occurs in the liver and kidney where an enzyme, a glutathione-insulin reductase, splits the disulfide bridges. Insulin destruction does not seem to be regulated; the plasma regulation of insulin levels occurs by changes in the rate of secretion. Plasma insulin has a half-life of about 5 to 10 minutes.

Glucose transport into cells is facilitated by a family of at least five glucose transporters.[8,46,88] The transporters are similar in structure but have different characteristics. Similar transporters, found primarily in erythrocytes and brain but also in many other tissues, have a low *Km* (1–2 mM glucose). A higher *Km* (15 mM glucose) transporter is dominant in the liver and beta cells. A third transporter, whose activity is regulated by insulin, is dominant in muscle and adipose tissue. Insulin increases the activity of this glucose transporter by causing the movement of additional glucose transporters from intercellular vesicles to the plasma membrane.

The mechanism of insulin action has been studied extensively but remains to be completely defined. We do know that insulin binds to a receptor, that the gene for the receptor is located on chromosome 19, and that this gene can produce several variations of the insulin receptor in different tissues.[77] The proreceptor protein undergoes several posttranslational modifications, including proteolytic cleavage into two alpha and two beta subunits. Several mutations in the receptor associated with rare forms of insulin-resistant diabetes have been described.[87] The intercellular component of the receptor has tyrosine kinase activity which phosphorylates the tyrosine residues on the receptor itself[89] and as yet unidentified proteins.[47] In addition, some of the effects of insulin appear to be mediated by decreases in cAMP. Other effects may involve an as yet incompletely characterized inositol glycan intercellular messenger.[56,74] The effects of insulin appear to involve enzyme dephosphorylation and phosphorylation and regulation of gene transcription.[63]

EFFECTS OF INSULIN AND COUNTERREGULATORY HORMONES

Insulin

Insulin is the primary hormone of the fed state. The overall effects of insulin are to promote glucose oxidation and storage (both as glycogen and fat), to promote protein synthesis, and to decrease the utilization of fat for energy. In adipose tissue, insulin increases the transport of glucose across the cell membrane and promotes both glucose oxidation and conversion into triglycerides. Insulin also promotes the uptake and storage of serum lipids and inhibits lipolysis. The inhibition of lipolysis in adipose tissue is mediated by an inhibition of adenyl cyclase, which reduces the concentration of cAMP. In muscle, insulin stimulates the uptake of glucose and its oxidation as well as the storage of glycogen; it also increases amino acid uptake and protein synthesis. Insulin does not have direct effects on glucose transport in the liver. However, it increases both glucose oxidation and glycogen synthesis and it inhibits glycogen breakdown and gluconeogenesis. Insulin appears to have no direct effect on the central nervous system.

Growth Hormone

Growth hormone is antagonistic to insulin in that it decreases glucose uptake and oxidation and increases lipolysis. Like insulin, however, it promotes protein synthesis.

Adrenocorticotropic Hormone (ACTH) and Cortisol

ACTH stimulates lipolysis in adipose tissue in vitro, but the physiologic importance of this effect is unknown. Cortisol promotes protein breakdown. It also stimulates gluconeogenesis in the liver (by increasing the production of several key gluconeogenic enzymes).

Glucagon

The primary effect of glucagon is to increase hepatic glucose production. It does this by both stimulating glycogen breakdown and promoting gluconeogenesis. Glucagon also stimulates lipolysis in adipose tissue. It probably does not have a direct effect on muscle metabolism. The effects of glucagon are primarily mediated by its activation of adenyl cyclase.

Catecholamines

Catecholamines increase glycogen breakdown in both muscle and liver and increase lipolysis in adipose tissue.

EPIDEMIOLOGY AND ETIOLOGY OF TYPE I DIABETES

The incidence of type I diabetes varies by age, race, geographic region, and season. Onset of type I diabetes has a bimodal age pattern, with one peak occurring between 10 and 14 years and another occurring in the fifth decade.[45] Adult patients have a longer symptomatic period prior to diagnosis, and better preservation of residual beta cell function, but there are no clear differences in the clinical syndrome.

Type I diabetes is most common in whites, particularly in persons of Northern European descent. The highest incidence occurs in Scandinavia.[54] Type I diabetes is relatively less common in blacks, Hispanics, and Asians, in descending order of incidence. A significant percentage of black patients have a type of diabetes that is different from typical type I diabetes; it is more strongly inherited (with a dominant inheritance pattern) but associated with incomplete insulin deficiency.

The onset of type I diabetes is seasonal: it peaks in the winter months, both in the Northern and Southern Hemispheres.[20,23,31,35] This pattern has been offered as evidence of a viral etiology; however, it also may be related to the seasonal pattern of higher blood glucose values in normal persons during the winter months.[58,85]

Although there is some evidence suggesting an increase in the incidence of diabetes in the United States in the 20th century, no clear temporal trends have been noted in studies covering the 1960s, 1970s, and 1980s.[40,55]

An important genetic component for type I diabetes is indicated by the approximately 50% concordance among monozygotic twins.[86] Clearly, however, type I diabetes is dependent upon environmental factors for its expression. At least one of the genes associated with type I diabetes is located on the short arm of chromosome 6 in the region of the HLA-DR or HLA-DQ locus.[76] It is not clear if this genetic factor associated with type I diabetes is part of the HLA locus or a closely linked locus. In whites, type I diabetes is more common in individuals who are HLA-DR3, -DR4, or both, and less common in persons who are HLA-DR2. Whites that have an aspartic acid at residue 57 of the DQ β chain are much less likely to have diabetes than those who have an alanine, serine, or glycine at position 57.[30] However, this one residue site does not completely explain diabetes susceptibility, as was once thought. In fact, persons with some HLA-DR types who have HLA-DQ aspartic acid at position 57 may have a relatively high risk of developing diabetes.[6] In addition, in the Japanese population, susceptibility of type I diabetes is associated with different HLA-DR types (HLA-DR4 and -DR9) which are not associated with aspartic acid at position 57 of the DQ β chain.[5] Despite the recognition of a strong association between the diabetes gene(s) and the HLA locus, the mutation(s) that causes diabetes is not clearly defined.

The environmental factors that may trigger diabetes in genetically susceptible persons are even less well understood. Viruses are often suggested as a possibility. Congenital rubella syndrome is associated with a high incidence of type I diabetes.[61] Coxsackievirus has similarly been suggested as a possible cause of type I diabetes.[4,17,51,94]

It has become clear that the mechanism of beta cell destruction in type I diabetes results from autoimmune damage.[28,29] In recently diagnosed patients, 70% to 80% have measurable islet cell antibodies.[57,59] There is also evidence of cellular autoimmune attacks. Islet cell antibodies may appear years before detectable islet cell dysfunction which suggests that the autoimmune damage is often insidious.[27,79] Studies of immunosuppression with cyclosporine suggest that this drug can slow the autoimmune destruction, but current therapy cannot completely arrest the process. Presumably, more specific immunotherapy might arrest the diabetes at an early phase.

KETOACIDOSIS

Pathophysiology

The acute effects of diabetes are due to a lack of insulin. The failure to secrete insulin results in an inability to oxidize glucose in muscle and adipose tissue. With insulin deficiency amino acids are released from the breakdown of protein. The amino acids are converted to glucose and glycogen in the liver, a process that continues despite hyperglycemia. Hyperglycemia results from decreased glucose oxidation, increased glucose production, and continued glucose intake. The hyperglycemia, in turn, leads to glycosuria when the renal threshold for glucose is exceeded. The glycosuria accounts for many of the classic symptoms of diabetes. The polyuria and polydipsia result from the osmotic diuresis caused by glycosuria. Dehydration occurs when fluid intake does not compensate for urine losses. Once vomiting occurs, dehydration develops rather rapidly. An untreated patient with diabetes may excrete glucose equivalent to 1,500 calories or more a day. The attempt to make up for lost calories results in polyphagia. Long-term weight loss is attributable to loss of calories; short-term weight loss is due to dehydration.

The lack of insulin causes excessive release of free fatty acids from adipose tissue. The free fatty acids are oxidized in the liver, but the rate of oxidation of free fatty acids exceeds the rate of oxidation of acetylcoenzyme A (acety-CoA) in the citric acid cycle. The accumulating acetyl-CoA is converted to ketone bodies, acetoacetate, and β-hydroxybutyrate. The formation of ketone bodies results in the production of hydrogen ion. The metabolism of triglycerides to free fatty acid and ketone bodies thus involves the release of hydrogen ion.

$$\text{Triglycerides} \rightarrow 3 \text{ fatty acids} + 3 \text{ H}^+$$

$$\text{Fatty acid (palmitate)} \rightarrow 4 \text{ ketone bodies} + 3 \text{ H}^+$$

The acidosis produced by ketosis is, in part, directly reversible and, in part, reversible only by compensatory mechanisms.[3] With correction of the ketoacidosis, the production of H^+ can be reversed either by reconversion of ketone bodies to triglyceride or by their complete oxidation.

$$\text{Ketone body} + \text{H}^+ \rightarrow \text{triglycerides}$$

$$\text{Ketone body} + \text{H}^+ \rightarrow 4 \text{ CO}_2$$

This accounts for the correction of the acidosis that usually occurs in patients with ketoacidosis once therapy is begun.

The nonreversible part of the acidosis results from the excretion of acetoacetate and β-hydroxybutyrate in the urine. A physiologic pH of urine acetoacetate and β-hydroxybuterate exists both as a free acid and as the salt. Some of the excreted acetoacetate and β-hydroxybutyrate is accompanied by sodium or potassium. In effect, the ketone body is eliminated but the H^+ remains. This H^+ cannot be eliminated by a reversal of the process by which it was produced. However, it can be eliminated by the usual mechanisms for eliminating acid, such as excretion with phosphate or ammonia.

The accumulation of H^+ results in total body depletion of potassium.[82] As H^+ accumulates, it partially replaces K^+ as the intracellular ion. Potassium is lost from the cells into the serum and is subsequently cleared by the kidney. The potassium depletion is accentuated by losses due to intercellular dehydration, tissue protein breakdown, and vomiting. The total body depletion of potassium is present despite normal (or even elevated) serum potassium levels prior to therapy. The H^+ accumulation also results in an increased renal excretion of phosphate during ketoacidosis.[7] This, in part, accounts for the hypophosphatemia that may develop during ketoacidosis therapy. Another cause of hypophosphatemia during therapy is the rapid increase in phosphorylated intermediates of glycolysis once insulin is given.

Total body depletion of sodium is common in ketoacidosis. Loss of sodium is due to the osmotic diuresis and vomiting. Since water is also lost, the serum sodium is often normal in ketoacidosis, but if the loss of either sodium or water is greater than the loss of the other, either hyponatremia or hypernatremia may be present, depending upon the balance of these factors. Two factors may markedly affect the measured serum sodium in ketoacidosis. First, the hyperglycemia will reduce the "normal" serum sodium. For each 100-mg/dL increase in the blood glucose, the serum sodium will be depressed by 1.6 mEq/L.[48] Thus, a normal serum sodium in a patient with a blood glucose of 1,100 mg/dL would be 140 mEq/L (normal sodium) −1.6 × 10 (observed glucose minus normal glucose divided by 100), or 124 mEq/ L. Second, a few patients with ketoacidosis have significant hyperlipidemia. Hyperlipidemia will appear to depress the serum sodium because the lipid fraction of the serum does not contain electrolytes.

The cause of coma that may accompany ketoacidosis is unknown. It is likely the result of the combination of ketosis, acidosis, hyperosmolality, and dehydration. Ketoacidosis is also frequently accompanied by abdominal pain; but signs of peritoneal irritation are absent. This pain often seems to be due to soreness of the accessory respiratory muscles caused by hyperventilation.

Treatment

General Measures

The treatment of ketoacidosis should be directed toward correction of the biochemical abnormalities discussed above. Initial evaluation should include a careful history and physical examination. Initial laboratory studies should include a complete blood count, urinalysis, and determination of electrolytes, glucose, blood urea nitrogen (BUN), serum acetones, and blood acid-base status, and, in very sick patients, serum phosphate and osmolality. A flow sheet that includes these laboratory tests, intake and output, and insulin dosage should be kept. In general, the serum glucose should be measured about every 2 hours, while the serum electrolytes, acetone, and blood pH should be measured every 3 to 4 hours.

Insulin

For the treatment of ketoacidosis, 0.1 unit/kg body weight of insulin is given IV followed by an infusion of 0.1 unit/kg/hr. To administer a constant infusion, 3 mL of 25% albumin is added to 250 mL of normal saline. (The albumin will minimize the binding of insulin to tubing.) Twenty units of regular insulin are added to 100 mL of this solution to yield a final concentration of 0.2 unit/mL of insulin. An infusion pump should be used to assure a constant rate of infusion. The insulin solution should be changed every 6 hours.

The constant infusion of insulin should be continued until the acidosis is corrected and the serum bicarbonate is greater than or equal to 15 mEq/L. It is not unusual for the blood sugar to fall well before the acidosis is cleared. A fall in the blood glucose to near normal is not an indication that insulin therapy should be discontinued; rather it is an indication to give IV glucose. Normalizing the blood glucose level is not the only, or even the primary, goal of therapy of ketoacidosis. The primary goal is to correct the acidosis, ketosis, and dehydration. Once this is accomplished, insulin should be given every 4 to 6 hours subcutaneously, depending upon the blood glucose and acetone.

Once the acetone is completely cleared, patients with established diabetes can be given their usual daily insulin dose. An appropriate starting dose for patients with newly diagnosed diabetes is 0.5 U/kg/day, with approximately two thirds in the morning and one third in the evening, divided into one-third regular and two-thirds NPH insulin.

Fluid and Electrolyte Management

The patient should receive about 20 mL/kg of either normal saline or Ringer's lactate solution over the first hour. This should be increased, and plasma added, if necessary, for the rare patient in shock. This initial fluid bolus need not contain glucose or potassium.

Volume

Fluid should be continued at a rate of about 4,000 mL/m²/day. This should be considered only the first approximation. Often, a faster rate will be required to keep up with continued polyuria. The objective is to replace the deficit over about 24 hours. The deficit is best estimated from acute weight loss, but if this is unknown, it can be estimated by clinical examination.

Fluid Content

Initial fluid should be normal saline or Ringer's lactate solution without glucose. Once the blood glucose level has fallen to about 250 to 300 mg/dL, 5% dextrose and half-normal saline solution should be used.

Potassium

Potassium should be added in a concentration of 30 to 40 mEq/L to all IV fluids after the initial bolus. Potassium should be given 50% as potassium chloride and 50% as potassium phosphate. Frequent monitoring of the serum potassium is indicated.

Bicarbonate

It is not necessary to give bicarbonate, unless the blood pH is severely depressed (less than 7.1), since the pH will be corrected as ketones are metabolized.[49] Very low blood pH values are treated because of the adverse effects of severe acidosis. Partial correction of the acidosis will make the patient more comfortable (by decreasing the drive for hyperventilation). On the other hand, correcting the pH to normal with bicarbonate will result in alkalosis as the ketones are metabolized. Rapid administration of bicarbonate can increase the intercellular acidosis in the brain. This occurs because bicarbonate binds with H^+, thereby decreasing the respiratory drive and elevating the serum carbon dioxide. This CO_2 then diffuses rapidly into the brain and disassociates into HCO_3^- and H^+. Since bicarbonate diffuses into the brain only slowly, the immediate effect is to increase the intercellular H^+ concentration.

When bicarbonate is given, the formula is body weight (kg) × 0.15 (estimated bicarbonate = 0.6 ÷ 4 for a 25% correction) × the base excess (with a maximum of 50 mEq of bicarbonate over any 2-hour period). The acid-base status is reevaluated; this dose is repeated if the pH remains below 7.1.

Occasionally patients with type I diabetes will present with severe hyperglycemia and dehydration but without severe ketosis or acidosis. This condition, called *hyperglycemic nonketotic coma*, is seen in infants and retarded children (presumably because they are unable to drink to thirst and therefore become dehydrated before acidosis develops). Treatment is similar to that for ketoacidosis, except that replacement should be slower (over 48 hours or longer) and the serum osmolarity should be decreased slowly. This condition has a higher mortality rate in the few pediatric patients reported.

Cerebral Edema

The major cause of morbidity and mortality in pediatric patients with ketoacidosis is sudden neurologic deterioration due to cerebral edema.[26] This problem is most common in young patients with new-onset diabetes. Computed tomography (CT) scans of patients in ketoacidosis indicate that some brain swelling is common in all patients.[53] Recent reviews of large series of cases of severe cerebral edema fail to reveal any clear association with any aspect of therapy.[72] Excessive fluid administration and rapid decreases in serum osmolarity should be avoided on a theoretical basis.[41] A therapeutic program that aims at judicious, steady correction of the metabolic abnormalities in diabetic ketoacidosis, without overcorrection, is appropriate. The clinical signs of significant cerebral edema often begin after 12 to 24 hours in patients with an otherwise unremarkable course. Diagnosing incipient deterioration is difficult. Initial symptoms, such as headache and lethargy, are common in ketoacidosis and alone do not justify intervention. Clear signs, such as pupillary dilatation or inequality, blood pressure instability, bradycardia, apnea, or seizures, should be viewed with alarm. Intervention should include raising the patient's head, hyperventilation, and IV mannitol in a dose of 1 to 2 g/kg.

Preventing Ketoacidosis

Ketoacidosis can develop at the time of diabetes onset or in patients with known diabetes. Preventing ketoacidosis at the onset of diabetes requires making the diagnosis before ketoacidosis develops. This requires that the family consult with the physician for early symptoms of diabetes and that the physician make the appropriate diagnosis.

Once diabetes is established, the risk of ketoacidosis is known. Almost all further episodes of ketoacidosis are due to major deviations in therapy, such as missed insulin injections.[38,75,90] Even one episode of ketoacidosis in a patient with established diabetes should be taken as an indication of either major knowledge deficits or a significant deviation from prescribed therapy.

Ketosis, and even mild ketoacidosis, can result from unavoidable variations (variable insulin absorption in standard therapy) or from intercurrent illness, especially in small children. Families should be instructed to monitor ketonuria (at any sign of illness or persistent high blood sugar) and seek consultation in the case of moderate or large ketonuria, or nausea or vomiting.[18] Patients with hyperglycemia and moderate to large ketonuria should be given extra regular insulin (10%–25% of their total daily dose) every 3 to 4 hours plus juices as tolerated until the ketonuria is resolved. If the family and therapist understand this process, ketoacidosis requiring IV therapy will be rare.

The incidence of ketoacidosis in patients with diabetes is highest in adolescents, particularly at 14 to 15 years of age.[37] It is more prevalent in patients from underprivileged, unstable families. It is important to make it clear to the patient and family that ketoacidosis is secondary to skipped insulin shots. A comprehensive treatment approach that addresses the complex psychosocial issues that interfere with this basic aspect of therapy is essential.

LONG-TERM MANAGEMENT

Complications and Control

The central question in diabetes management remains scientifically unanswered almost 70 years after the first clinical use of insulin. Can improved control prevent or delay the complications of diabetes?

On a theoretical level, evidence is accumulating which suggests that the complications of diabetes are a consequence of hyperglycemia. Glucose reacts with structural macromolecules, particularly proteins and DNA, forming cross-links and altering their structure and function. For example, glycosylation of β-lipoproteins can impair their degradation. This may account for the hypercholesterolemia of poorly controlled diabetes and may, in turn, explain the increased risk of myocardial infarction, stroke, and claudication in patients with diabetes. Mechanisms other than glycosylation may account for some complications. For example, diabetic cataracts result from conversion of glucose to sorbitol, which contributes to osmotic disruption of the lens.[34] Increased tissue sorbitol and decreased *myo*-inositol may contribute to diabetic neuropathy.

Glucose may also be toxic to beta cells.[73] Elevated levels of glucose in early type I diabetes and throughout the course of type II diabetes may contribute to beta cell damage and further insulin deficiency. This hypothesis indicates that it may be especially important to control the blood glucose in patients wtih residual insulin secretion.

Conclusive evidence that clinically achievable improvements in diabetes control can delay or prevent the complications of diabetes is lacking. Several retrospective studies have shown a clear association between good control and reduced complications.[19,24] Since these studies are retrospective, they cannot discount the possibility that patients with an inherent ability to achieve good control are inherently less likely to develop complications. A multicenter study currently under way, the Diabetes Control and Complications Trial, is designed to prospectively determine the effects of intensive management on diabetes outcome.[25]

In the meantime, theoretical and retrospective evidence strongly suggests that improved control will at least delay the complications. Moreover, the degree of control necessary for a significant impact on complications appears to be achievable. With that premise, it follows that medical management of diabetes becomes a matter of balancing the desire for low (normal or nearly normal) blood glucose levels against the risk of insulin reactions. The risk of severe insulin reaction varies among patients and, in the individual patient, may be different at different times.

The following factors increase the risk of insulin reactions and shift the balance toward maintaining somewhat higher blood glucose levels to avoid reactions (see Table 9–1):

TABLE 9–1.

Factors That Increase the Risk of Severe Insulin Reaction

1. Hypoglycemia unawareness
2. Young age (<5–6 yr)
3. Sleeping
4. When impaired function may cause consequences (e.g., driving)
5. Patients receiving full insulin replacement—no endogenous production of insulin

1. *Hypoglycemia unawareness syndrome* is often related to a decreased catecholamine response to hypoglycemia and thus an absence of adrenergic symptoms.[11,14,22] This may be a complication of poor control and a recurrent problem in some patients.

2. *Age*: Most children younger than 5 or 6 years of age cannot recognize and respond to the symptoms of a hypoglycemia.[32,39] Hypoglycemia may also be more likely to cause neurologic damage during this period of brain development.

3. *Sleep vs. awake*: Most patients in a sleep state will not awaken and recognize the early symptoms of hypoglycemia. A disproportionate number of severe insulin reactions occur when patients are asleep[9]

4. *Individuals who are alone or driving*: The consequences of a severe reaction (should it occur) are increased when the patient is alone or driving. On the other hand, pregnancy increases the desirability of good control and patients who continue to have residual insulin secretion can often achieve very good control without much risk of insulin reaction.

Diabetes control requires a complex balance among insulin, food, and exercise. With present methods, ideal control is not achievable. Even near normal blood glucose control requires very demanding patient participation that is not sustainable by many patients. Diabetes programs need to be practical, manageable, and achievable. Therefore, they should be individualized as much as possible within the bounds of reasonable control. For pediatric patients, this often means changing expectations at different developmental stages. For example, the family of a toddler may be willing to do blood tests four to five times a day. That child, in early adolescence, may only test once or twice a day, but with maturity he or she may be willing to follow a more demanding schedule.

"Honeymoon" Period

One major factor determining diabetes control is the capability of the patient to secrete some insulin.[60] For patients that produce substantial insulin, this capability may make nearly ideal control possible. Those patients who can secrete even small amounts of insulin seem to have more stable blood glucose control.

Insulin is normally released from stored insulin. A high blood glucose level may exhaust these stores. On the other hand, normal blood glucose levels may allow the pancreas to replenish insulin stores. Thus, in patients who retain some ability to secrete insulin, high blood glucose levels may make control more difficult and low blood glucose levels may make control easier. This can be seen clinically in children who have consistent good control and who may suddenly develop persistent high blood glucose levels. Often, if aggressive increases in insulin restore low blood glucose levels, consistent good control may resume. Since good control begets good control and a high blood glucose may itself damage beta cells, a continuation of a significant dose of insulin with a target of near-normal blood glucose levels may be a reasonable goal during the "honeymoon" period.

Compliance

In addition to retention of the ability to secrete insulin, the most important factor in achieving good control is the ability of the patient to follow a treatment plan. Even the simplest treatment plan demands considerable patient participation and adaptation. Some patients, particularly during adolescence, find it difficult to make the necessary adjustments.[66] Some patients may not follow the basics, such as consistently taking insulin. Pressure by their family and physician to produce good blood glucose levels may contribute to deception such as fabrication of blood glucose test results.[36,91] Peer pressure and a desire to conform may also contribute to deviations from diet and schedule.

It is important to recognize not only when compliance is the problem but also to appreciate that the causes of noncompliance lie in our inability to manage diabetes without making considerable demands on patients and their families. This recognition must be balanced with the desire to avoid making overwhelming demands on the patient. Nevertheless, the physician can modify the requirements only so much. For example, some consistent pattern of insulin administration is essential. To the extent possible, however, the physician should adjust the diabetes program so that the recommended therapy is only as much as the patient is capable of sustaining. Theoretically, the patient and family should make informed decisions as to the best program for themselves. In practice, however, many patients will look to the physician for guidance.

Insulin and Insulin Absorption

The absorption of insulin given subcutaneously is far from consistent and is influenced by a number of factors (see Table 9-2).[10,33,42,52,70,95] Patients need to learn proper injection techniques, so that insulin injections are as consistent as possible. Inadvertent intramuscular injection can significantly hasten insulin absorption and shorten the duration of action. Intramuscular injection may result when the subcutaneous tissue is not pinched. In our clinic, we recommend against patients' self-injecting their own arm (the traditional lean against the wall may be inadequate) without help from others to pinch their subcutaneous tissue. Likewise, insertion of the needle should not be perpendicular to the skin of thin young children whose available pinched subcutaneous tissue is scanty. Failure to release the pinch prior to withdrawing the needle may result in pressure forcing the insulin out of the injection site.

Insulin absorption also varies by injection site. Frequent injection in the same area may result in hypertrophy, which can impair insulin absorption. Insulin absorption also varies by anatomic region, with decreasing rapidity of absorption in the abdomen, arms, thighs, and buttocks, in that order. A rotation pattern in which all injections at any one time of the day are given into areas with similar insulin absorption may improve absorption regularity. Insulin absorption may be increased by exercise.

TABLE 9–2.

Insulin Absorption

Increased rapidity of absorption
    Human NPH insulin
    IM injection
    Abdomen and arms vs. legs and buttocks
    Exercise
    Massage of site
    Jet injectors
    Regular vs. NPH or Lente insulin
    Increased room and body temperature
Decreased rapidity of absorption or action
    Injection into hypertrophied area
    Intradermal injection
    Premixing regular with NPH or Lente insulin
    Large insulin volume
    Insulin antibodies

TABLE 9–3.

Insulin Preparations

Insulin Type	Activity (hr)		
	Onset	Peak	Duration
Regular	0.5	2–4	5–8
Semilente	0.5–1.0	4–6	8–12
NPH	2–4	6–10	12–24
Lente	2–4	6–10	12–24
Ultralente	3–4	12–20	24–36

Therefore, avoiding areas of exercising muscle may be indicated for some patients (e.g., avoiding the thighs when running). Giving insulin 30 to 50 minutes prior to meals can significantly reduce postprandial hyperglycemia.[92]

Loss of insulin potency may contribute to poor control. Patients and families should be warned that excessive heat or freezing may damage insulin. A single bottle of insulin may be sufficient to provide months of insulin therapy for a very young child. The expiration date is intended to provide a safe limiting date for insulin that is not being used regularly. In my practice, I recommend that a vial of insulin be used for 6 weeks to 2 months.

Insulin is also available in several different forms that affect the duration of action (see Table 9–3). The most common insulin regimens are combinations of regular insulin with NPH or Lente insulin, usually given twice a day. Human insulin, when converted to NPH, does appear to dissolve more rapidly than animal insulins in the NPH form.[80]

Early-Morning Hyperglycemia

High blood glucose levels in the morning are a common problem. Since the risk of severe insulin reactions is increased at night, it is desirable to have glucose levels at the high end of the acceptable range. For most patients, nighttime activity levels are consistent. The early-morning blood glucose levels should therefore be more consistent than the daytime levels. Hormonal changes, particularly a physiologic increase in growth hormone in the 2 to 3 hours prior to awakening, contribute to an increase in glucose levels—the dawn phenomenon.[2,12,16,43] High blood glucose levels in the morning may also be due to a decrease in circulating insulin levels (as a result of rapid insulin absorption). Insufficient duration of insulin action is frequent in young children receiving NPH insulin prior to an early dinner.

Traditionally, it was felt that early-morning hyperglycemia was often due to a rebound from nocturnal hypoglycemia (the Somogyi reaction).[71,83] Recent studies in which nocturnal hypoglycemia was purposely induced found no rebound hyperglycemia; they cast doubt on the importance of rebound hyperglycemia.[13] Rapid insulin absorption may be a more likely explanation of low blood glucose levels in the early evening, with high levels later as insulin dissipates.

Monitoring and Measuring in Diabetes Control

Monitoring and recording of blood glucose levels at sufficiently frequent intervals will allow for an adjustment of the insulin dose. For most children and adolescents, testing one to four times a day provides sufficient information to make insulin adjustments. Many patients do well with a system in which their dose of regular insulin is self-adjusted according to a scale based on the capillary blood glucose level.[81] To obtain accurate results of capillary blood glucose, the procedure must be followed closely. Therefore, thorough patient and family instruction is important. The physician should also recognize that daily testing is demanding and be alert to the possibility that reported results may not reflect glucose levels accurately. Insulin adjustment (see Figure 9–2) should maintain blood glucose levels as low as possible without unduly increasing the risk of insulin reaction.

Periodic measurement of glycohemoglobin or hemoglobin A_{1c} levels allows objective assessment of long-term control.[44,62] In some patients, nonglucose factors (high fetal hemoglobin, hemoglobin S or C, hemolytic anemia) may distort the glycohemoglobin value.[1,93] In these patients, glycosylated albumin or fructosamine may provide a better objective measure of control.[50] Glycohemoglobin levels vary considerably from one laboratory to another because of differences in methodology. Table 9–4 lists a reasonable assessment of control for children with diabetes, based upon the percentage elevation in the glycohemoglobin above the highest normal value in nondiabetic children.

Patients with type I diabetes have a higher incidence of thyroiditis which may result in hypothyroidism. Some physicians recommend annual thyroid tests in all patients. Another approach is to measure antimicrosomal and antithyroglobulin antibodies in all patients and obtain annual thyroid tests in patients with positive antibodies and only clinically monitor thyroid function in antibody-negative patients. Annual measurement of cholesterol and cholesterol fractionation allows adjustment of fat intake if indicated. In adolescents, annual measurement of urinary microalbumin may allow early detection of renal involvement. An annual eye examination is also indicated for adolescents. Periodic blood pressure measurement is indicated; an el-

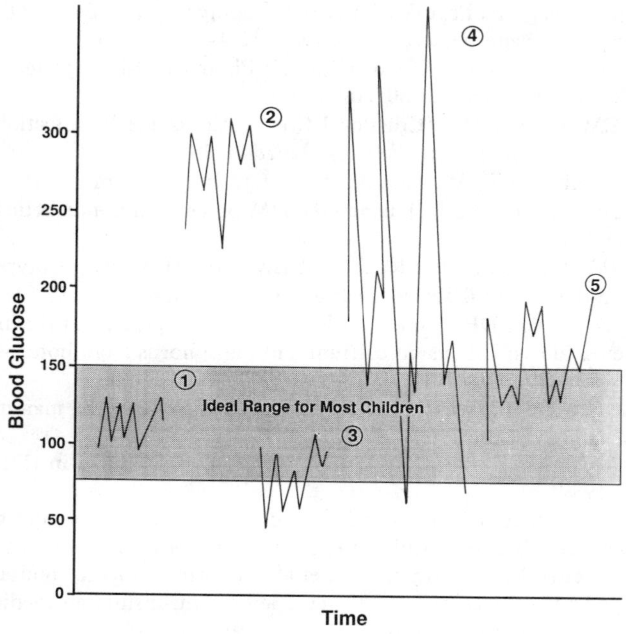
Blood Glucose
300
250
200
150
100
50
0
Time
Ideal Range for Most Children
①
②
③
④
⑤
1. Ideal control - Rarely possible except during honeymoon period
2. Poor control - More insulin needed
3. Low blood glucose - Reduce dose
4. Marked fluctuations - work on consistency diet, exercise, insulin absorption
5. Good control for most patients - 1/2 tests in ideal range.

FIG 9–2.
Blood glucose control.

TABLE 9–4.
Glycohemoglobin and Assessment of Control

Glycohemoglobin	Control Level	Percentage of Patients*
<10% higher†	Excellent	20
10%–20% higher	Very good	19
20%–30% higher	Good	21
30%–40% higher	Fair	20
40%–50% higher	Poor	12
>50% higher	Very poor	16

*Percentage of author's patients aged 12 to 20 years with a diabetes duration of at least 1 year in each control level.
†As compared with the highest normal in nondiabetic persons.

evated blood pressure significantly increases the risk of diabetic nephrotoxicity and should be treated.

REFERENCES

1. Allen DB, MacDonald MJ: Artifacts in glycosylated hemoglobin values in pediatric patients. *J Pediatr*, 1986; 109:655.

2. Altiea JA, Creagh F, Page M; Early-morning hyperglycemia in IDDM: Acute effects of cholinergic blockade. *Diabetes Care* 1989; 12:443.

3. Androgue JH, Wilson H, Boyd AE, et al: Plasma acid-base pattern in diabetic ketoacidosis. *N Engl J Med* 1982; 307:1603.

4. Asplin CM, Cooney MK, Crossley JR, et al: Coxsackie B4 infection and islet cell antibodies 3 years before overt diabetes. *J Pediatr* 1982; 101:398.

5. Awata T, Kuzuya T, Matsuda A, et al: High frequency of aspartic acid at position 57 of HLA-DQ beta-chain in Japanese IDDM patients in nondiabetic subjects. *Diabetes* 1990; 39:266.

6. Baisch JM, Weeks P, Giles R, et al: Analysis of HLA-DQ genotypes and susceptibility in insulin-dependent diabetes mellitus. *N Engl J Med* 1990; 322:1836.

7. Becker DJ, Bryon DR, Steranka BH; Phosphate replacement during treatment of diabetic ketoacidosis; Effects on calcium and phosphorus from homeostasis. *Am J Dis Child*, 1983; 137:240.

8. Bell GI, Kayano T, Buce JB, et al: Molecular biology of the mammalian glucose-transporters. *Diabetes Care* 1990; 13:198.

9. Bergada I, Suissa S, Dufresne J, et al: Severe hypoglycemia in IDDM children. *Diabetes Care* 1989; 12:239.

10. Berger M, Cuppers HJ, Hegner H, et al: Absorption kinetics and biologic effects of subcutaneously injected insulin preparations. *Diabetes Care* 1982; 5:77.

11. Bolli G, DeFeo P, Compagnucci P, et al: Abnormal glucose counter-regulation in insulin-dependent diabetes mellitus; Interaction of anti-insulin antibodies and impaired glucagon and epinephrine secretion. *Diabetes* 1983; 32:134.

12. Bolli GB, Gerich JE: The "dawn phenomena" — a common occurrence in both non-insulin-dependent and insulin-dependent diabetes mellitus, *N Engl J Med* 1984; 310:746.

13. Bolli GB, Gottesman IS, Campbell PJ, et al: Glucose counterregulation and waning of insulin in the Somogyi phenomena (posthypoglycemic/hyperglycemia). *N Engl J Med* 1984; 311:1214.

14. Bolli GD, Dimitriadis GD, Pehling GB, et al: Abnormal glucose counter-regulation after subcutaneous insulin in insulin-dependent diabetes mellitus. *N Engl J Med* 1984; 310:1706.

15. Campbell IL, Hellquist LND, Taylor KW: Insulin biosynthesis and its regulation. *Clin Sci* 1982; 62:449.

16. Campbell PJ, Bolli GM, Cryer PE, et al: The pathogenesis of the dawn phenomenon in patients with insulin-dependent diabetes mellitus: Accelerated glucose production and impaired glucose utilization due to nocturnal surges in growth hormone secretion. *N Engl J Med* 1985; 312:1473.

17. Champsaur HS, Bottazzo GF, Bertrams J, et al: Virologic, immunologic, and genetic factors in insulin-dependent diabetes mellitus. *J Pediatr* 1982; 100:15.

18. Chase HP, Garg SK, Jelley DH: Diabetic ketoacidosis in children and the role of outpatient management. *Pediatr Rev* 1990; 11:297.

19. Chase HP, Jackson WE, Hoops SL, et al: Glucose control and the renal and retinal complications of the insulin-dependent diabetes. *JAMA* 1989; 261:1155.

20. Christau B, Kromann H, Andersen 00, et al: Incidence, seasonal, and geographic patterns of juvenile onset insulin dependent diabetes mellitus in Denmark. *Diabetologia* 1977; 13:281.

21. Cook DL, Satin LS, Ashford MLJ, et al: ATP-sensitive channels in the pancreatic beta cells. Spare-channel hypothesis. *Diabetes* 1988; 37:495.

22. Cryer PE: Decreased sympathochromaffin activity in IDDM. *Diabetes* 1989; 38:405.

23. Dahlquist G, Gustavsson KH, Holmgren G, et al; The incidence of diabetes mellitus in Swedish children 0–14 years of age. *Acta Paediatr Scand* 1982; 71:7.

24. D'Antonio JA, Ellis D, Doft BH, et al: Diabetic complications in glycemic control: The Pittsburgh Perfective Insulin-Dependent Diabetes Cohort Study. Status report after 5 years of IDDM. *Diabetes Care* 1989; 12:694.

25. DCCT Research Group: Diabetes Control in Complications Trial (DCCT): Results of feasibility study. *Diabetes Care.* 1987; 10:1.

26. Duck SC, Wyatt DT: Factors associated with brain herniation in the treatment of diabetic ketoacidosis. *J Pediatr* 1988; 133:10.

27. Eisenbarth GS: Type I diabetes mellitus, a chronic autoimmune disease. *N Engl J Med* 1986; 314:1360.

28. Eisenbarth GS: Genes, generator of diversity, glycoconjugates, and autoimmune beta cell insufficiency in type I diabetes. *Diabetes* 1987; 36:355.

29. Eisenbarth GS: Type I diabetes. Clinical implications of autoimmunity. *Hosp Pract* 1987; 167.

30. Erlich HA, Bugawan TL, Scharf F: HLA-DQ beta sequenced polymorphism and genetic susceptibility to IDDM. *Diabetes* 1990; 39:96.

31. Fleegler SM, Rogers RD, Drash A, et al: Age, sex, and season of onset of juvenile diabetes in different geographic areas, *Pediatrics* 1979; 63:174.

32. Frank M, Link J, Daneman D, et al: The young child with diabetes; Challenges of diagnosis and management. *Clin Diabetes* 1986; 4:125.

33. Frid A, Ostman J, Linde D: Hypoglycemia risks during exercise and after intramuscular injection of insulin in thigh. *Diabetes Care* 1990; 13:473.

34. Gabbay KH: The sorbitol pathway and the complications of diabetes. *N Engl J Med* 1973; 288:831.

35. Gambel BR, Taylor KW: Seasonal incidence of diabetes mellitus. *Br Med J* 1969; 3:631.

36. Glasgow AM: Little deceits often repeat: Detecting false blood glucose reports. *Diabetes Care* 1987; 10:791.

37. Glasgow AM, Altieri ME: The epidemiology of readmissions of children with diabetes to a children's hospital, in Ahmed PL, Ahmed N (ed): Coping With Juvenile Diabetes. Springfield, Ill, Charles C Thomas, Publisher, 1985, p 358.

38. Golden J, Herrold A, Orr D: An approach to prevention of recurrent diabetic ketoacidosis in the pediatric population. *J Pediatr* 1985; 107:195.

39. Golden MP, Russell BP, Ingersol GM, et al: Management of diabetes mellitus in children younger than 5 years of age. *Am J Dis Child* 1985; 139:448.

40. Hamman RF, Cay EC, Cruickshank KJ: Colorado IDDM registry. Incidence and validation of IDDM in children ages 0–17 years. *Diabetes Care* 1990; 13:499.

41. Harris GD, Fiordalisi I, Harris WL, et al: Minimizing the risks of brain herniation during treatment of diabetic ketoacidemia: A retrospective and prospective study. *J Pediatr* 1990; 117:22.

42. Haycock P: Insulin absorption: Understanding the variables. *Clin Diabetes* 1986; 4:101.

43. Hirsch IB, Smith LJ, Havlin CE, et al: Failure of nocturnal hypoglycemia to cause daytime hyperglycemia in patients with IDDM. *Diabetes Care* 1990; 13:133.

44. Jovanovic L, Peterson CM: The clinical utility of glycosylated hemoglobin. Am J Med 1981; 70:331.

45. Karjalainen J, Salmela P, Ilornen J, et al: Comparison of childhood and adult type I diabetes mellitus. *N Engl J Med* 1989; 320:881.

46. Kasanicki MA, Pilch PF: Regulation of glucose-transporter function. *Diabetes Care* 1990; 13:219.

47. Kasuga M, Izumi T, Tobe K, et al: Substrates for insulin-receptor kinase. *Diabetes Care* 1990; 13:317.
48. Katz MA: Hyperglycemia induced hyponatremia-calculation of expected serum sodium depression. N Engl J Med 1973; 289:843.
49. Kaye R: Diabetic ketoacidosis—the bicarbonate controversy. *J Pediatr* 1975; 87:156.
50. Kemp SS, Creech RH, Horn TR: Glycosylated albumin and transferrin: Short-term markers of blood glucose control. *J Pediatr* 1984; 105:394.
51. King ML, Shaikh A, Bidwell D, et al: Coxsackie B virus specific IgM responses in children with insulin dependent (juvenile-onset, type I) diabetes mellitus, *Lancet* 1983; 1:1397.
52. Kolendorf K, Bojsen J, Deckert T: Clinical factors influencing the absorption of I_{125} NPH insulin in diabetic patients. *Horm Metab Res* 1983; 15:274.
53. Krane EJ, Rockoff MA, Wallman JK, et al: Subclinical brain swelling in children during treatment of diabetic ketoacidosis. *N Engl J Med* 1985; 312:1147.
54. Krolewski AS, Warram JH, Rand LI, et al: Epidemiologic approach to the etiology of type I diabetes mellitus and its complications. *N Engl J Med* 1987; 317:1390.
55. Laporte RE, Fishbein HA, Drash AL, et al; The Pittsburgh Insulin-Dependent Diabetes Mellitus (IDDM) Registry. The incidence of insulin-dependent diabetes mellitus in Allegheny County, PA (1965–1976). *Diabetes* 1981; 30:279.
56. Larner J: Insulin-signaling mechanisms. Lessons from the Old Testament of glycogen metabolism and the New Testament of molecular biology. *Diabetes* 1988; 37:262.
57. Lendrum R, Walker G, Gambel DR: Islet-cell antibodies in juvenile diabetes mellitus of recent onset. *Lancet* 1975; 1:880.
58. MacDonald NJ, Liston L, Carlson I: Seasonality in glycosylated hemoglobin in normal subjects. *Diabetes* 1987; 36:265.
59. MacLaren NK, Huang SW, Sogh J: Antibody to cultured human insulinoma cells and insulin dependent diabetes. *Lancet* 1975; 2:997.
60. Madsbad S; Prevalence of residual beta cell function and its metabolic consequences in type I (insulin-dependent) diabetes. *Diabetetologia* 1983; 24:141.
61. Menser NA, Forrest JM, Bransby RD: Rubella infection in diabetes mellitus. Lancet 1978; 1:57.
62. Nathan DM, Singer DE, Hurzthal K: The clinical information value of the glycosylated hemoglobin assay. *N Engl J Med* 1984; 310:341.
63. O'Brien RM, Granner DK: PEPCK genes as a model of inhibitory effects of insulin on gene transcription. *Diabetes Care* 1990; 13:327.
64. Orci L: Macro-micro-domains in the endocrine pancreas. *Diabetes* 1982; 31:538.
65. Orci L, Malatsse-Lagae F, Razazzola M, et al: A morphological basis for intercellular communication between alpha and beta cells in the endocrine pancreas. *J Clin Invest* 1975; 46:1066.
66. Orr DP, Eccles T, Lawlor R: Surreptitious insulin administration in adolescents with insulin-dependent diabetes mellitus. *JAMA* 1986; 256:3227.
67. Pfeifer MA, Halter JD, Porte D: Insulin secretion in diabetes mellitus. *Am J Med* 1981; 70:579.
68. Rajan AF, Aguilar-Bryan L, Nelson DA, et al: Ion channels and insulin secretion. *Diabetes Care* 1990; 13:340.
69. Rasmussen H, Zawalich KC, Ganesan S, et al: Physiology and pattern physiology of insulin secretion. *Diabetes Care* 1990; 13:655.
70. Ronnemaa T, Koivisto DA: Combined effect of exercise and ambient temperature of insulin absorption and postprandial glycemia in type I patients. *Diabetes Care* 1988; 11:769.

71. Rosenbloom AL, Giordano BP: Chronic overtreatment with insulin in children and adolescents. *Am J Dis Child* 1977; 131:881.

72. Rosenbloom AL: Intracerebral crisis during treatment of diabetic ketoacidosis, *Diabetes Care* 1990; 13:22.

73. Rossetti L, Giaccari A, Defronza RA: Glucose toxicity. *Diabetes Care* 1990; 13:610.

74. Saltiel AR: Second messengers of insulin action. *Diabetes Care* 1990; 13:244.

75. Schade DS, Drumm DA, Duckworth WC, et al: Etiology of incapacitating, brittle diabetes. *Diabetes Care* 1985; 8:12.

76. Segall M: HLA and genetics of IDDM. Holism vs. reductionism? *Diabetes* 1988; 37:1005.

77. Seino S, Seino M, Bell GI: Human insulin-receptor gene. *Diabetes* 1990; 39:129.

78. Selden RF, Skoskiewicz MJ, Russell PS, et al: Regulation of insulin-gene expression: Implications for gene therapy. *N Engl J Med* 1987; 317:1067.

79. Sirkanta S, Ganda OP, Jackson RA, et al: Type I diabetes mellitus in monozygotic twins: Chronic progressive beta cell dysfunction. *Ann Intern Med* 1983; 99:320.

80. Skyler JS: Human insulin of recombinant DNA origin: Clinical potential. *Diabetes Care* 1982; 5:181.

81. Skyler JS, Skyler DL, Seigler DE: Algorithms for adjustment of insulin dosage by patients who monitor blood glucose. *Diabetes Care* 1981; 4:311.

82. Soler NG, Bennett MA, Dixon K, et al: Potassium balance during treatment of diabetic ketoacidosis with special reference to the use of bicarbonate. *Lancet* 1972; 2:665.

83. Somogyi M: Exacerbation of diabetes by excess insulin action. *Am J Med* 1959; 26:169.

84. Steiner DF, Oyer PE: The biosynthesis of insulin and a probable precursor of insulin by a human islet cell adenoma. *Proc Natl Acad Sci USA* 1967; 57:473.

85. Suarez L. Barrett-Connor E: Seasonal variation in fasting plasma glucose levels in man. *Diabetalogia* 1982; 22:250.

86. Tattersall RB, Pyke DA: Diabetes and identical twins. *Lancet* 1972; 2:1120.

87. Taylor SI, Kadowaki T, Kadowaki H, et al: Mutations in insulin-receptor gene in insulin-resistant patients. *Diabetes Care* 1990; 13:257.

88. Thornes B, Charron MJ, Lodish HF: Molecular physiology of glucose transporters. *Diabetes Care* 1990; 13:209.

89. Wente SR, Rosen OM: Insulin-receptor approaches to studying protein kinase domain. *Diabetes Care* 1990; 13:280.

90. White K, Kolman ML, Wexler P, et al: Unstable diabetes in unstable families: A psychosocial evaluation of diabetic children with recurrent ketoacidosis. *Pediatrics* 1984; 73:749.

91. Wilson DP, Endres RK: Compliance with blood glucose monitoring in children with type I diabetes mellitus. *J Pediatr* 1986; 108:1022.

92. Witt MS, White NH, Santiago JV: Role of sight and timing of the morning insulin injection in type I diabetes. *J Pediatr* 1983; 103:528.

93. Yatscoff RW, Tezaarwerk GJM, Clarson CL: Interference of fetal hemoglobin and labile glycosylated hemoglobin with measurement of glycosylated hemoglobin. *Clin Chem* 1983; 29:543.

94. Yoon JW, Austin M, Onodera, T, et al: Virus-induced diabetes mellitus. Isolation of a virus from the pancreas of a child with diabetic ketoacidosis. *N Engl J Med* 1979; 300:1173.

95. Zinman B: The physiologic replacement of insulin: An elusive goal. *N Engl J Med* 1989; 321:363.

Chapter 10

Hypoglycemia

Allen M. Glasgow

Glucose is the body's main energy substrate. Although muscle and other nonneural tissues oxidize fat and amino acids, the brain and other neural tissues oxidize glucose as a preferred substrate. Only after prolonged fasting is the brain able to obtain part of its energy needs from the oxidation of ketones. Moreover, the energy produced from ketone oxidation only provides a maximum of 50% of the brain's energy needs. It is, therefore, essential for the body to maintain a glucose concentration sufficient for normal cerebral function.

While glucose is essential, it also can be a toxin. Glucose reacts spontaneously with a wide variety of proteins to form glycosylated derivatives. Glycohemoglobin is the prototypical derivative of this process. Glucose also forms covalent links with DNA. Glycosylation of protein and DNA is the major mechanism of glucose toxicity. Since a toxin is the body's chief source of energy, elaborate mechanisms exist to maintain a sufficient but not excessive supply.

The body glucose pool is subject to widely different rates of glucose input and consumption during the fed and fasted states. The need to maintain sufficient but not excessive glucose concentrations may be the teleologic explanation for the evolutionary development of elaborate mechanisms for regulating the blood glucose concentration. For example, the glucose concentration is more stable and regulated than the concentration of other energy substrates, amino acids and fats.

Abnormalities in the substrates, metabolic pathways, and hormones that contribute to glucose regulation lead to hypoglycemia if a minimal glucose concentration is not maintained and lead to diabetes mellitus if blood glucose concentrations become excessive.

DEFINITION

The lowest normal blood glucose is widely regarded as 40 mg/dL.[81] People with normal glucose control mechanisms may, in special circumstances, have blood glucose concentrations below 40 mg/dL. Some examples include children fasting for more than 36 hours, adults fasting for more than 72 hours, or individuals exercising to exhaustion. Blood glucose concentrations below 40 mg/dL are also common in asymptomatic small-for-date infants, premature infants, and term neonates in the first 2 to 3 days of life. This may be regarded as "normal" in that it is usually a transient problem which does not require extensive evaluation. However, blood glucose concentrations in this range may adversely affect brain development, even in asymptomatic infants. Therefore, blood glucose should be maintained in excess of 40 mg/dL in infants.

The brain appears to adapt to the prevailing glycemic level.[32] Patients with chronic hypoglycemia may tolerate a blood glucose level well below 40 mg/dL. Patients with chronic hyperglycemia may develop symptoms at blood glucose levels above 40 mg/dL.

In most clinical situations, a diagnosis of hypoglycemia should be based on the combination of (1) symptoms consistent with hypoglycemia; (2) a relatively low blood glucose level; and (3) prompt relief of symptoms when the blood glucose level is raised. In some complex situations, such as prolonged severe hypoglycemia, Reye's syndrome, or maple syrup urine disease, the symptoms may not respond rapidly to a correction of the hypoglycemia.

Glucose levels are dependent upon both the source of the blood sample and the method of measurement. Plasma glucose levels are approximately 15% greater than whole blood glucose levels. Capillary and arterial blood glucose levels are approximately 10% higher than venous levels. The difference among capillary, arterial, and venous levels is greatest at low glucose levels. Since glucose can be consumed in shed blood, the specimen must either be rapidly tested (usually within 30 minutes) or an inhibitor of glycolysis, such as fluoride, must be added to the specimen. Measurement of glucose levels is most accurate when performed in a laboratory. Blood glucose estimates are also performed via portable meters and reagent strips. When properly used, information obtained from the meters and strips can be very valuable. However, such methods should never be relied upon for diagnosis of hypoglycemia or to make major therapy decisions.[11,52]

REGULATION OF BLOOD GLUCOSE CONCENTRATION

Blood glucose concentration is a reflection of the balance between glucose input into the circulation and glucose extraction from blood. Glucose input includes sugars and carbohydrates in the diet, glucose release from glycogen stores, and gluconeogenesis (the production of glucose from noncarbohydrate precursors). Pathways of glucose extraction include glucose storage as glycogen, glucose conversion to lipid, and glucose oxidation. Glucose oxidation consists of a low level of obligate glucose oxidation, primarily by neural tissues, and highly variable glucose oxidation by muscle, adipose, and other tissues.

Fed State

During the fed state, glucose input consists of dietary intake. Dietary carbohydrates are hydrolyzed to simple sugars in the upper intestine. Nonglucose simple sugars, such as fructose and galactose, are rapidly converted to glucose in the liver. The rise in blood glucose stimulates insulin release and suppresses glucagon release. These hormonal changes and the increase in the concentration of blood glucose result in an inhibition of glucose production from glycolysis and gluconeogenesis. Glucose is stored as glycogen in the liver and muscle. It is oxidized in the muscle and adipose tissue and converted to lipid in the liver and adipose tissue. Insulin stimulates amino acid incorporation into protein and fatty acids incorporation into triglycerides.

Fasting State

During periods of fasting, the source of energy shifts from the oxidation of glucose to the oxidation of fat. After relatively short periods of fasting, the insulin level falls and the oxidation of glucose in insulin-sensitive tissues is markedly reduced. Glycogenolysis serves to maintain the blood glucose concentration for several hours. During the early part of a fast, the brain continues to obtain its energy requirements from the oxidation of glucose. As the fast continues, the brain oxidizes ketones, which may eventually supply 50% of the brain's energy needs.[19] The brain's ability to oxidize ketones appears to be directly related to the level of circulating ketones and does not involve an adaptation or a hormonally regulated change. The formed elements of the blood and peripheral neural tissues also oxidize glucose, but these tissues mainly oxidize glucose anaerobically to lactate, which is recycled to glucose in the liver using energy derived from fat.[25]

The maintenance of a normal blood glucose during fasting is dependent on both the ability to produce adequate glucose (glycolysis and gluconeogenesis) and the ability to utilize alternative sources of energy via fatty acid oxidation.

APPROACH TO THE DIFFERENTIAL DIAGNOSIS OF HYPOGLYCEMIA

Table 10–1 is an extensive list of the causes of hypoglycemia in infants and children. It is often convenient to divide the differential diagnosis into three age categories: (1) transient neonatal hypoglycemia (usually confined to the first 1 or 2 weeks of life); (2) persistent neonatal and infantile hypoglycemia; and (3) hypoglycemia in older children (generally after 2 years of age).

Transient neonatal hypoglycemia is common in premature and small-for-gestational-age infants, as well as in infants who are stressed.[40,79] Infants of diabetic mothers and infants with erythroblastosis also have transient hyperinsulinemia. Usually, these neonates are treated to avoid hypoglycemia without the need to engage in a diagnostic evaluation. However, if the hypoglycemia is persistent (beyond 7–10 days of life), or if the infant requires large amounts of intravenous (IV) glucose (greater than 5–6 mg/kg/min), and is not known to be the child of a diabetic mother, a diagnostic evaluation is indicated.

It is helpful to distinguish between persistent hypoglycemia in infants under 2 years of age vs. older children because the relative frequency of the underlying causes is different in the two age groups. A high percentage of infants with hypoglycemia have hyperinsulinemia or an enzyme or hormonal deficiency. Children who first develop hypoglycemia when older are less likely to have a specific cause for their hypoglycemia and are more likely to have ketotic hypoglycemia (which has no clearly defined defect). Even though up to 95% of children who first have hypoglycemia after the age of 2 years have ketotic hypoglycemia, it is possible for almost any of the disorders that cause hypoglycemia to present after this age.

Another clinically useful distinction is made between hypoglycemia due to increased glucose utilization and hypoglycemia due to decreased glucose production. Infants with increased glucose utilization often require IV glucose at a rate greater than 5 to 6 mg/kg/min to maintain normoglycemia. Infants who require a large glucose intake to maintain a normal blood glucose are likely to have hyperinsulinemia.

Although the list of disorders that can cause hypoglycemia in childhood is extensive, most will fall into one of five broad categories: (1) ketotic hypoglycemia; (2) hyperinsulinemia; (3) counterregulatory hormone deficiency; (4) a defect in glycolysis-gluconeogenesis; and (5) a defect in fatty acid oxidation. The first diagnostic step is to determine which of these categories is most likely. Patients with a disorder in one of these five categories often present with hypoglycemia as a primary problem. Most causes of hypoglycemia not in the five categories are either readily apparent (e.g., hypoglycemia in a child with diabetes on insulin therapy, hypoglycemia in severe liver disease, hypoglycemia in a child receiving bolus nasogastric feedings) or are part of a complex clinical picture (e.g., Reye's syndrome, galactosemia, methylmalonic acidemia, and maple syrup urine disease). Occasionally one of these disorders will present with hypoglycemia as a primary, relatively isolated finding.

Initial diagnostic testing should determine which of the five major categories is most likely in a child with hypoglycemia.[85] This distinction is usually possible from measurements of the plasma glucose, serum insulin, cortisol, growth hormone, lactate, and β-hydroxybutyrate (see flow chart, Fig 10–1). The plasma glucose is measured to confirm hypoglycemia and to have a simultaneous glucose level to aid in interpreting the other tests. In the presence of hypoglycemia, the insulin level should be unmeasurable (or nearly so). If the insulin is high (above 6 units/mL), hyperinsulinemia is likely. If the growth hormone is not above 8 ng/mL or the cortisol is not above 20 μg/mL in the presence of hypoglycemia, a hormonal deficiency is suggested. If the lactate is elevated, a defect in gluconeogenesis is indicated. Normally, β-hydoxybutyrate will rise when a child is fasted and becomes hypoglycemic.[101,119] A relatively low level is found in hyperinsulinemia because insulin inhibits fatty acid mobilization and patients with hyperinsulinemia usually become hypoglycemic rapidly before ketosis develops. Hypoketonemia is also expected in patients with defects in fatty acid

TABLE 10–1.

Causes of Hypoglycemia in Infants and Children*

Age	Major Categories	Primary Diagnosis
Neonatal (transient), 0–7 days	Exact cause unknown	More common in small-for-date, fetal distress, and sick newborns
	Hyperinsulinism	Infant of diabetic mother
		Erythroblastosis
		Discontinuation of IV glucose
Neonatal (persistent), infancy, and early childhood, 0–2 yr	Hyperinsulinism	Islet cell hyperplasia
		Nesidioblastosis
		Islet cell adenoma
		Leucine sensitivity
		Beckwith's syndrome
	Glycogen storage disease	Glycogen synthetase deficiency
		Debrancher deficiency
		Phosphorylase deficiency
		Phosphorylase kinase deficiency
		Glucose-6-phosphatase deficiency
	Defect in gluconeogenesis	Fructose-1, 6-diphosphatase deficiency
		Pyruvate carboxylase deficiency
		Phosphoenolpyruvate carboxykinase deficiency
	Hormone deficiency	Growth hormone deficiency
		Cortisol deficiency
		ACTH deficiency
		Congenital adrenal hyperplasia
		Glucagon deficiency
		Thyroid hormone deficiency
	Defect in fatty acid oxidation	Primary carnitine deficiency
		Ethyl malonic adipic aciduria
		Glutamic aciduria
		β-Hydroxy-β-methylglutaryl-CoA dehydrogenase deficiency
		Medium-chain acyl-CoA dehydrogenase deficiency
		Long-chain acyl-CoA dehydrogenase deficiency
		Long-chain acyl-CoA carnitine transferase deficiency
		Long-chain 3-OH-acyl-CoA dehydrogenase deficiency
		Short-chain 3-OH-acyl-CoA dehydrogenase deficiency
	Miscellaneous	Galactosemia
		Fructose intolerance
		Maple syrup urine disease
		Propionic acidemia
		Methylmalonic acidemia
		Acetoacetyl-CoA thiolase deficiency
		Other organic acidemias
		Salicylate intoxication
		Alcohol intoxication
		Reye's syndrome
		Jamaican vomiting sickness
		Hepatitis
		Massive nonpancreatic tumors
		Malnutrition
Older children, 1–18 yr	Hyperinsulinism	Secondary to therapy of diabetes
		Islet cell adenoma
		Malicious insulin or oral hypoglycemic administration
	Ketotic	Due to insufficient substrate (alanine)
		Due to epinephrine deficiency
	Miscellaneous	See above
	Nonfasting hypoglycemia	Misplaced IV line
		Postgastrectomy
		Pyloroplasty, etc.
		Functional reactive (?)

*→ = appropriate level; ↑ = increased level; ↓ = decreased level; → ↑ = appropriate or increased.
†Hypoglycemia in these patients is usually only part of a complex disorder.

Hepatomegaly	Insulin	Hormones	Lactate	β-Hydroxybutyrate	Pathophysiology
No	→	→	→	→	↓ Production ↑ Utilization
No	↑	→	→	↓	↑ Utilization
No (usually)	↑	→	→	↓	↑ Utilization
Yes (marked)	→	→	→ ↑ Depends on disorder	→	↓ Production
Yes (marked)	→	→	↑	↓	↓ Production
No	→	Affected hormone ↓	→	→	Uncertain
Yes (mild–moderate)	→	→	↑ →	↓	↓ Production ↑ Utilization
		Variable†			
No	↑ May include nonhuman insulin	→	→	↓	↑ Utilization
No	→	→	→	→	↓ Production
No	→	↓ Epinephrine	→	→	↓ Production
No	↑	→	→	↓	↑ Utilization

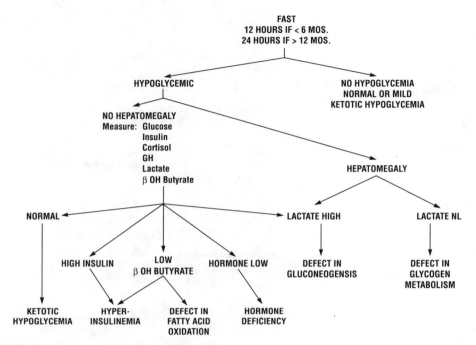

FIG 10–1.
Flow chart for differential diagnosis of hypoglycemia.

oxidation. If the child has hypoglycemia with appropriate hormone, lactate, and β-hydroxybutyrate levels, then ketotic hypoglycemia is the likely diagnosis.

Traditionally, every hypoglycemic child (except neonates) has received a diagnostic evaluation including a fast. However, patients with defects in fatty acid oxidation may suffer a cardiac arrest during a fasting stress. Therefore, although fasting is a useful diagnostic procedure, it must be done with care. Older children (greater than 2 years) with a single episode of hypoglycemia after a fasting stress may not need to have a diagnostic fast. An alternative approach is to first exclude a defect in fatty acid oxidation (by measuring serum carnitine, urine acylcarnitines after a carnitine load, and urine acylglycines) and then instruct the family on ways of avoiding future fasting stress. The key hormones and substrates (insulin, growth hormone, cortisol lactate, and β-hydroxybutyrate) can be measured when and if the hypoglycemia recurs.

Several other screening tests (Table 10–2) may be useful in some patients. These tests are not needed in every patient. They may be indicated if the clinical findings suggest a diagnosis for which the test is helpful. Finally, a number of specific tests, such as the glucagon response test, fructose tolerance test, growth hormone stimulation, adrenocorticotropic hormone (ACTH) assay, ACTH response test, enzyme assay, serum amino acids, and urine carnitine clearance, should be reserved for patients in whom a specific diagnosis is likely. Historically, a glucose tolerance test was often performed on children suspected of having hypoglycemia; however, this test is rarely helpful.

GLYCOGEN AND GLYCOLYSIS

Glycogen is a polymer of approximately 20,000 to 30,000 glucose units. It is stored in the liver, where it serves as a reservoir of glucose which can then be released to maintain the blood glucose. Glycogen is also stored in muscle, where it serves as a reservoir of glucose for muscle cell use. A single glycogen molecule, called a *b* particle, has a treelike structure with glucose units in a straight 1, 6 linkage and branch points with a 1, 4 linkage.[99] Multiple *b* particles aggregate to form *a* particles.

The pathways for glycogen synthesis and degradation are shown in Figure 10–2. Glycogen synthesis and degradation in the liver are highly regulated and seem to be sensitive to the level of blood glucose as well as the concentration of several hormones, particularly glucagon and insulin.[47,49] Most of the regulation of glycogen synthesis results from changes in the activity of glycogen synthase, which exists in an active *a* form (dephosphorylated) and an inactive *b* form (phosphorylated). Similarly, glycogen breakdown is regulated by the activity of phosphorylase, which exists in an active *a* form (phosphorylated) and an inactive *b* form (dephosphorylated). A cyclic adenosine monophosphate (cAMP)–dependent protein kinase phosphorylates and inactivates glycogen synthase. It also phosphorylates and activates phosphorylase kinase which, in turn, phosphorylates and activates phosphorylase. The net result is that increases in the level of cAMP (increased by glucagon and epinephrine, decreased by insulin) inhibit glycogen synthesis and stimulate glycogen degradation. High glucose levels increase the inactivation of phosphorylase. Phosphorylase *a*, the active form of phosphorylase, inhibits the enzyme that activates glycogen synthetase. High glucose levels release this inhibition, and thereby increase the activation of glycogen synthetase. The phosphorylase enzyme in muscle is genetically distinct from the liver enzyme. In addition, the control of glycogen synthesis and degradation in muscle is less dependent than in the liver on the circulating glucose and hormones and thus less dependent on the fed or fasted state and more dependent on muscle activity.

TABLE 10–2.

Supplementary Tests in Hypoglycemia

Glucagon	Low in glucagon deficiency
Plasma or urine epinephrine, norepinephrine	Low in adrenal medullary insufficiency
Urine organic acids	Increased in organic acidemias
Urine acylcarnitines after carnitine load	Abnormal in organic acidemias and defects in fatty acid oxidation
Serum carnitine	Low in organic acidemias and defects in fatty acid oxidation
Serum uric acid	High in defects in gluconeogenesis and fatty acid oxidation
Serum cholesterol, triglycerides	High in defects in gluconeogenesis and fatty acid oxidation
Plasma free fatty acids	In hypoketonemic patients should be low in hyperinsulinemia, high in defects in fatty acid oxidation
Urine suberylglycine, hexanoylglycine, and phenylproponylglycine	High in medium-chain acyl-CoA dehydrogenase deficiency

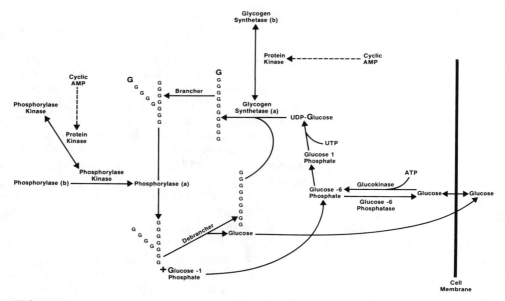

FIG 10–2.
Pathways for glycogen synthesis and degradation. *Cyclic AMP* = cyclic adenosine monophosphate, *UDP* = uridine diphosphate, *UTP* = uridine triphosphate; *ATP* = adenosine triphosphate.

GLUCONEOGENESIS

The substrates for gluconeogenesis are lactate, glycerol, and amino acids. The major source of lactate is anaerobic glycolysis. Glucose is oxidized to lactate in peripheral tissues, and the lactate is reconverted to glucose in the liver with the consumption of noncarbohydrate energy sources. In this overall process, the tissues that can oxidize only glucose are supported by noncarbohydrate energy sources, and there is no net consumption of glucose.

Glycerol is released from triglycerides and may account for as much as one third of glucose production. The major substrates for gluconeogenesis are amino acids that are released primarily from muscle. Many amino acids in muscle are partially metabolized before they are released. Alanine is the predominant amino acid released from muscle during fasting. Gluconeogenesis is frequently limited by the amount of available substrate. The major enzymatic control point for gluconeogenesis and glycolysis occurs at the interconversion of fructose-6-phosphate and fructose-1,6-diphosphate. During glucose oxidation, phosphofructokinase catalyzes the conversion of fructose-6-phosphate to fructose-1,6-diphosphate. Fructose-1,6-diphosphatase catalyzes the reverse reaction in the gluconeogenic direction. The activity of these two enzymes, and therefore the balance between glycolysis and gluconeogenesis, is controlled by the intracellular level of fructose-2,6-diphosphate.[31] Fructose-2,6-diphosphate is produced from or converted to fructose-6-phosphate by fructose-2,6-diphosphatase. The direction in which this bifunctional enzyme is active depends on its own phosphorylation. High insulin levels cause dephosphorylation of this enzyme, increasing fructose-2,6-diphosphate levels, activating phosphofructokinase, and producing glycolysis. High glucagon levels increase cAMP. cAMP activates cAMP-dependent kinase, which phosphorylates the enzyme, thereby decreasing fructose-2,6-diphosphate levels and, in turn, activating fructose-1,6-diphosphatase.

Two other steps in glycolysis are physiologically irreversible. The glycolytic step for conversion of phosphoenolpyruvate to pyruvate is reversed in the gluconeogenic direction by two enzymes, pyruvate carboxylase and phosphoenolpyruvate carboxykinase. Pyruvate kinase, the glycolytic enzyme, is phosphorylated and inactivated by a cAMP-dependent kinase. It is also activated by fructose-1,6-diphosphate, which accumulates when glycolysis predominates. The synthesis of phosphoenolpyruvate carboxykinase is increased by a cAMP-dependent mechanism. Glucose-6-phosphatase catalyzes the conversion of glucose-6-phosphate to glucose. This step is common to both glycogenolysis and gluconeogenesis.

FATTY ACID OXIDATION

Fatty acid oxidation contributes to the maintenance of normal blood glucose by providing an alternative source of energy in tissues that can oxidize fatty acids and by providing the necessary energy for gluconeogenesis in the liver. The fatty acid oxidation pathway is shown in Figure 10–3. Fatty acids are first converted to fatty acid acyl-coenzyme A (CoA).[70] Medium- and short-chain CoA derivatives can cross the mitochondrial membrane directly. Long-chain fatty acyl-CoA is converted to the carnitine derivative by the enzyme carnitine palmitoyl transferase (CPT).[12] The fatty acylcarnitine is then transported into the mitochondria by carnitine translocase. The fatty acylcarnitine is reconverted to fatty acyl-CoA by mitochondrial CPT. CPT is a highly regulated enzyme. Malonyl CoA is a potent inhibitor of CPT activity.[73] Insulin inhibits, and glucagon and epinephrine stimulate this process by changing malonyl CoA levels.[72] Control of the activity of CPT determines whether fatty acids will be oxidized or converted to triglycerides for storage. Further oxidation of fatty acyl-CoA procedes via a repeating four-step cycle that releases two carbon acetyl-CoA units.[12] The four steps in this process are catalyzed by acyl-CoA dehydrogenase, enol-CoA hydratase, 3-hydroxyacyl-CoA dehydrogenase, and 3-ketoacyl-CoA thiolase. At least two of these activities are catalyzed by different enzymes, depending on the chain length. There are three acy-CoA dehydrogenases: long (chain length greater than 12), medium (chain length 6–12), and short (chain length 4–6).[108] Recent evidence suggests that there are two 3-hydroxyacyl-CoA dehydrogenases (a long and a short) with overlapping chain length activities.[42] The first oxidation in this cycle, the acyl-CoA dehydrogenase step, results in the reduction of electron transport factor protein (ETF). ETF is reoxidized when electrons are transported to the respiratory chain in a reaction catalyzed by ETF ubiquinone oxidoreductase. In muscle and adipose tissue, the acetyl-CoA generated in fatty acid oxidation is further oxidized to carbon dioxide in the citric acid cycle. Most of the acetyl-CoA in the liver is converted to ketones. Acetoacetate and β-hydroxybutyrate are exported to other tissues, including the brain, for oxidation. Production of ketones involves several steps, including one catalyzed

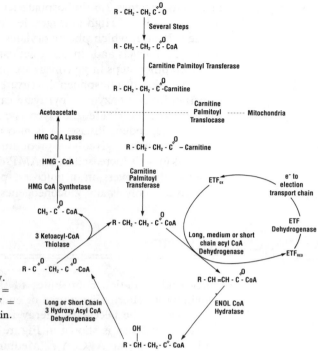

FIG 10–3.
Fatty acid oxidation pathway.
CoA = coenzyme A, *HMG* =
hydroxymethylglutaryl, *ETF* =
electron transfer factor protein.

by the enzyme hydroxymethylglutaryl-CoA dehydrogenase. The subsequent oxidation of ketones requires the enzyme acetoacetyl-CoA thiolase.

The only clear function of carnitine is in the oxidation of long-chain fatty acids.[12] However, it may also be important in buffering elevations in the concentration of a number of acyl-CoA derivatives derived from amino acid and fat metabolism. Many short-chain acyl CoAs appear to inhibit metabolic processes. When acyl-CoAs accumulate, they may be converted to the carnitine derivative and then excreted.

Carnitine is produced in the liver from trimethyllysine released from methylated lysine residues in protein.[12,42,64,88] It is also widely available in the diet.[75] Carnitine is transported into tissues by an active process that maintains tissue levels 20 to 50 times higher than plasma levels.[117] Muscle, both skeletal and cardiac, and the liver are especially rich in carnitine.

GLYCOGEN STORAGE DISEASE AND DEFECTS IN GLUCONEOGENESIS

Glucose-6-phosphatase deficiency (glycogen storage disease type I, von Gierke's disease) is the prototypical hepatic glycogen storage disease associated with hypoglycemia. Affected children have short stature, cherubic doll-like features (see Fig 10–4 of patient with type III glycogen storage disease), marked hepatomegaly, enlarged kidneys, hypoglycemia, lactic acidosis, hyperlipidemia, hyperuricemia, and frequent nose bleeds (Table 10–3). In most patients, the disorder is caused by a genetic deficiency of glucose-6-phosphate. However, some patients (type Ib) have a functional deficiency of glucose-6-phosphatase because of a defect in the transport of glucose-6-phosphatase into the endoplasmic reticulum, the site of active glucose-6-phosphatase.[77,100] Patients with the type Ib variant suffer from the additional clinical problem of neutropenia and frequent pyrogenic infections.[3,61,63]

The clinical features of glucose-6-phosphatase deficiency are due to the inhibition of both glycolysis and gluconeogenesis in the liver. Hypoglycemia is a result of the direct inhibition of the usual pathways of hepatic glucose production, although patients with this disorder can produce some glucose via alternative pathways. Lactic acidosis is the result of an inability to convert lactate generated in the periphery to glucose, and an increased lactate production in the liver from glucose, galactose, and fructose. Hyperlipidemia results from increased release of free fatty acids owing to low insulin, high glucagon levels, and an inhibition of fatty acid oxidation at the level of carnitine palmitoyl transferase because of high malonyl-CoA levels. Fatty acids are therefore shunted into excess very low-density lipoprotein (VLDL) production. Hypoketonemia results from impaired fatty acid oxidation. The hyperuricemia is due to lactic acid inhibition of urate excretion and excess urate production, which is most likely a result of low hepatic inorganic phosphate.[98]

The defect in glycogenolysis and glucogenogenesis is functionally most important during fasting. Hypoglycemia exaggerates the peripheral fasting state thereby resulting

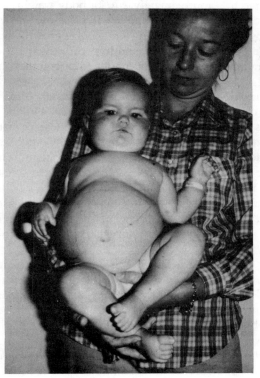

FIG 10–4.
Child with debrancher deficiency (type III GSD). Note cherubic doll-like facies, marked hepatomegaly.

TABLE 10–3.

Findings in Hepatic Glycogen Storage Diseases*

	Type I	Type III	Type VI
Short stature	Very common	Some	Few
Cherubic facies	Common	Some	Some
Hypoglycemia	Very common	Common	Few
Large liver	Very common	Very common	Very common
Large kidney	Very common	None	None
Epistaxis	Common	Few	None
Muscle weakness	None	Some	None
Lactic acidosis	Common	Few	None
Hyperlipidemia	Common	Common	Few
Hyperuricemia	Some	Few	None
Proteinuria	Some	None	None
Infections	Only type Ib	None	None

*Type I = glucose-6-phosphatase deficiency; type III = debrancher deficiency; type VI = phosphorylase, phosphorylase kinase deficiencies; Very common = almost all; common = well over 50%; some = about 50%; few = less than 50%; none = not usually seen.

in a chronic low-insulin, high-glucagon state. The aim of therapy is to achieve a chronic normoglycemic fed state. This can be achieved at night through continuous nocturnal nasogastric infusion of high-glucose formula[18,38,102] or by bedtime ingestion of uncooked cornstarch[23] (approximately 2 g/kg body weight). During the day, frequent feeding of a diet high in glucose and low in galactose and fructose will maintain a fed state. Therapy should be adjusted to maximize growth and minimize hypoglycemia, hyperlipidemia, lactice acidosis, and hyperuricemia. Patients should be monitored for liver adenomas (which may degenerate to carcinoma)[55] and progressive renal impairment.[22]

Debranching enzyme (amylo-1,6-glucosidase) *deficiency* (type III glycogen storage disease) is similar to glucose-6-phosphatase deficiency, but the features are usually less severe.[30,97] This defect does not impair gluconeogenesis so lactate can be converted to glucose, and fatty acid oxidation is not impaired. Consequently, lactic acidosis, hyperlipidemia, and hyperuricemia[74] are less of a problem. The disease, however, does affect muscle glycogen metabolism; clinical muscle weakness and pain may present a problem for some patients.[105,106]

Phosphorylase deficiences (type VI) and phosphorylase kinase deficiency[2,66] cause hepatomegaly and, occasionally, hypoglycemia, but do not cause lactic acidosis or hyperuricemia. In some kindred, phosphorylate kinase deficiency is inherited as an X-linked disorder.[66]

Treatment for debrancher deficiency is similar to the treatment for glucose-6-phosphatase deficiency, but usually requires less stringent measures. Typically, treatment is not needed for phosphorylase deficiency or phosphorylase kinase deficiency. *Branching enzyme deficiency* (type IV) is associated with progressive hepatosplenomegaly, cirrhosis, hypotonia, and, occasionally, hypoglycemia.[39] *Glycogen synthetase deficiency*[5,68,82] is a very rare cause of hypoglycemia and ketosis.

Fructose-1,6-diphosphatase deficiency[8,87], *Fructose aldolase deficiency*[78] and *galactosemia* also cause hypoglycemia, lactic acidosis, hyperlipidemia, and hyperuricemia.

In contrast to patients with glycogen storage disease, patients with these disorders appear more acutely ill. Symptoms include failure to thrive, acute liver dysfunction, and renal tubular acidosis. Treatment consists of avoiding the offending sugar, and in the case of fructose-1,6-diphosphatase deficiency, a frequent feeding diet. A few patients with hypoglycemia secondary to *deficiency of phosphoenolpyruvate carboxykinase*[53,115] or *pyruvate carboxylase* have been reported, but a clear clinical picture has not emerged.

DISORDERS OF FATTY ACID OXIDATION

Defects in fatty acid oxidation were first described relatively recently.[12] *Medium-chain acyl-CoA dehyrogenase deficiency* is the prototypical and most common defect in fatty acid oxidation.[34,89,110] Patients with this defect usually have episodic encephalopathy, which is often associated with hypoglycemia, and mild-to-moderate hepatic dysfunction (a Reye's syndrome–like presentation with elevated transaminase levels, mild hyperammonemia, and prolongation of the prothrombin time, but without hyperbilirubinemia). In some cases, the encephalopathy may cause sudden unexplained death.[28] The episodes are usually induced by fasting. The IV infusion of glucose usually results in rapid correction of the hypoglycemia and mild acidosis. During acute episodes (and inconsistently when well) patients excrete increased urinary levels of dicarboxylic acids and medium-chain acylcarnitines. Urine and serum ketone bodies are low. Increased urinary suberylglycine, hexanoylglycine, and phenylpropionylglycine are apparently found consistently and are specific to this disease.[90] Patients with this disorder also tend to have low levels of serum and tissue carnitine, probably secondary to increased urinary carnitine losses.[28] Muscle weakness may also occur. Treatment consists of avoiding fasting. A high-carbohydrate diet and carnitine replacement may also be of some benefit.

Long-chain acyl-CoA dehydrogenase deficiency causes a similar, but more severe, clinical syndrome with hypoglycemia and hepatic dysfunction at an earlier age than in medium-chain acyl-CoA dehydrogenase deficiency. Patients with this disorder also have severe muscle weakness and a cardiomyopathy.[41]

Two patients, who subsequently have been demonstrated to have *long-chain 3-hydroxyacyl-CoA dehydrogenase deficiency*, also had the triad of hypoketotic hypoglycemia with hepatic dysfunction, muscle weakness, and cardiomyopathy.[34,42] A diet high in medium-chain triglycerides resulted in marked clinical improvement. *Primary carnitine deficiency* is due to a defect in the cellular uptake and renal transport of carnitine.[113] Patients with primary carnitine deficiency have hypoketonemic hypoglycemia with hepatic dysfunction and muscle weakness.

A single patient with *carnitine palmitoyl transferase deficiency* only involving the liver presented with hypoketotic hypoglycemia and hepatic dysfunction.[15] Another apparently separate disorder of carnitine palmitoyl transferase deficiency involving muscle usually presents as rhabdomyolysis and muscle pain after prolonged exercise.[83,95]

β-Hydroxy β-methylglutaryl-CoA lyase deficiency, which impairs ketogenesis but not fatty acid oxidation, also causes hypoketotic hypoglycemia.[29,120] *Multiple acyl-CoA dehydrogenase deficiency*, which may be due to either a deficiency of ETF or ETF dehydrogenase, has a variable clinical presentation. Severe cases, also called *glutaric acidemia type II,* have profound acidosis, coma, and hypoglycemia shortly after birth.[36,86] Dysmorphic features may be present.[35] The severe form is lethal. A milder form, also called *ethylmalonic adipic aciduria*, causes psychomotor delay, hypotonia, and episodic hypoketonemic hypoglycemia that is precipitated by fasting.[45]

Short-chain acyl-CoA dehydrogenase deficiency similarly causes psychomotor retardation, episodic coma, and acidosis. However, it is usually not associated with hypoglycemia. To the extent that the mode of inheritance is understood, all of the disorders of fatty acid oxidation appear to be autosomal recessive.

The diagnosis of disorders of fatty acid oxidation is complicated by the lack of a single simple screening test. Hypoketonemia is suggestive, but a simple urine ketone test may be misleading because other accumulating organic acids may give a false-positive reaction. Patients with many of these disorders have low serum and tissue carnitine with high acylcarnitine. Some disorders lead to the excretion of abnormal urine organic acids; the dicarboxylic acids, adipic, suberic, and sebacic, are most common but least specific. Others produce a typical profile of urine acylcarnitines during the acute phase or after a carnitine load.[93] Medium-chain acyl-CoA dehydrogenase deficiency is associated with a consistent and specific increase in urine suberylglycine, hexanoylglycine, and phenylpropionyl glycine.[90]

Patients with most of these disorders improve and do not suffer from hypoglycemia if protected from fasting stress.[33] A diet high in medium-chain triglycerides may help patients with a defect limited to long-chain fatty acid oxidation. Carnitine, 100 mg/kg, is specifically indicated in primary carnitine deficiency and may help patients with other disorders as well. Therapy for multiple acyl-CoA dehydrogenase deficiency and short-chain acyl-CoA dehydrogenase deficiences is not very satisfactory.

Disorders of Ketone Oxidation

Defects in the oxidation of ketones due to β-ketothiolase deficiency[27,92] cause hyperketonemic hypoglycemia.

HYPERINSULINEMIA

Hyperinsulinemia causes the most severe form of hypoglycemia, and usually presents between birth and the first 3 months of life. In this age group, hyperinsulinemia is usually secondary to diffuse beta cell hyperplasia or nesidioblastosis,[121] but there are scattered reports of adenoma.[7,17]

Normally, the exocrine tissue of an infant is less well organized into islets than that of older children and adults; insulin, glucagon, and somatostatin-producing cells may be seen scattered singly or in small clumps among the acinar cells. Some infants with clinical hyperinsulinemia appear to have an increased mass of insulin-producing cells (i.e., nesidioblastosis). However, others cannot be clearly differentiated from normal on the basis of pathologic examination of the pancreas.

Neonates and infants with hyperinsulinemia usually have severe hypoglycemia. Many patients cannot tolerate even 1 or 2 hours of fasting; others become hypoglycemic while supported with routine IV glucose treatment. Most babies with hyperinsulinemia are large for their age.

In older children, hyperinsulinemia is almost always due to an adenoma. This disorder is rare in the pediatric age range and is relatively common in adults. In older children, the symptoms of hypoglycemia may be pedestrian, consisting of weakness and dizziness after fasting or exercise. Obesity is common.

The diagnosis of hyperinsulinemia is dependent on the demonstration of an abnormally high serum insulin concentration and coexistent hypoglycemia. In the presence of hypoglycemia, a serum insulin level of less than 6 μU/mL is expected. However, clinical findings often suggest this diagnosis. If glucose consumption is normal, an IV infusion of glucose at a rate of 5 mg/kg/hr should maintain normoglycemia. There is little but hyperinsulinemia that will cause hypoglycemia in the face of a steady glucose infusion at this rate or greater.[6]

Patients with hyperinsulinemia have unexpectedly low levels of serum β-hydroxybutyrate if they are fasted until they become hypoglycemic.[109,118] This has been attributed to the inhibition of fatty acid mobilization by the elevated insulin, but it may reflect, in part, the short fast tolerated by these patients. Patients with hyperinsulinemia are also reported to have abnormally low levels of branched-chain amino acids during hypoglycemia.[21]

The general course of hyperinsulinemia in infants is one of improvement. Some infants with significant hypoglycemia will improve markedly if they can be maintained with medical therapy.[65] Intravenous glucose and infusions of glucagon and somatostatin[109] can be used temporarily while the infant is switched to therapy that can be maintained at home. Practical long-term therapy includes frequent feedings, continuous nasogastric feedings (either 24 hours or only at night), nighttime cornstarch, daily injections of zinc glucagon[96] or a long-acting somatostatin analogue,[50,57] and diazoxide in a dose of 8 to 12 mg/kg. A low protein diet (because protein stimulates insulin secretion) may help some patients.[122] Therapy with corticosteroids is usually avoided. Recurrent hypoglycemia can cause permanent neurologic damage. In the past, the prognosis for these infants was poor.[112] Therefore, it is important to ensure that the therapy will consistently maintain normoglycemia. If normoglycemia cannot be maintained, or if the patient cannot be withdrawn from IV therapy, surgical exploration and a 70% pancreatectomy are indicated. Some authors recommend more extensive initial surgery. Following surgery, medical management with diet and diazoxide may still be needed. Many patients who are treated medically gradually improve and medical therapy can be withdrawn.[37] Others remain dependent on medical therapy with significant dietary restrictions and have side effects, such as obesity and excess hair, from diazoxide. Some of these patients have required late surgery so that medical therapy can be withdrawn.[37] Hypoglycemia caused by hyperinsulinemia may occur as part of a more extensive disorder. Beckwith's syndrome (omphalocele, macroglossia, and gigantism)[94] and cerebrohepatorenal syndrome[84] are associated with hyperinsulinemia.

Hypoglycemia may also be due to surreptitious or malicious insulin or oral hypoglycemic administration.[9] The clinical course of patients who have received exogenous insulin is characterized by severe hypoglycemia that rapidly and completely resolves once the source of insulin is removed. Insulin administration is associated with very high serum insulin levels, and low C peptide levels, and, in some cases, circulating nonhuman insulin.[10] Pentamidine, used to treat *Pneumocystis carinii* pneumonia, can cause hyperinsulinemia.[4,107] Severe hypoglycemia due to insulin receptor antibodies[111] has been reported.

KETOTIC HYPOGLYCEMIA

Ketotic hypoglycemia probably accounts for 90% of the hypoglycemia in children older than 2 years of age. Typically, hypoglycemia first occurs around 1½ to 5 years of age. After 8 or 9 years of age, hypoglycemia in children with this disorder is uncommon. Many children with ketotic hypoglycemia are small and thin for their age and many were small-for-gestational-age at birth. Attacks often include neurologic symptoms, ranging from lethargy to seizures and coma; they most commonly occur in the morning. There is usually a history suggesting decreased food intake the previous day. An early-morning seizure in any child should suggest ketotic hypoglycemia.

The cause of ketotic hypoglycemia is unclear. One theory is a deficient release of substrate from muscle for gluconeogenesis, particularly alanine.[46] Children with this disorder have low serum alanine levels. They also have an appropriate rise in serum glucose if given an infusion of alanine during hypoglycemia.[80] Another possibility is a deficient catecholamine response to hypoglycemia.[16,60] Adrenal medullary unresponsiveness to hypoglycemia, or Zetterstrom syndrome, a common diagnosis in the 1960s, was diagnosed on the basis of the failure of urinary epinephrine to increase in the 3 hours after insulin-induced hypoglycemia. The clinical features of this disorder are identical with what is now known as *ketotic hypoglycemia*. A recent study found that about 50% of the patients who would otherwise fulfill the criterian for ketotic hypoglycemia had a reduced plasma epinephrine response to hypoglycemia.[43,44]

Since almost any child will become hypoglycemic after a 24- to 36-hour fast, ketotic hypoglycemia may be simply one end of the normal spectrum rather than a distinct disorder.[26,103] Often, the distinction between ketotic hypoglycemia and normalcy remains unclear.

The diagnosis of ketotic hypoglycemia is usually based on the response to fasting. Children with ketotic hypoglycemia will typically become hypoglycemic in 12 to 24 hours and will have a "normal" hormonal and metabolic response to fasting. Normal children will become hypoglycemic in 24 to 36 hours. Children who have had clinical episodes of hypoglycemia, but who do not become hypoglycemic during a 24-hour fast, probably have a mild form of ketotic hypoglycemia.

The treatment consists of ensuring that prolonged periods of fasting do not occur. Most important is the provision of a bedtime snack every night. During intercurrent illnesses, the child should be given carbohydrate-rich liquids. Parents should be taught to test for urine ketones, so that they can tell when hypoglycemia is likely to occur. It has been suggested that this diagnostic label should be discarded.[104] However, it remains useful as a label to identify children who need to be protected from fasting.

Glucagon Deficiency

Only two well-documented cases of children with hypoglycemia secondary to glucagon deficiency have been reported.[62,114] Both patients presented with hypoglycemia in the neonatal period and both developed refractory hypoglycemia. This may be one disorder other than hyperinsulinemia that is refractory to routine IV glucose therapy. Both patients had low plasma immunoreactive glucagon and both responded well to daily injections of zinc protamine glucagon. The family history of one patient suggested a heritable disorder.

Counterregulatory Hormone Deficiency

Deficiency of growth hormone or cortisol (either primary or secondary to ACTH deficiency) is a fairly common cause of hypoglycemia.[54,56,58] Hypoglycemia due to a deficiency of one of these counterregulatory hormones usually presents in the first year of life. Many patients will not present with other symptoms (short stature, small phallus,[69] hyperpigmentation, masculinization, or adrenal crisis) suggesting a pituitary or adrenal problem. (These disorders are discussed in more detail in Chapters 3 and 6). As discussed above, some patients with ketotic hypoglycemia may have a deficient catecholamine response to hypoglycemic stress. Propranolol therapy, which inhibits the metabolic response to catecholamines, may also cause hypoglycemia.[71,116]

Reactive Hypoglycemia

Hypoglycemia may occur because of a misplaced central IV catheter that delivers large amounts of glucose to the pancreas.[76] It may also occur in children who have had pyloric surgery,[91] and in children with a nasogastric or gastrostomy tube[1] (particularly if the tip of the tube slips below the pylorus and bolus feeds are given). Much has been written about patients with "reactive" hypoglycemia after a normal meal. Many endocrinologists doubt that "reactive" hypoglycemia exists.[13,51,67] Some patients may have postprandial symptoms on the basis of something other than hypoglycemia.[20] However, many patients with this syndrome have a strong psychological component.

REFERENCES

1. Allen DB: Postprandial hypoglycemia resulting from nasogastric tube malposition. *Pediatrics* 1988; 81:582.
2. Alvarado LJF, Gasca-Centeno E, Greir RE: Hepatic phosphorylase B kinase deficiency with normal enzyme activity in leukocytes. *J Pediatr* 1988;113:865.
3. Ambruso DR, McCabe ERB, Anderson D: Infectious and bleeding complications in patients with glycogenosis Ib. *Am J Dis Child* 1985; 119:691.
4. Anderson R, Boedicker M, Ma M, et al: Adverse reactions associated with pentamidine isethionate in AIDS patients: Recommendations for monitoring therapy. *Drug Intell Clin Pharm* 1986; 20:862.

5. Ansley-Green A, Williamson DM, Gitzelmann R: Hepatic glycogen synthetase deficiency: Definition of syndrome from metabolic and enzyme studies in a 9-year-old girl. *Arch Dis Child* 1977; 52:573.

6. Antunes JD, Geffner ME, Lippie BM, et al: Childhood hypoglycemia: Differentiating hyperinsulinemic from nonhyperinsulinemic causes, *J Pediatr* 1990; 116:105.

7. Balsam MJ, Baker L, Bishop HC, et al: Beta cell adenoma in a child with hypoglycemia controlled with diazoxide. *J Pediatr* 1972; 80:788.

8. Baker L, Wingrad AI: Fasting hypoglycemia in metabolic acidosis associated with deficiency of hepatic fructose-1,6-diphosphatase activity. *Lancet* 1977; 2:13.

9. Bauman WA, Yalow RF: Child abuse, parenteral insulin administration, *J Pediatr* 1981; 99:588.

10. Bauman WA, Yalow RF: Hyperinsulinemic hypoglycemia, Differential diagnosis by determination of the species of circulating insulin. *JAMA* 1984; 252:2730.

11. Belsey R, Morrison JI, Whitlow KJ, et al: Managing bedside glucose testing in the hospital. *JAMA*. 1987; 258:1634.

12. Bieber LL: Carnitine. *Ann U Rev Biochem* 1988; 57:261.

13. Blonde L, Riddick FA: Hypoglycemia, the undisease, *South Med J* 1976; 69:1262.

14. Bougneres PF, Lamdier F, Garnier P, et al: Treatment of insulin excess by continuous subcutaneous infusion of somatostatin and glucagon in an infant. *J Pediatr* 1985; 106:792.

15. Bougrneres PF, Saudubray JM, Marsac C, et al: Fasting hypoglycemia resulting from hepatic carnitine palmitoyl transferase deficiency. *J Pediatr* 1981; 98:742.

16. Broberger O, Zetterstrom R: Hypoglycemia with an inability to increase the epinephrine secretion in insulin-induced hypoglycemia. *J Pediatr* 1961; 59:215.

17. Bruist NRM, Campbell JR, Castro A, et al: Congenital islet cell adenoma causing hypoglycemia in a newborn. *Pediatrics* 1971; 47:605.

18. Burr IM, O'Niel JA, Karzon DT, et al: Comparison of the effects of total parenteral nutrition, continuous nasogastric feeding, and portacaval shunt on a patient with type I glycogen storage disease. *J Pediatr* 1974; 85:1792.

19. Cahill GF: Starvation in man. *N Engl J Med* 1970; 282:668.

20. Chalew SA, McLaughlin JV, Mercey JH, et al: The use of plasma epinephrine response in the diagnosis of idiopathic postprandial syndrome. *JAMA* 1984; 251:612.

21. Chaussain JL, Georges P, Gendrel D, et al: Serum branch-chain amino acids in a diagnosis of hyperinsulinemia in infancy. *J Pediatr* 1980; 96:923.

22. Chen YT, Coleman RA, Scheinman JI, et al: Renal disease in type I glycogen storage disease. *N Engl J Med* 1988; 318:7.

23. Chen YT, Cornblath M, Sidbury JB: Cornstarch therapy in type I glycogen storage disease. *N Engl J Med* 1984; 310:171.

24. Coates PM, Hale DE, Stanley CA, et al: Genetic deficiency of medium chain acyl-coenzyme-A dehydrogenase: Studies in cultured skin fibroblasts and peripheral mononuclear leukocytes. *Pediatr Res* 1985; 19:672.

25. Coy CF: Mammalian carbohydrate metabolism. *Physiol Rev* 1931; 11:143.

26. Dahlquist G, Gentz J, Hagenfeldt L, et al: Ketotic hypoglycemia of childhood—a clinical trial of several unifying etiological hypotheses. *Acta Paediatr Scand* 1979; 68:649.

27. DeGroot CJ, Luit-De Haan G, Hulstaert CE, et al: A patient with severe neurologic symptoms and acetyl-CoA thiolase deficiency. *Pediatr Res* 1977; 11:1112.

28. Duran M, Hofkamp M, Rhead WJ, et al: Sudden child death in healthy affected family members with medium chain acyl-CoA dehydrogenase deficiency. *Pediatrics* 1986; 78:1052.

29. Faull K, Bouton P, Halpren B, et al: Patient with a defect in leucine metabolism. *N Engl J Med* 1976; 294:1013.
30. Forbes GB: Glycogen storage disease. Report of a case with abnormal glycogen structure in liver and skeletal muscle. *J Pediatr* 1953; 42:645.
31. Foster DW: From glycogen to ketones and back. *Diabetes* 1984; 33:1188.
32. Gjedde A, Crone C: Blood-brain glucose transfer: Repression in chronic hyperglycemia. *Science* 1981; 214:456.
33. Glasgow AM, Eng G, Engel AG: Systemic carnitine deficiency simulating recurrent Reye syndrome. *J Pediatr* 1980; 96:889.
34. Glasgow AM, Engel AG, Bier DM, et al: Hypoglycemia, hepatic dysfunction, muscle weakness, cardiomyopathy, free carnitine deficiency and long chain acyl carnitine excess responsive to medium chain triglyceride diet. *Pediatr Res* 1983; 17:319.
35. Goodman SI, Reale M, Berlow F: Glutaric acidemia type II: A form with deleterious intrauterine effects. *J Pediatr* 1983; 102:411.
36. Goodman SI, Stene DO, McCabe ERB, et al: Glutaric acidemia type II: Clinical, biochemical, and morphologic considerations. *J Pediatr* 1982; 100:946.
37. Grant DB, Dunger DB, Burns EC: Long-term treatment with diazoxide in childhood hyperinsulinemia. *Acta Endocrinol [(suppl)] (Copenh)* 1986; 279:340.
38. Greene HL: Glycogen storage disease. *Semin Liver Dis* 1982; 2:291.
39. Greene HL, Ghishan FK, Brown B, et al: Hypoglycemia in type IV glycogenosis: Hepatic improvement in two patients with nutritional management. *J Pediatr* 1988; 112:55.
40 Gutverlet RL, Cornblath M: Neonatal hypoglycemia revisited, 1975. *J Pediatr* 1976; 58:10.
41. Hale DE, Batchel ML, Coates PM, et al: Long chain acyl-CoA dehydrogenase deficiency: An inherited cause of nonketotic hypoglycemia. *Pediatr Res* 1985; 19:666.
42. Hale DE, Thorp C, Brast K, et al: The L-3-hydroxyacyl-CoA dehydrogenase deficiency, in Tanaka K, Coates PM (eds): *Fatty acid oxidation: Clinical, Biochemical, and Molecular Aspects*. New York, Alan R Liss, 1990.
43. Hansen RL, Levy MN, Kerr DS: Differential diagnosis of hypoglycemia in children by responses to fasting and to deoxyglucose. *Metabolism* 1983; 32:960.
44. Hansen RL, Levy MN, Kerr DS: The 2-deoxyglucose test as a supplement to fasting for detection of childhood hypoglycemia. *Pediatr Res* 1984; 18:490.
45. Harpey JP, Charpentier C, Coude M, et al: Sudden infant death syndrome and multiple acyl-coenzyme A dehydrogenase deficiency, ethylmalonic-adipic or systemic carnitine deficiency. *J Pediatr* 1987; 110:881.
46. Haymond MW, Pagliara AS: Ketotic hypoglycemia. *Clin Endocrinol Metab* 1983; 12:447.
47. Hems DA, Whitton PD: Control of hepatic glycogenolysis, *Physiol Rev* 1980; 60:1.
48. Henderson LM, Nelson PG, Henderson L: Mammalian enzymes of trimethyl-lysine conversion to trimethylaminobutyrate. *Fed Proc* 1982; 41:2843.
49. Hers H, Vanhoff F, deBarsy T: Glycogen storage diseases, Scriver CR, Beaudet AL, Sly WS, et al (eds): in *Metabolic Basis of Inherited Diseases*. New York, McGraw-Hill Book Co, 1989.
50 Hirsch HJ, Loo F, Evans N, et al: Hypoglycemia of infancy and nesidioblastosis. Studies with somatostatin. *S Engl J Med* 1977; 296:1323.
51. Hogan MJ, Service FJ, Charbrough SW, et al: Oral glucose tolerance test compared with a mixed meal in the diagnosis of reactive hypoglycemia. A caveat on stimulation. *Mayo Clin Proc* 1983; 58:491.
52. Holtrop PC, Madison KA, Kiechle Fl, et al: A comparison of chromogen test strip

(chemstrip bG) and serum glucose values in newborns. *Am J Dis Child* 1990; 144:183.

53. Hommes FA, Bendien K, Elema JD, et al: Two cases of phosphoenolpyruvate car-boxykinase deficiency. *Acta Paediatr Scand* 1976; 65:233.

54. Hopwood NG, Forsman PJ, Kenney FM, et al: Hypoglycemia in hypopituitary children. *Am J Dis Child* 1975; 129:918.

55. Howell RR, Stevenson RE, Ben-Menachem Y, et al: Hepatic adenomata with type I glycogen storage disease. *JAMA* 1976; 236:1481.

56. Hung W, Migeon CJ: Hypoglycemia in a 2-year-old boy with adrenocorticotropic hormone (ACTH) deficiency (probably isolated) and adrenal medullary unresponsiveness to insulin induced hypoglycemia. *J Clin Endocrinol Metab* 1968; 28:146.

57. Jackson JA, Hahn HB, Oltorf CE, et al: Long-term treatment of refractory neonatal hypoglycemia with long-acting somatostatin analog. *J Pediatr* 1987; 111:548.

58. Johnson JD, Hansen RC, Albritton WL, et al: Hypoplasia of the anterior pituitary in neonatal hypoglycemia. *J Pediatr* 1973; 82:634.

59. Knight J, Garvin PJ, Danis RK, et al: Nesidioblastosis in children. *JAMA* 1980; 115:880.

60. Koffler H, Schubert WK, Hug G: Sporadic hypoglycemia: Abnormal epinephrine response to the ketogenic diet or to insulin. *J Pediatr* 1971; 78:448.

61. Koletzko B, Wendel U, Bremer HJ: Lithium for treatment of neutropenia in glycogen storage disease type Ib. *J Pediatr* 1986; 110:902.

62. Kollee LA, Monnens LA, Cejka V, et al: Persistent neonatal hypoglycemia due to glucagon deficiency. *Arch Dis Child* 1978; 53:422.

63. Koven NL, Clark MN, Cote CS, et al: Impaired chemotaxis and neutrophil (polymor-phonuclear leukocyte) function in glycogenosis type Ib. *Pediatr Res* 1986; 20:438.

64. LaBadie J, Dunn WA, Aronson NN: Hepatic synthesis of carnitine from protein bound trimethyl-lysine. *Biochem J* 1976; 160:85.

65. Landau H, Perlman N, Meyer S, et al: Persistent neonatal hypoglycemia due to hyperinsulinemia: Medial aspects. *Pediatrics* 1982; 70:440.

66. Lederer B, VanHoos F, Van Dew BG: Glycogen phosphorylase and its converter enzymes in hemolysates of normal human subjects and of patients with type VI glycogen-storage disease. *Biol Chem J* 1975; 147:23.

67. Levine R: Hypoglycemia. *JAMA* 1974; 230:462.

68. Louis GH, Spencer-Peet J, Stuart KM: Infantile hypoglycemia due to inherited deficiency of glycogen synthetase in liver. *Arch Dis Child* 1963; 38:40.

69. Lovinger DL, Kaplan SL, Grumbach MM: Congenital hypopituitarism associated with neonatal hypoglycemia and microphallus: Four cases secondary to hypothalamic hormone deficiency. *J Pediatr* 1975; 87:1171.

70. Mahler HR, Wakil FJ, Bock RM: Studies on fatty acid oxidation I. Enzymatic activation of fatty acids. *J Biol Chem* 1953; 204:453.

71. McBride JT, McBride MC, Viles PH: Hypoglycemia associated with propranolol. *Pediatrics* 1973; 51:1085.

72. McGarry JD, Foster DW: Hormonal control of ketogenesis. *Arch Intern Med* 1977; 137:495.

73. McGarry JD, Leatherman GF, Foster DW: Carnitine palmitoyltransferase I. The site of inhibition of fatty acid oxidation by malonyl-CoA. *J Biol Chem* 1978; 253:4128.

74. Mineo I, Kono N, Hara N, et al: Myogenic hyperuricemia, a common pathophysio-logic feature of glycogenosis type III, V, and VII. *N Engl J Med* 1987; 317:75.

75. Mitchel ME. Carnitine metabolism in human subjects I. Normal metabolism. *Am J Clin Nutr* 1978; 31:293.

76. Nagel JW, Sims JF, Aplin CE, et al: Refractory hypoglycemia associated with a malpositioned umbilical artery catheter. *J Pediatr* 1979; 64:315.
77. Narisawa K, Otomo H, Igarashi Y, et al: Glycogen storage disease type Ib: Microsomal glucose-6-phosphatase system in two patients with different clinical findings. *Pediatr Res* 1983; 17:545.
78. Odievre M, Gentil C, Gautier M, et al: Hereditary fructose intolerance in childhood. *Am J Dis Child* 1978; 132:605.
79. Ogata ES: Carbohydrate metabolism in the fetus and neonate and altered neonatal glucose regulation. *Pediatr Clin North Am* 1986; 33:25.
80. Pagliara AS, Caul IE, Devivo DC, et al: Hypoalanemia, a concomitant of ketotic hypoglycemia. *J Clin Invest* 1972; 51:1440.
81. Pagliara AS, Karl IE, Haymond M, et al: Hypoglycemia in infancy and childhood part I. *J Pediatr* 1973; 82:365.
82. Parr J, Teree TM, Larner J: Symptomatic hypoglycemia, visceral fatty metamorphosis, and aglycogenosis in an infant lacking glycogen synthetase and phosphorylase. *J Pediatr* 1965; 35:770.
83. Patten DM, Wood JM, Harati Y, et al: Familial recurrent rhabdomyolysis due to carnitine palmitoyl transferase deficiency. *Am J Med* 1979; 67:167.
84. Patton RG, Cristie DL, Smith DW, et al: Cerebro-hepato-renal syndrome of Zellweger: Two patients with islet cell hyperplasia, hypoglycemia, and thymic abnormalities and comments on iron metabolism. *Am J Dis Child* 1972; 124:840.
85. Philip M, Bashan N, Smith CPA: An algorithmic approach to diagnosis of hypoglycemia. *J Pediatr* 1987; 110:387.
86. Przyrembl H, Wandel U, Becker K, et al: Glutaric aciduria type II: Report on a previously undescribed metabolic disorder. *Clin Chim Acta* 1976; 66:227.
87. Rallison ML, Meikle AW, Zigrang WD: Hypoglycemia in lactic acidosis associated with fructose-1,6-diphosphatase deficiency. *J Pediatr* 1979; 94:933.
88. Rebouche CJ: Sites and regulation of carnitine biosynthesis in mammals. *Fed Proc* 1982; 41:2848.
89. Rhead WJ, Amendt BA, Fritchman KS, et al: Dicarboxylic aciduria: Deficient (1-14C) octanoate oxidation and medium chain acyl-CoA dehydrogenase in fibroblasts. *Science* 1983; 221:73.
90. Rinaldo P, O'Shea JJ, Coates PM, et al: Medium-chain acyl-CoA dehydrogenase deficiency: Diagnosis by stable-isotope dilution measurement of urinary n-hexanoylglycine and 3-phenylpropionylglycine. *N Engl J Med* 1988; 319:1308.
91. Rivkees SA, Crawford JD: Hypoglycemia pathogenesis in children with dumping syndrome. *Pediatrics* 1987; 80:937.
92. Robinson BH, Sherwood WG, Taylor J, et al: Acetyl-CoA thiolase deficiency: A cause of severe ketoacidosis in infancy simulating salicylism. *J Pediatr* 1979; 95:228.
93. Roe CR, Millington DAM, Boham TP, et al: Diagnostic and therapeutic implications of medium chain acetyl carnitine in medium chain acetyl-CoA dehydrogenase deficiency. *Pediatr Res* 1985; 19:666.
94. Roe TF, Kershnar AK, Weitzman JJ, et al: Beckwith's syndrome with extreme organ hyperplasia. *Pediatrics* 1973; 52:372.
95. Roff NS, Hoppel CL: Partial muscle carnitine palmitoyl transferase-A deficiency. Rhabdomyolysis associated with transiently decreased muscle carnitine content after ibuprofen therapy. *JAMA* 1987; 257:62.
96. Rose FR, Chrousos G, Cornblath M, et al: Management of postoperative nesidioblastosis with zinc protamine glucagon and oral starch. *J Pediatr* 1986; 108:97.

97. Rosenfeld EL, Popoza IA, Chibisov IV: Some cases of type III glycogen storage disease, *Clin Chim Acta* 1976; 67:123.
98. Rowe TF, Kogut MD: The pathogenesis of hyperuricemia in glycogen storage disease, type I. *Pediatr Res* 1977; 11:664.
99. Ryman BE: The glycogen storage diseases. *J Clin Pathol* 1974; 8:106.
100. Sann L, Mathieu M, Borgeois J, et al: In vitro evidence for defective activity of glucose-6-phosphatase in type Ib glycogenosis. *J Pediatr* 1980; 96:691.
101. Saudubray JM, Marsac C, Limal JM, et al: Variation in plasma ketone bodies during a 24-hour fast in normal and in hypoglycemic children: Relationship to age. *J Pediatr* 1981; 98:904.
102. Schwenk WF, Haymond MW: Optimal rate of enteral glucose administration in children with glycogen storage disease type I. *N Engl J Med* 1986; 314:682.
103. Senior B: Ketotic hypoglycemia: A tale (tail) of Gauss. *J Pediatr* 1973; 82:555.
104. Senior B, Sideghi-Nejad A: Hypoglycemia: A pathophysiologic approach. *Acta Paediatr Scand [suppl]* 1989; 352:1.
105. Slomim AE, Coleman RA, Moses WS: Myopathy and growth failure in the debrancher enzyme deficiency: Improvement with high-protein nocturnal enteral therapy. *J Pediatr* 1984; 105:906.
106. Slomim AE, Weisberg C, Benke P, et al: Reversal of debrancher deficiency myopathy by the use of a high-protein nutrition. *Ann Neurol* 1982; 11:420.
107. Stahl-Bayliff CM, Kalman CM, Laskin LL: Pentamidine-induced hypoglycemia in patients with the acquired immune deficiency syndrome. *Clin Pharmacol Ther* 1986; 39:271.
108. Stanley CA: New genetic defects in mitochondrial fatty acid oxidation and carnitine deficiency. *Adv Pediatr* 1987; 34:59.
109. Stanley CA, Baker L: Hyperinsulinemia in infancy: Diagnosis by demonstration of abnormal response to fasting hypoglycemia. *Pediatrics* 1976; 57:702.
110. Stanley CA, Hale DE, Coates PM, et al: Medium-chain acyl-CoA dehydrogenase deficiency in children with nonketotic hypoglycemia and low carnitine levels. *Pediatr Res* 1983; 17:877.
111. Taylor SI, Grunberger G, Marcus-Samules B, et al: Hypoglycemia associated with antibodies to the insulin receptor. *N Engl J Med* 1982; 307:1422.
112. Thomas CG, Underwood LE, Carney CN, et al: Neonatal and infantile hypoglycemia due to insulin excess: New aspects of diagnosis and surgical management. *Ann Surg* 1977; 185:505.
113. Treem RW, Stanley CA, Finegold DN, et al: Primary carnitine deficiency due to a failure of carnitine transport in kidney, muscle, and fibroblasts. *N Engl J Med* 1988; 319:1331.
114. Vidnes J, Oyasaeter S: Glucagon deficiency causing severe neonatal hyperglycemia in a patient with normal insulin secretion. *Pediatr Res* 1977; 11:943.
115. Vidnes J, Slovik O: Gluconeogenesis in infancy and childhood. III: Deficiency of the extramitochondrial form of hepatic phosphoenolpyruvate carboxykinase in a case of persistent neonatal hypoglycemia. *Acta Paediatr Scand* 1976; 65:307.
116. Wells TG, Ulftrom RA, Nevins TE: Hypoglycemia in pediatric renal allograft recipient. *J Pediatr* 1988; 113:1002.
117. Willner JH, Ginsburg F, Dimauro S: Active transport of carnitine in the skeletal muscle. *Neurology* 1978; 28:721.
118. Wolffdorf JI, Fadeghi-Nejad A, Senior B: Ketonuria does not exclude hyperinsulinemia or hypoglycemia. *Am J Dis Child* 1984; 138:168.

119. Wolfsborf JI, Sadeghi-Nejad A, Senior B: Fat-derived fuels during a 24 hour fast in children. *Eur J Pediatr* 138; 141, 1982.
120. Wysocki SJ, Hannel R: 3-Hydroxy-3-methylglutaryl-coenzyme A lysase deficiency: A review. *J Inherit Metab Dis* 1986; 9:225.
121. Yakovac WC, Baker L, Hummeler K: Beta cell nesidioblastosis in idiopathic hypoglycemia of infancy. *J Pediatr* 1971; 79:226.
122. Zuniga O, Golden MP, Sargeant DT, et al: Persistent leucine sensitivity following partial pancreatectomy and diazoxide treatment. *Am J Dis Child* 1983; 137:393.

Chapter 11

Childhood Obesity

Val Abbassi

Obesity is one of the most common nutritional disorders of childhood. Despite the accumulation of a vast body of knowledge regarding the etiology, metabolic derangements, and long-term consequences, the pathophysiology eludes understanding and treatment for the most part remains ineffective. Experimental and clinical studies have implicated a multifactorial basis for human obesity with contributions from genetic, environmental, psychosocial, metabolic, and hormonal factors. As a result of these complex etiologic factors, simple approaches to therapy have uniformly met with failure, and short-term gains have been difficult to maintain over long periods of time. An evident characteristic of human obesity is its prevalence as the most common nutritional disorder in developed countries and its relative lack of existence in underdeveloped countries. Based on the diagnostic criteria employed, as many as 25% of children in the United States are considered obese.[13] This is not to incriminate nutrition as the sole etiologic factor in the development of human obesity, but to imply its prominent role as a prerequisite.

DEFINITION

Obesity exists when total body fat is increased in relation to body weight. Increased adiposity may be assessed by measurement of subcutaneous skinfold thickness in specific anatomic sites, by total body weight in excess of 120% of ideal weight for height, or by determination of body mass index (BMI = weight/height squared). In the pediatric age group, triceps skinfold thickness correlates well with the degree of adiposity.[41] By definition, obesity is present when triceps skinfold thickness exceeds the 85th percentile of the normative data (Table 11–1). Inappropriate calipers and

TABLE 11–1.

Triceps Fatfold Percentiles for Whites and Blacks*

Midpoint Age (yr)	No.	Percentile Values					No.	Percentile Values				
		5	15	50	85	95		5	15	50	85	95
		White Males						**White Females**				
1	138	5	7	9	13	15	175	6	7	9	12	15
2	173	5	7	10	13	14	166	6	7	10	13	15
3	209	6	7	9	12	14	163	6	7	10	12	14
4	206	5	6	9	12	14	215	5	7	10	12	14
5	259	5	6	8	12	16	231	6	7	10	13	16
6	263	5	6	8	11	15	255	6	7	10	12	15
7	310	4	6	8	11	14	272	6	7	10	13	17
8	301	5	6	8	12	17	266	6	7	10	15	19
9	285	5	6	9	14	19	282	6	7	11	17	24
10	313	5	6	10	16	22	275	6	8	12	19	24
11	292	6	7	10	17	25	267	7	8	12	20	29
12	293	5	7	11	19	26	267	6	9	13	20	25
13	265	5	6	10	18	25	227	7	9	14	23	30
14	206	5	6	10	17	22	183	8	10	15	22	28
15	179	4	6	9	19	26	197	8	11	16	24	30
16	163	4	5	9	20	27	186	8	10	15	23	27
17	141	4	5	8	14	20	141	9	12	16	26	31
20	539	4	5	10	18	25	828	9	12	17	25	31
30	675	4	6	11	21	28	1,144	9	12	19	29	36
40	613	4	6	12	22	28	917	10	14	22	32	39
50	604	5	7	12	22	28	906	11	15	23	34	42
60	572	5	7	11	20	26	753	11	15	22	32	40
70	489	5	7	11	18	25	700	11	14	21	29	35
80	232	4	7	11	18	25	286	10	12	19	26	33
		Black Males						**Black Females**				
1	161	5	6	9	13	15	147	6	7	9	12	15
2	175	6	7	9	13	16	212	5	6	9	13	15
3	217	5	7	9	12	15	188	5	6	9	12	15
4	261	5	6	8	12	14	219	5	6	8	12	13
5	247	4	5	7	11	13	264	5	6	8	11	14
6	265	4	5	7	10	13	271	4	5	8	12	14
7	266	4	5	7	10	13	304	5	6	8	13	15

Continued.

TABLE 11–1. —Cont'd

Midpoint Age (yr)	No.	Percentile Values					No.	Percentile Values				
		5	15	50	85	95		5	15	50	85	95
		Black Males						Black Females				
8	250	3	4	7	10	15	270	5	6	8	13	17
9	290	3	4	7	12	18	283	5	6	9	15	22
10	252	4	5	7	12	17	276	4	6	10	15	21
11	239	4	5	8	15	20	279	5	6	11	18	28
12	266	4	5	8	14	21	272	6	7	11	19	24
13	226	4	5	8	16	26	266	5	7	11	21	27
14	233	3	4	7	15	24	236	6	8	14	24	31
15	190	4	4	7	15	23	206	7	9	14	22	28
16	163	4	4	7	14	19	203	6	9	14	22	27
17	112	3	5	8	13	16	146	7	8	15	23	31
20	267	3	5	7	14	23	587	7	10	17	26	33

*From Garn SM, Clark DC: *Pediatrics* 1976; 54:443. Used by permission.

inexperience may introduce a great degree of variability in measuring skinfold thickness. However, the technique is simple to learn and with some practice the variability can be avoided.

ETIOLOGY

Obesity, in its most common form, results from the conversion of excessively retained calories to fat. What is not known, however, is the mechanism of this diversion. Excessively retained calories may result from excessive consumption or from reduced expenditure. Multiple systems are involved in the physiologic regulation of energy balance in the body. The development of obesity is related to dysregulation of these sytems of energy homeostasis in an integrated and interrelated fashion.

Factors In Energy Homeostasis
- Eating behavior
- Energy expenditure
- Metabolic factors
- Hormonal factors
- Psychosocial and environmental factors
- Genetic factors

The role of each system is reviewed briefly.

Eating Behavior

Eating behavior results from a complex interplay of internal and external factors. Eating is usually initiated by hunger and terminated by a feeling of satiety. Experimental and clinical observations have identified the existence of two brain centers. One that evokes hunger is located in the lateral hypothalamic nuclei and another that signals satiety is located in the ventromedial hypothalamic nuclei. These brain centers are influenced by a variety of afferent and efferent pathways. Afferent pathways include neurosensory (smell), metabolic (glucose), and hormonal (cholecystokinin, insulin). Efferent pathways from thalamic centers include vagal and sympathetic nerve tracts as well as many neuroendocrine axes such as the hypothalamic-adrenal or hypothalamic-thyroid glands.[42] The effects of lesion or stimulation of hypothalamic nuclei leading to altered eating behavior in experimental animals are summarized in Table 11–2. Altered eating behavior or compulsive eating is a constant feature of certain types of human obesity, e.g., the hypothalamic syndrome or Prader-Willi syndrome. However, hyperphagia is not constantly present in idiopathic childhood obesity. Factors related to eating behavior and implicated in the development of obesity include the speed of eating, gorging, and preferential taste for sweet or fatty foods. In addition to hypothalamic centers for appetite and satiety, other centers such as central and hepatic glucoreceptors may be involved in eating behavior.[42]

Energy Expenditure

Energy expenditure equals the amount of energy required to maintain basic or resting metabolic rate (RMR), various physiologic functions such as digestion, thermoregulation, and growth, and the amount of energy for physical activity.

Resting metabolic rate, although increased in human obesity, when expressed per unit of lean body mass is not different from nonobese individuals.[39] Decreased thermogenesis in response to food ingestion has been reported in obese children[34] and in obese adults.[3] In obese adults decreased thermogenesis in response to glucose infusion persists even after weight loss and has been considered as evidence for a predisposition to development of obesity.[3] However, this observation has not been confirmed by all investigators and the question of reduced thermogenic response to food ingestion as an etiologic factor in human obesity remains unresolved.

It is generally assumed that obesity results from excessive consumption of calories. In addition, the reduced level of the energy cost of physical activity may further contribute to retention of calories, and increased adiposity. In one study of childhood obesity, in a small number of obese boys caloric intake was found excessive, but the energy cost of physical activity was comparable to control subjects.[46] In a study of

TABLE 11–2.

Effects of Hypothalamic Stimulation or Destruction on Feeding Behavior and Metabolism in Animals

	Lateral Hypothalamus	Ventromedial Hypothalamus
Stimulation	Hunger, glycogen synthesis	Satiety, glycogenolysis
Destruction	Hypophagia, hypometabolic state	Hyperphagia, hyperinsulinism

infants born to lean and overweight mothers, on the other hand, a significant reduction in energy expenditure was present prior to onset of obesity.[40] As an alternative to reduced rate of energy expenditure as a risk factor for body weight gain, a theory of altered set-point for body weight and adiposity but normal energy homeostasis has been proposed.[29]

Metabolic Factors

White adipose tissue is the site of storage of fat in the body. Adipocytes derive from mesenchymal tissue and appear in the fetus at about the 15th week of gestation.[30] The number and size of adipocytes increase throughout gestation. During the last trimester of pregnancy the amount of fetal body fat increases to 12% to 15% of body mass at term. Although postnatal increment in body fat is mostly via cell hypertrophy, adipocyte number increases in late infancy and during the adolescent period.[31] At the time of puberty, body fat content decreases in boys to about 17% while the percentage increases to 26% in girls. In obese children the number and size of adipocytes continue to increase with advancing obesity.[31] There is a maximum size for the adipocyte though the number seems limitless. The source of the seemingly limitless supply of adipocytes is a matter of speculation.

Ninety percent of the adipose tissue content is composed of triglycerides which are constantly formed (lipogenesis) and broken down to fatty acids and glycerol (lipolysis). The rate-limiting step in these processes is the activity of hormone-sensitive lipase (HSL). Agents that stimulate cyclic adenosine monophosphate (cAMP) formation (β_1-adrenergic agonists) will increase lipolysis and those that inhibit cAMP production (β_2-adrenergic agonists) promote lipogenesis.[19]

Epinephrine and norepinephrine, mixed adrenergic agonists, are the major hormones that influence these catecholamine-responsive processes. Depending on the concentration of these hormones and tissue responsiveness, lipolysis or lipogenesis is stimulated. In a study of adult obese men, depression in sympathetic and parasympathetic activity was found to correlate with percentages of body fat. Specifically, the plasma concentration of epinephrine and norepinephrine was inversely related to body fat.[37] In limited in vitro studies of adipose tissue from infants and children, the lipogenic process was preferentially operative, favoring the accretion of fat in the child.[33]

Insulin and adenosine are also important regulators of lipogenesis and lipolysis. Insulin acts at several sites to promote lipogenesis. These include increased glucose uptake by adipocytes, stimulation of lipoprotein lipase (LPL), and inhibition of HSL. Adenosine, derived from cAMP metabolism, has a direct antilipolytic effect on adipocytes.[42]

Hormonal Factors

Insulin

Hyperinsulinemia is a consistent feature of obesity. Impaired glucose tolerance and the insulin-glucose ratio both indicate peripheral insulin resistance.[12] On the other hand, amino acid transport, activation of LPL, and antilipolysis is not affected.[27] Under these circumstances (i.e., hyperinsulinemia) lipogenesis is stimulated and lipolysis is inhibited, favoring further increase in lipid storage.

Thyroxine

The thyroid hormones thyroxine (T_4) and triiodothyronine (T_3) play a pivotal role in energy homeostasis. Because of this prominent role, hypothyroidism is invariably included in the differential diagnosis and hormone therapy with T_4 is frequently considered in obese patients. Except for T_3 concentration, which may be increased in obese children owing to increased peripheral conversion, baseline levels of T_4, T_3, and thyroid-stimulating hormone (TSH) are normal.[26] Other changes may include hyporesponsiveness of thyroid to TSH and decreased nuclear T_3 receptors.[10] All these changes are reversible with weight loss, and are therefore considered secondary rather than primary.

Cortisol

Hypercortisolism is frequently suspected in the presence of obesity, despite its rare incidence in the pediatric age group. Plasma cortisol concentration, free and bound; circadian rhythm; and urinary excretion are all normal in obese children. Cortisol production and cortisol turnover rates are increased.[43] Mean 24-hour concentrations of adrenal sex steroids, including dihydroepiandrosterone (DHEA), androstenedione, and testosterone, are increased in obese children.[23] Corticosteroids play a permissive role in the expression of obesity in various genetic models of animal obesity.[6] Whether the same is true in human obesity is not known.

Growth Hormone

Both resting and stimulated levels of growth hormone (GH) are diminished in obese subjects.[28] This abnormality is completely reversible by weight loss. Despite low concentrations of GH, the level of somatomedin C (SM-C) is normal or increased.[4] The increased production of SM-C, attributable to hyperinsulinemia, may explain the accelerated growth invariably observed in obese children. In addition, elevated levels of SM-C may, on the basis of negative feedback, inhibit pituitary responsiveness to growth hormone–releasing hormone (GHRH) and spontaneous GH secretion.[32]

Hypogonadism

Hypogonadism is a concomitant feature of several syndromes presenting with obesity. In idiopathic childhood obesity the serum testosterone level in prepubertal boys is comparable to age-matched lean controls. However, the testicular response to human chorionic gonadotropin (hCG) is diminished.[11] Puberty is not delayed and indeed may be advanced because of accelerated growth and bone maturation. In postpubertal girls obesity may be associated with polycystic ovaries, hirsutism, and menstrual irregularities (Stein-Leventhal syndrome). In this disorder the serum level of luteinizing hormone (LH) is usually increased as well as the levels of some of the androgens.[2] Sex hormone–binding globulin is decreased in obese children.[16]

Psychosocial and Environmental Factors

Prenatal and postnatal factors exert important influences on the incidence of subsequent obesity. Babies born to mothers with gestational diabetes are larger and fatter and have a higher incidence of subsequent obesity.[45] Feeding practices beyond the neonatal period have not been related to the subsequent development of obesity.

Formula-fed infants are longer and larger compared with exclusively breast-fed infants but do not show an increased susceptibility to subsequent development of obesity.[20]

Environmental factors that have been implicated in the development of obesity, in addition to nutrition, include urban vs. rural environment, and geographic location. Family variables also play an important role. Those associated with increased risk of childhood obesity include parental obesity, socioeconomic class, parental education, parental age, birth order, and family size.[14]

Genetic Factors

The role of genetics in human obesity has been investigated in monozygous and dizygous twins and in adoptees. These studies have revealed a significantly higher concordance rate among monozygous twins compared with dizygous twins for skinfold thickness, fat mass, and fat distribution.[7] Also, there is a significant correlation of BMI among female adoptees with their biologic rather than adoptive mothers.[44]

Although these studies imply genetic susceptibility, specific genetic markers have not been located as yet. In one study, HLA-B18 antigen was found in 37% of obese members of one family.[21]

CLASSIFICATION

Childhood obesity can be classified into three major categories:

1. Idiopathic or common childhood obesity
2. Obesity secondary to metabolic or hormonal derangement
   a. Endocrine disorders associated with obesity
      (1). Hypothalamic syndrome
      (2). Cushing's syndrome
      (3). Hypothyroidism
      (4). Pseudohypoparathyroidism
      (5). GH deficiency
      (6). Polycystic ovary syndrome
      (7). Insulinoma, hyperinsulinism
   b. Drugs associated with obesity
      (1). Glucocorticoids
      (2). Amitriptyline (tricyclic antidepressant)
      (3). Cyproheptadine
      (4). Phenothiazine
      (5). Estrogen
      (6). Progesterone (medroxyprogesterone)
      (7). Lithium
3. Obesity associated with certain genetic syndromes
   a. Prader-Willi syndrome
   b. Laurence-Moon-Biedl syndrome

c. Cohen syndrome
d. Carpenter's syndrome
e. Pseudohypoparathyroidism
f. Turner's syndrome
g. Alström's syndrome

Subclassifications of obesity based on fat distribution into android and gynecoid types, as in adult obesity, has not been attempted in the pediatric age group. Most children with common childhood obesity tend to have a generalized distribution of fat with no predilection for abdominal, truncal, or gluteal areas.

CLINICAL EVALUATION

Evaluation of a child presenting with obesity should include a thorough medical and, if necessary, psychosocial evaluation. The medical evaluation should include a complete history and physical examination. Special attention should be paid to all areas that may have a contributing role in the development of obesity. Physical examination should include anthropometric measurements: height and weight, arm span, upper-lower segment ratio, and triceps skinfold thickness. The phenotypic designation of fat distribution, i.e., android (truncal) vs. gynecoid (gluteal, femoral), is usually replaced by truncal vs. generalized-type obesity (Fig 11–1). A significant accumulation

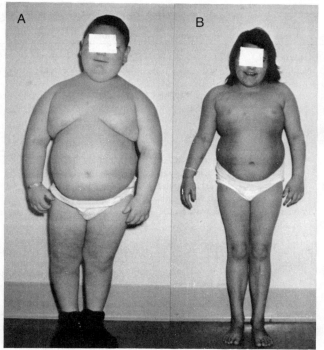

FIG 11-1.
A, 6½-year-old-boy with generalized idiopathic childhood obesity; height at 75th percentile, weight greater than 95th percentile.
B, 9³⁄₁₂-year-old-girl with truncal idiopathic childhood obesity; height at 25th percentile, weight at 90th percentile.

of fat in the upper truncal region (chest, supraclavicular, and upper posterior cervical) along with a significant reduction in growth velocity assume diagnostic significance.

The diagnosis of obesity, without etiologic consideration, could be made on the basis of triceps skinfold thickness greater than 85% for age, BMI, and weight for height in excess of 120%.

The clinical differential diagnosis of obesity could be based on the presence or absence of short stature, mental retardation, and dysmorphic features. Common childhood obesity is a simple diagnosable condition on clinical grounds, with no need for laboratory confirmation. If growth is affected, in the absence of mental retardation, two conditions should be considered and ruled out by appropriate laboratory tests: hypothyroidism and Cushing's syndrome. Hypothyroidism is much more common than Cushing's syndrome and could present with a relative lack of recognizable findings.[1] Cushing's syndrome, on the other hand, is a much more difficult diagnosis to substantiate. Drug-related obesity is uncommon in children and the presence of mental retardation and dysmorphic features would indicate syndromic obesity (Table 11–3). A formal evaluation of food intake, although often unrevealing, may be helpful in subsequent dietary planning.

Laboratory measures are not necessary for the purpose of diagnosis. However, lipid profile and glucose tolerance should be evaluated to identify the individuals at risk. A random blood sample for chemistry profile and a urinalysis should be obtained.

TABLE 11–3.
Cardinal Features of Syndromes of Obesity and Mental Retardation

Feature	Prader-Willi	Laurence-Moon-Biedl	Cohen	Carpenter's	Alström's	Pseudohypo-parathy-roidism
Obesity	Generalized	Generalized	Truncal	Truncal	Truncal	Generalized
Mental retardation	Mild–moderate	Mild	Mild	Slight	Absent	Moderate to severe
Gonadal function	Primary hypogonadism	Primary hypogonadism	Normal hypogonadism	Secondary hypogonadism	Male hypogonadism	Intact
Stature	Short–normal	Short–normal	Normal	Normal–short	Short	Short
Craniofacial abnormalities	Narrow bifrontal diameter	None	High nasal, bridge, high arched palate, low-set ears	Acrocephaly Flat nasal bridge,	None	Moon facies
Extremities	Small hands and feet	Polydactyly, syndactyly	Narrow hands and feet, genu valgum	Polydactyly, syndactyly	None	Small hands and metacarpal shortening
Other features	Hypotonia, behavior problems	Retinitis pigmentosa	Hypotonia	Cranio-synostosis	Sensory nerve deafness, blindness diabetes mellitus	Hypocalcemic seizures, basal ganglia and metastatic calcifications
Inheritance	Sporadic, ⅔ have defective chromosome 15	Autosomal recessive	Autosomal recessive	Autosomal recessive	Autosomal recessive	Variable

If abnormalities of lipid or glucose are detected, fasting blood for evaluation of lipids or a formal 2- to 3-hour glucose tolerance test should be performed.

MORBIDITY

In addition to the psychosocial stigmata of obesity, important consequences include conditions that are age-related such as orthopedic complications and those that persist into adulthood.

- Hypertension
- Hyperlipidemia
- Orthopedic (slipped capital femoral epiphyses, Blount disease)
- Dermatologic (acanthosis nigricans, furunculosis, intertrigo)
- Psychosocial dysfunction
- Persistence into adulthood
- Hypoventilation syndrome

The most serious consequence of childhood obesity is the high incidence of persistence into adult life of its concomitants hypertension and hyperlipidemia.[35] Obesity, hyperlipidemia, and hypertension are major risk factors for the development of adult coronary heart disease. As a result, the obese individual has a higher incidence of coronary heart disease and a shorter life span.

The obesity-hypoventilation syndrome (pickwickian syndrome) is a life-threatening complication of morbid obesity in children. Its clinical presentation is characterized by somnolence, hypoventilation, congestive heart failure, and plethora in the extremely obese child. Laboratory findings include hypercapnea, hypoxia, decreased vital capacity and ventilatory minute volume, and cardiac enlargement. Hospitalization is often required for urgent supportive therapy in such children.

TREATMENT

Effective medical treatment of idiopathic childhood obesity is a difficult task if not an impossible one. Long-term follow-up studies of weight-reduced obese children have invariably demonstrated a return to pretreatment weight after several years.[25] In addition, significant morbidity and mortality attributable to low calorie diets have been reported.[42] Considering the limitations of the therapeutic approaches, the goals of therapy should be realistic, attainable, and amenable to long-term maintenance. The essential components of any program include diet, exercise, and behavior modification.[42] Since most obese children come from obese families, it is important that parents be included in the treatment plan. Studies have shown more effective weight reduction and more favorable treatment outcomes when parents are included in such treatment plans.[9]

Diet should contain adequate calories and essential nutrients to allow for normal growth and prevent nutritional deficiencies. There is no advantage in limiting the nutrient-derived calories from carbohydrate or from fat. Therefore, the diet should be balanced in terms of carbohydrate, protein, and fat content. The appropriate number of dietary calories can be approximated from the number of calories consumed daily minus the number of calories calculated from the rate of daily weight gain. Such a diet may not be conducive to immediate weight loss; however, over a period of time it will reduce the weight-height ratio and the degree of adiposity.

Exercise is the most effective method of increasing caloric expenditure. An exercise program suitable for age and one that is easy to adhere to should be implemented.[18] Exercise for a minium of 20 minutes, three times weekly, of an intensity to expend 300 calories per session is required to affect weight loss.[24] A variety of exercises, such as brisk walking, jogging, cycling, swimming, and aerobic dancing, are effective and easy to implement.

Behavior modification has been shown to be an effective complement to the diet and exercise program. Several techniques such as self-monitoring, contingency management, and contracting have been used with various rates of success.[17]

Pharmacologic and surgical approaches to childhood obesity have been limited to exceptional and unusual circumstances. Progesterone has been used in children suffering from hypoventilation syndrome with short-term success, improving ventilation and contributing to weight loss.[36] The long-term effects, however, are not known. Various hormones, including chorionic gonadotropins, thyroid hormones, and GH, have been used in adult obesity.[47] Only thyroid hormones have been used in obese children. Because of lack of effectiveness and significant side effects such as hypercalciuria and osteoporosis, hormone use in idiopathic childhood obesity should be avoided.

Appetite suppressant drugs have not been found effective in chronic weight control in adults, and should not be used in children.[5]

PREVENTION

In view of the limited effectiveness of therapeutic intervention, consideration of preventive measures seems appropriate. However, limited preventive interventional observations have been made. In one study aimed at prevention of obesity in infants, skimmed milk, precooked cereal, and fresh fruits were given to 80 infants from 3 months of age.[38] In a second study, a school-based program, utilizing nutrition education, behavior modification, and physical activities, was implemented.[8] Both studies have reported success in preventing obesity in infants and inducing weight loss in school-age children. Large-scale family or community-based preventive programs such as these have not been attempted and their successful claims remain in need of further evaluation.

Although the characteristic behavioral and biochemical features of childhood obesity are not known, children at risk could be identified on the basis of family variables associated with the development of obesity.[14] In addition, television viewing has been shown to be a significant risk factor in childhood and adolescent obesity.

Children and adolescents reportedly devote 22 to 36 hours per week of their time to television viewing.[15] This period of inactivity not only reduces caloric expenditure but may also increase caloric intake associated with snacking, particularly of the high calorie foods advertised on television.

Physicians responsible for the care of children should identify those at risk prior to the development of obesity and provide appropriate counseling as well as dietary and other measures as deemed necessary. Whether such preventive measures will be effective in preventing the development of obesity remains unknown.

REFERENCES

1. Abbassi V, Aldige C: Clinical recognition of juvenile hypothyroidism in the early stage. *Clin Pediatr* 1980, 19:782.
2. Baird DT, et al: Pituitary ovarian relationships in polycystic ovary syndrome. *J Clin Endocrinol Metab* 1977, 45:798.
3. Bessard T, et al: Energy expenditure and post prandial thermogenesis in obese women before and after weight loss. *Am J Clin Nutr* 1982; 38:680.
4. Binet E, et al: Serum somatomedin activity in obese children. *Pediatr Adolesc Endocrinol* 1976; 1:153.
5. Bray GA: Treatment of obesity with drugs and invasive procedures, Bray GA (ed): *Obesity in America*. US Department of Health and Human Services (NIH), Publication No 79-359, 1979, pp 179–305.
6. Bray GA: Obesity—A disease of nutrient or energy balance? *Nutr Rev* 1987; 45:33.
7. Brook CGD, et al: Influence of heredity and environment in determination of skinfold thickness in children. *Br Med J* 1975; 3:719.
8. Brownell KD, Kaye FS: A school-based behavior modification. Nutrition education and physical activity program for obese children. *Am J Clin Nutr* 1982; 35:277.
9. Brownell KD et al: Treatment of obese children with and without their mothers: Changes in weight and blood pressure. *Pediatrics* 1983; 71:515.
10. Burman KD, Latham KR, Dzuh YY: Solubilized nuclear thyroid hormone receptors in circulating human mononuclear cells. *J Clin Endocrinol Metab* 1980; 51:106.
11. Cacciari E: Effect of obesity on the hypothalamic pituitary gonadal function in childhood. *Acta Paediatr Scand* 1977; 66:345.
12. Chiumello G, et al: Relationship between obesity, chemical diabetes, and beta pancreatic function in children. *Diabetes* 1969; 18:238.
13. Dietz WH: Childhood obesity: Susceptibility, cause and management. *J Pediatr* 1983; 103:676.
14. Dietz WH: Prevention of childhood obesity. *Pediatr Clin North Am* 1986; 33:823.
15. Dietz WH, Gortmaker SL: Do we fatten our children at the TV set? Television viewing and obesity in children and adolescents. *Pediatrics* 1975; 75:807.
16. Dunkel L, et al: Low levels of sex hormone-binding globulin in obese children. *J Pediatr* 1985; 107:95.
17. Epstein LH, et al: Childhood obesity. *Pediatr Clin North Am* 1985; 32:363.
18. Epstein LH, et al: Effect of diet and controlled exercise on weight loss in obese children. *J Pediatr* 1985; 107:358.
19. Fain JN, Garcia-Sainz JA: Adrenergic regulation of adipocyte metabolism. *J Lipid Res* 1983; 24:945.
20. Fomon SJ, et al: Indices of fatness and serum cholesterol at age eight years in relation to feeding and growth during early infancy. *Pediatr Res* 1984; 18:1233.

21. Fumerone F, Apfelbaum M: Association between HLA-18 and family obesity syndrome (letter). *N Engl J Med* 1981; 305:645.

22. Garn SM, Clark DC: Trends in fatness and the origins of obesity. *Pediatrics* 1976; 57:443.

23. Gemazzani AR, et al: Adrenal and gonadal steroid in obese prepubertal girls. *J Clin Endocrinol Metab* 1978; 47:974.

24. Gilles ME, et al: A clinical review of obesity. *Med Rounds* 1989; 2:223.

25. Ginsberg-Fellner F, Knittle J: Weight reduction in young obese children: I. Effect on adipose tissue cellularity and metabolism. *Pediatr Res* 1981; 15:1381.

26. Glass AR: Endocrine aspect of obesity. *Med Clin North Am* 1989; 73:139.

27. Howard BV, et al: The antilipolytic action of insulin in obese subjects with resistance to its glucoregulatory action. *J Clin Endocrinol Metab* 1984; 58:544.

28. Josefsberg Z, et al: Growth hormone response to insulin tolerance test and arginine stimulation in obese children and adolescents. *Pediatr Adolesc Endocrinol* 1976; 1:146.

29. Keesey RE: A set point theory of obesity, in Brownell KD, Forety JP (eds): *Handbook of Eating Disorders: Physiology, Psychology and Treatment of Obesity, Anorexia and Bulimia*. New York, Basic Books, 1981, pp 63–87.

30. Knittle JL: Adipose tissue development in man, in Faulkner F, Tanner JM (eds): *Human Growth*. Vol 2: *Postnatal Growth*. New York, Plenum Press, 1978, pp 295–315.

31. Knittle JL, et al: The growth of adipose tissue in children and adolescents. *J Clin Invest* 1979; 63:239.

32. Loche S, et al: Reduced growth hormone response to growth hormone releasing hormone in children with simple obesity: Evidence for somatomedin-C mediated inhibition. *Clin Endocrinol* 1987; 27:145.

33. Marcus C, et al: Changes in catecholamine-induced lipolysis in isolated human fat cells during the first year of life. *J Clin Invest* 1987; 79:1812.

34. Molnar DP, et al: Food induced thermogenesis in obese children. *Eur J Pediatr* 1985; 144:27.

35. Mossberg HO: 40-year follow-up of overweight children. *Lancet* 1989; 2:491.

36. Orenstein DM, et al: Progesterone treatment of the obesity hypoventilation syndrome in a child. *J Pediatr* 1977; 90:477.

37. Peterson HR, et al: Body fat and the activity of the autonomic nervous system. *N Engl J Med* 1988; 318:1077.

38. Pisacano JC, et al: An attempt at prevention of obesity in infancy. *Pediatrics* 1978; 61:360.

39. Ravussin EB, et al: Twenty-four hour energy expenditure and resting metabolic rate in obese, moderately obese and control subjects. *Am J Clin Nutr* 1982; 35:566.

40. Roberts SB, et al: Energy expenditure and intake in infants born to lean and overweight mothers. *N Engl J Med* 1988; 318:461.

41. Roch AF, et al: Grading body fatness from limited anthropometric data. *Am J Clin Nutr* 1981; 34:2831.

42. Rosenbaum M, Leibel RL: Pathophysiology of childhood obesity. *Adv Pediatr* 1988; 35:73.

43. Slavnov VN, Epshtein EV: Somatotropic, thyrotopic, and adrenocorticotropic functions of the anterior pituitary in obesity. *Endocrinologie* 1977; 15:213.

44. Stunkard AJ, et al: An adoption study of human obesity. *N Engl J Med* 1988; 314:193.

45. Vohr BR, et al: Somatic growth of children of diabetic mothers with reference to birth size. *J Pediatr* 1980; 97:196.

46. Waxman M, Stunkard AJ: Caloric intake and expenditure of obese boys. *J Pediatr* 1980; 96:187.

47. Weintraub M, Bray GA: Drug treatment of obesity. *Med Clin North Am* 1989; 73:237.

Chapter 12

Hyperlipidemia

Val Abbassi

Major advances have been made in our understanding of the biochemistry and metabolism of plasma lipids and lipoproteins. As a result, the pathophysiology of several important lipid disorders has been elucidated. In addition, hypercholesterolemia, because of its implications for adult coronary heart disease (CHD), has received increasing attention. Public awareness and routine screening for hypercholesterolemia have led to an increase in the number of case findings in the pediatric age group and the need for appropriate diagnosis and management. This chapter is devoted to the description of the lipid disorders that primarily involve cholesterol and triglyceride metabolism. Because of its importance, hypercholesterolemia as a major risk factor in CHD is discussed separately.

BIOCHEMISTRY AND PHYSIOLOGY

Lipoproteins are the secretory products of enterocytes and hepatocytes and the intravascular metabolism of these products. The major functions of the lipoproteins include transport of triglycerides and cholesterol from the intestine and liver to other tissues, and transport of excess cholesterol produced by other tissues to the liver for secretion as bile acids.

Five major classes of lipoproteins are present in plasma: chylomicrons, very low-density lipoproteins (VLDL), low-density lipoproteins (LDL), intermediate-density lipoproteins (IDL), and high-density lipoproteins 2 and 3 (HDL_2, HDL_3). For the purpose of transport, solubility, and enzymatic hydrolysis, plasma lipoproteins are uniquely packaged in spherical structures containing a core made of triglyceride and cholestryl esters and an outer shell consisting of phospholipids, free cholesterol, and a specific protein.[28] Some of the characteristics of the lipoproteins are presented in Table 12–1.

The protein constituents of plasma lipids serve several important physiologic functions including lipoprotein biosynthesis, activation of lipolytic enzymes, and interaction with cellular receptors.[8] These proteins are known as apolipoproteins or apoproteins (apo). Some of their characteristics are outlined in Table 12–2.

LIPOPROTEIN METABOLISM

Chylomicrons originate in the absorptive intestinal cells (Fig 12–1). They are the largest lipoprotein particles circulating and the major vehicle for transport of dietary triglycerides and cholesterol.[25] They contain apo B, C, and E. Lipoproteins secreted by hepatocytes are of two major forms, VLDL[51] and HDL.[24] Some HDL is also produced by the intestine. These lipoproteins are subject to major metabolic degradation and exchange by several important lipolytic enzymes including lipoprotein

TABLE 12–1.

Some Characteristics of Plasma Lipoproteins*

Lipoprotein	Origin	Major Apoprotein Constituent	Core Lipid	Function	Destination
Chylomicron	Intestine	B,C,E	TG	Transport of dietary TG	Liver and TG storage cells
VLDL	Liver	B,C,E	TG, cholesterol	Transport of endogenous TG	TG storage and TG metabolizing cells
LDL	Intravascular	B	Cholesterol esters	Transport of hepatic and intravascular cholesterol	Peripheral tissue and liver
HDL	Liver, intestine, vascular	A-I, A-II	Cholesterol esters	Transport of cholesterol from peripheral tissues	Liver, adrenals, gonads

*TG = triglycerides.

TABLE 12–2.

Source, Lipoprotein Distribution, and Major Functions of Apolipoproteins

Apolipoprotein	Source	Lipoprotein Distribution	Function
A-I	Liver	Chylomicron, VLDL, HDL	Enzyme activation
B-48	Intestine	Chylomicron	Lipoprotein synthesis
B-100	Liver	VLDL, LDL	Enzyme activation, receptor binding*
C-I,C-II	Liver	Chylomicron, VLDL, LDL, HDL	Enzyme activation, receptor binding*
E	Liver	Chylomicron, VLDL, LDL, HDL	Receptor binding†

*LDL receptor.
†Chylomicron remnant receptor binding.

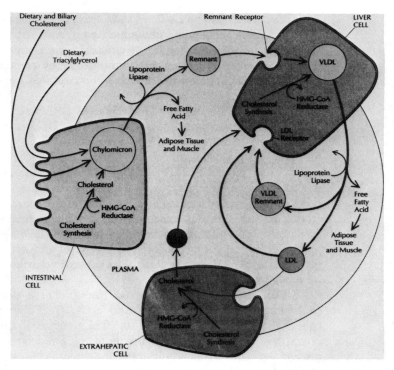

FIG 12-1.
Pathways of lipoprotein metabolism. Chylomicron synthesized and released by intestinal cell is converted to free fatty acids and chylomicron remnant. Chylomicron remnant is taken into circulation and under the influence of lipolytic enzymes lipoprotein lipase and lecithin-cholesterol acyltransferase it is metabolized and converted to HDL and LDL. HMG = CoA = hydroxymethylglutaryl coenzyme A. (From Dietschy JM: *Hosp Pract* 1990; (June) 67, Used by permission.)

TABLE 12-3.
Lipolytic Enzymes: Their Origin and Site of Action

Enzyme	Tissue of Origin	Site of Action
Lipoprotein lipase	Adipose tissue Striated muscle Pulmonary capillary bed Lactating breast	Chylomicron, LDL
Hepatic lipase	Hepatocytes	VLDL, IDL, HDL
Lecithin-cholesterol acyltransferase	Hepatocytes	HDL (nascent)

lipase (LPL)[15], hepatic lipase (HL),[30] and lecithin-cholesterol acyltransferase (LCAT).[17] The tissue of origin and site of action of these enzymes are presented in Table 12–3.

LPL is synthesized by parenchymal cells of various tissues (see Table 12–3). Following release it localizes to the luminal surface of the vascular endothelial cells.

LPL is activated by apo C-II and hydrolyzes chylomicrons to release monoglycerides, free fatty acids (FFA), and chylomicron remnant. Apolipoprotein B-48 is necessary for biosynthesis and secretion of chylomicrons from the intestinal epithelial cells. Apolipoprotein E serves as a recognition site by chylomicron remnant receptor on liver cells, and is responsible for receptor-mediated uptake of chylomicron remnant from plasma.

VLDLs are also subject to hydrolysis by LPL which removes triglycerides leaving IDL. With further modification by HL, the IDL is converted to LDL in plasma.[51] The LDL thus derived from hydrolysis of VLDL is the major transport lipoprotein for cholesterol. Further metabolism of LDL is via the LDL receptor-mediated process.[6] The hepatocyte LDL receptor is synthesized in endoplasmic reticulum, transported to the Golgi apparatus, and subsequently inserted into specific regions of the cell membrane called *coated pits*. The LDL receptor interacts with apo B-100 of the LDL particle. The LDL-receptor complex thus formed enters the cell by the process of endocytosis and fuses with liposomes. The LDL particle dismounts from the receptor and is hydrolyzed to free cholesterol and amino acids that enter the cytoplasmic pool. LDL receptor is recycled and returned to the coated pits where it becomes functional once again.

HDL is secreted by liver and intestine in a discoid "nascent HDL" form containing mostly phospholipid and apo A-I. These particles grow into mature spherical particles by incorporating free cholesterol from cell membranes of peripheral tissues and from other lipoproteins. The liver enzyme LCAT mediates this process by converting cholesterol to cholesteryl ester and incorporating it into the core of the HDL particle. Thus, it has been hypothesized that HDL is the vehicle for reverse transport of cholesterol from peripheral tissues to the liver. Two subclasses of HDL are predominantly present in human plasma: HDL_2, a lipid-rich particle, and HDL_3, a smaller and denser form. The significance of HDL concentration in relation to CHD has been established by epidemiologic as well as interventional studies.[24]

Hormonal Influence on Lipoprotein Metabolism

Several hormones influence hepatic intracellular metabolism of FFA, triglycerides, and cholesterol. Insulin and glucagon exert a mutually and interrelated controlling mechanism in this respect. In periods of substrate excess (absorptive state) and high insulin concentration, FFA are rapidly cleared by the liver from circulation and converted to triglycerides. At the same time fatty acid oxidation is suppressed. In the postabsorptive state, both substrate and insulin levels fall and glucagon level rises. Triglyceride synthesis is halted and FFA are shunted into mitochondria for oxidation and energy production. Steroid hormones[49] and estrogen[37] also increase the rate of triglyceride synthesis. Progesterone and testosterone have an opposite effect.[48] Triiodothyronine (T_3) enhances mitochondrial oxidation of long-chain fatty acids.[5]

In addition to their intracellular effects, hormones influence the activity of lipolytic enzymes as well as the activity and expression of lipoprotein receptor. These actions of hormones are summarized in Tables 12–4 and 12–5.

TABLE 12–4.

Hormonal Influence on Lipoprotein Metabolism by Liver Cells

	Stimulatory	Inhibitory
FFA oxidation	Thyroxine, glucagon	Insulin
Triglyceride synthesis	Insulin, glucocorticoid, estrogen	Glucagon, progesterone
LDL Receptor	Thyroxine, estrogen	Androgen

TABLE 12–5.

Hormonal Influence on Lipolytic Enzymes

	Stimulation of Synthesis	Inhibition of Synthesis
Lipoprotein lipase	Insulin, thyroxine, catecholamines, estrogen (adipose tissue)	β-blockers, prolactin (adipose tissue)
Hepatic lipase	Triiodothyronine, progesterone, androgen	Estrogen

TABLE 12–6.

Classification of Hyperlipoproteinemias

Lipoprotein Type	Primary Genetic Disorder	Lipoprotein Abnormality	Inheritance
I	Familial lipoprotein lipase deficiency	Increased chylomicrons	Recessive
IIa	Familial hypercholesterolemia	Increased LDL	Dominant
IIb	Familial combined hyperlipidemia	Increased LDL	Dominant
III	Familial type III hyperlipidemia	Increased LDL	Dominant
IV	Familial hypertriglyceridemia	Increased LDL	Dominant
V	Familial type V hyperlipidemia	Increased VLDL and chylomicrons	Dominant

Disorders of Lipoprotein Metabolism

Disorders of lipoprotein metabolism may be considered under two major categories: primary types, caused by genetic abnormalities of lipoprotein metabolism; and secondary types, caused by hormonal, metabolic disorders or drug interaction.

Genetic abnormalities of lipoprotein metabolism may lead to the development of hyper- or hypolipoproteinemias and may involve the synthesis of apoproteins, lipolytic enzymes, and lipoprotein receptors. Traditionally, genetic disorders, causing hyperlipoproteinemias are classified under five major types (Table 12–6). Since not all types have clinical expressions in the pediatric age group, only familial LPL deficiency, familial hypercholesterolemia, and familial combined hyperlipidemia will be discussed.

Secondary hyperlipidemias are more commonly encountered in pediatric age groups. They are caused by a variety of endocrine, metabolic, and other disorders (Table 12–7). Because of their significance, both in terms of diagnosis and manage-

TABLE 12–7.

Common Causes of Secondary Hyperlipidemias*

Cause	Hypercholesterolemia	Hypertriglyceridemia
Cushing's syndrome	+	+
Diet	+	
Drugs†		+
Glycogen storage disease	+	+ +
Hypothyroidism	+	+
Lipodystrophy		+
Nephrotic syndrome	+	
Obesity		+
Obstructive liver disease	+	
Porphyria	+	
Renal failure		+
Uncontrolled insulin-dependent diabetes	+	+ +

*+ = present; + + = predominant
†Alcohol, estrogens, β-blockers, hydrochlorothiazide.

ment, and their relevance, endocrinopathies as causes of hyperlipidemia must be diagnosed and appropriately treated.

FAMILIAL LIPOPROTEIN LIPASE DEFICIENCY (TYPE I HYPERLIPOPROTEINEMIA, HYPERCHYLOMICRONEMIA)

Familial LPL deficiency is a rare genetic disorder with autosomal recessive inheritance. The clinical manifestations, often presenting in childhood, are characterized by recurrent pancreatitis, eruptive xanthomas, hepatosplenomegaly, and lipemia retinalis.[31]

Clinical Presentation

The most common clinical manifestation of familial LPL deficiency is recurrent abdominal pain caused by pancreatitis. The most consistent characteristic of the pain is its recurrent nature. The attacks may be mild to severe, and may mimic a variety of intraabdominal crises associated with pain. These episodes are precipitated by a rise in plasma triglycerides to over 2,000 mg/dL, and may ultimately lead to pancreatic deficiency and the development of steatorrhea or diabetes, or both. Occasionally they may have a fatal outcome.

Eruptive xanthomas are cutaneous lesions of white-yellowish raised nodules, 1 to 4 mm in diameter, on an erythematous base, localized commonly to the buttocks, shoulders, and extensor surface of extremities. They contain chylomicron-like particles and macrophages filled with fat droplets. These lesions may fade and reappear as plasma lipids rise and fall.

Hepatosplenomegaly is often present in children with this disorder. The organomegaly is caused by accumulation of chylomicrons in histiocytes, macrophages, and Kupffer cells, and correlates with the fat content of the diet.

Lipemia retinalis is caused by intense hyperlipidemia in arteries and veins in the periphery of the retina, giving a milky appearance. In addition, lipid deposits and true retinopathy (hemorrhage and microaneurysms) may be present.

Diagnosis

The diagnosis can be made by simple observation of the patient's blood in a test tube. The appearance of blood, even after overnight fasting, is turbid, and on standing at 4°C separates into a creamy layer on top and a clear subnatant.

The concentration of triglycerides is markedly increased, ranging from 3 to 10 g/dL. Occasionally, higher values have been reported. Cholesterol concentration is usually in the normal range or only modestly increased. A useful diagnostic index is the ratio of cholesterol to triglycerides (in mg/dL) which is always less than 0.2 in this condition. The presence of excessive chylomicronemia could be assessed by electrophoresis or ultracentrifugation. The concentration of VLDL is usually normal, but LDL and HDL concentrations are suppressed.

The diagnosis should be confirmed by measurement of enzyme activity, although the dramatic lipid response to dietary restriction of fat is confirmatory. LPL activity may be assessed from postheparin plasma or adipose tissue obtained by needle biopsy.

Variant Forms

LPL requires the presence of apo C-II for its activation. In the absence of this apoprotein a clinical syndrome resembling familial LPL deficiency develops.[7] However, certain differences between LPL deficiency and apo C-II deficiency separate the two entities. Homozygous individuals with apo C-II deficiency usually present later in age with recurrent pancreatitis, lacking cutaneous manifestations of the LPL deficiency, as well as hepatosplenomegaly and lipemia retinalis. A third clinical type of hyperchylomicronemia caused by circulating inhibitors of LPL has been described.[32]

There is no apparent association between CHD and LPL deficiency or its clinical variants.

Treatment

Hypertriglyceridemia responds dramatically to restriction of dietary fat. However, the corresponding increase in carbohydrate intake leads to increased concentrations of VLDL. Therefore, the reduction in chylomicron to triglycerides is replaced by VLDL triglycerides and normal levels may not be attained. To some extent medium-chain triglycerides (MCT) may be substituted for other forms of fats in the diet. Lipid-lowering drugs have not been effective in the treatment of LPL deficiency.

FAMILIAL HYPERCHOLESTEROLEMIA (TYPE IIa HYPERLIPIDEMIA)

Familial hypercholesterolemia is the most common form of the genetic hyperlipo-proteinemias to become manifest in childhood. The basic genetic defect is a deficiency of LDL receptors on cell membranes leading to marked elevation of LDL cholesterol. It is inherited as an autosomal dominant trait.[22]

Clinical Presentation

In the homozygous state plasma cholesterol is above 500 mg/dL (Table 12–8). There-fore the LDH concentration is significantly increased to usually twice the level in heterozygotes. Xanthomas (deposition of cholesterol in tendons) appear before age 10 years, and atheromas (deposition of cholesterol in arteries) before age 20. Both parents have elevated blood levels of cholesterol. In the heterozygous form, serum cholesterol is between 350 and 550 mg/dL. The LDL concentration is increased. Only one parent has an elevated cholesterol level. Xanthomas appear late and vascular disease occurs in the fourth decade, peaking in the fifth and sixth decades.

The prevalence of heterozygous hypercholesterolemia is about 1 in 500, and of homozygous, about 1 in 1 million.

The primary genetic defect involves the function of the LDL receptor on the cell membrane. Three classes of mutations have been described, all attributable to mutant genes at the receptor loci. In one form the LDL receptor is absent (receptor-negative). In another form, transport of the LDL receptor to the cell surface is deficient (transport-deficient), and in the third form LDL binding is normal, but internalization does not occur.[9]

Lipoprotein Profile

In heterozygotes hypercholesterolemia is a constant finding. In large studies the range of plasma cholesterol is between 250 and 550 mg/dL with mean concentrations of about 350 mg/dL. In homozygotes the plasma cholesterol concentration is usually much higher, between 600 and 1200 mg/dL.

The excess cholesterol is entirely in the LDL fraction. Both the composition and

TABLE 12–8.
Clinical Characteristics of Familial Hypercholesterolemia in Homozygotes and Heterozygotes

	Homozygote	Heterozygote
Hypercholesterolemia	Present at birth	Present at birth
Level (mg/dL)	>600	250–550
Cut xanthomas	Present at birth or developing by age 4 yr	Begin to appear in 2nd or 3rd decade
Tendon xanthomas	Appear in childhood	Appear in 2nd and 3rd decade
Arcus corneae	Appears in childhood	Appears in 2nd and 3rd decade
Generalized atherosclerosis	Presents early in childhood	Appears in 2nd and 3rd decade
CHD	Before 30 yr	In 4th decade

the metabolism of LDL from homozygous and heterozygous individuals are nearly normal. The concentration of triglycerides is usually normal, although it may be slightly increased in homozygotes. The HDL cholesterol is slightly reduced in both homozygotes and heterozygotes for reasons that are not clear at present.

Prenatal Diagnosis

Prenatal diagnosis of homozygous familial hypercholesterolemia has been reported.[10] Neonatal diagnosis can be made by measurement of cord blood cholesterol if one of the parents is known to be affected. However, neonatal mass screening is not a reliable means of identifying the heterozygotes because the majority of newborn infants with elevated LDL cholesterol do not have familial hypercholesterolemia.[36]

Treatment

Heterozygous Hypercholesterolemia

The aim of therapy is to lower cholesterol by enhancement of the LDL receptor, by inhibition of intracellular cholesterol production, or by a combination of both. Cholestyramine and colestipol are nonabsorbable anion-exchange resins that bind bile acids in the intestinal lumen and prevent their reabsorption. Prevention of bile acid reabsorption apparently stimulates the production of an increased number of LDL receptors on liver cells, and enhances the fractional catabolic rate of cholesterol.[53] This type of therapy leads to a reduction of cholesterol concentration of 15% to 30%. Since the effectiveness of cholesterol removal may be compensated by an increase in cholesterol production by the liver, drugs that inhibit intracellular cholesterol production would be of value. Recently, two drugs have been introduced that are capable of blocking intracellular cholesterol production by inhibition of the rate-limiting enzyme hydroxymethylglutaryl coenzyme A (HMG-CoA) reductase. Compactin is a competitive inhibitor of HMG-CoA reductase with cholesterol-lowering capabilities.[61] Another drug, levostatin, a methylated form of compactin, has a higher potency in inhibiting HMG-CoA reductase.[58] Experimental studies have shown two mechanisms by which these drugs lower cholesterol.[58,61] They inhibit cholesterol synthesis by 50% and enhance the fractional clearance of LDL twofold.[3]

Other forms of therapy successful in heterozygous hypercholesterolemia include a combination of bile acid sequestrant and inhibitors of HMG-CoA reductase, and partial ileal bypass.[1] A low fat diet must be implemented along with pharmacotherapy (see Management of Hypercholesterolemia in Children).

Homozygous Hypercholesterolemia

In homozygous hypercholesterolemia, dietary and pharmacologic therapy is less successful. However, several approaches have been found effective in lowering plasma cholesterol. These incude intravenous alimentation,[59] portocaval shunt,[57] liver transplantation,[55] and continuous-flow cell separation to remove cholesterol by exchange.[33] Plasma exchange must be repeated at 2- to 3-week intervals to be effective. Whether the cholesterol-lowering approaches prevent the development of life-threatening atherosclerotic processes is not yet known.

FAMILIAL COMBINED HYPERLIPIDEMIA

Familial combined hyperlipidemia was first reported by Goldstein et al. among survivors of myocardial infarction.[23] It is an autosomal dominant disorder with an incidence of 1% to 2% in the general adult population. Other than elevated plasma cholesterol and triglycerides, the condition is asymptomatic in the pediatric age group. However, because of its association with increased risk for CHD, it should be recognized and treated in a manner similar to familial hypercholesterolemia. The diagnosis is based on elevated levels of cholesterol and triglycerides, elevated LDL-cholesterol or triglycerides, or both, in the parents, and a family history of premature CHD (occurring at less than 50 years of age).[12]

FAMILIAL TYPE III HYPERLIPIDEMIA

Familial type III hyperlipidemia is rarely expressed in individuals younger than 20 years of age, although occasional case reports have appeared. It is inherited as an autosomal dominant trait. The clinical presentation in adults is usually in the form of xanthoma in the palmar creases, premature atherosclerosis and CHD.

Diagnosis

The basic defect in this condition is not known. Serum cholesterol and triglycerides are elevated to the same degree. There is an accumulation of LDL which can be identified by ultracentrifugation. The response to treatment is favorable.[60]

APOLIPOPROTEIN DEFICIENCY DISORDERS

Abetalipoproteinemia

Abetalipoproteinemia is a rare autosomal recessive disorder characterized by absence of apo B–containing lipoproteins (chylomicrons, LDL, VLDL). The molecular basis of the disorder is unknown. Parents of an affected individual are normolipidemic.[26]

Clinical Presentation

In the neonatal period, poor feeding, vomiting, loose voluminous stools, and a picture of failure to thrive is present. Subsequent growth and psychomotor development is slow and severe ataxia may present before age 20 years. Neurologic manifestations include loss of stretch reflexes (posterior column degeneration of the spinocerebellar pathway), loss of position and vibratory senses (proprioceptive pathway), and a positive Romberg sign. Cerebellar signs, dysdiadochokinesia, dysmetria, scanning of speech, hypotonia, asthenia, and intention tremor are present. Retinitis pigmentosa is a constant finding. Night blindness and loss of visual acuity have variable presentation. Nystagmus is common and occasionally ptosis and ophthalmoplegia have been reported. Acanthocytosis is a predominant feature of abetalipoproteinemia. Acanthocytes are deformed red cells with severeal spikes protruding from the surface. The deformity is perhaps due to an abnormal ratio of phosphotidylcholine to sphingomyelin (1:06) in the red cell membrane, reflecting the abnormal plasma lipoproteins. Severe anemia is often present, but may have a nutritional basis.

Diagnosis

The constellation of fat malabsorption, retinitis pigmentosa, acanthocytosis, and neuromuscular manifestations should raise suspicion of abetalipoproteinemia. Plasma cholesterol and triglycerides are usually very low. Confirmation of the diagnosis requires demonstration of the absence of apo B in plasma.

Treatment

Administration of vitamin E has been successful in preventing the neurologic and retinal lesions, provided therapy is initiated during the first 18 months of life.[42] The recommended dose is 100 mg/kg/day of α-tocopherol. Dietary restriction of long-chain fatty acids is helpful in relieving the gastrointestinal manifestations. Substitution of fat-soluble vitamins A and D is not apparently required. With this type of therapy, retinal and neurologic manifestations have been delayed for as long as 10 years.[43]

Familial Hypobetalipoproteinemia

This is a rare genetic disorder with autosomal recessive transmission. The lipoprotein abnormality is similar to abetalipoproteinemia. However, LDL is detectable. In addition, concentrations of lipoproteins (LDL and VLDL) are low in heterozygous parents.[26]

Clinical Presentations

Gastrointestinal manifestations are related to fat malabsorption. Hepatic steatosis may be present. Neurologic manifestations are limited to absent deep tendon reflexes. Pigmentary retinopathy has been described. Acanthocytes are present and red blood cells demonstrate lipoprotein abnormality. Growth failure does not occur when the nutritional deficiencies are corrected.[56]

Diagnosis

The plasma cholesterol concentration is low and usually below 100 mg/dL. The triglyceride concentration is less than 50 mg/dL. LDL and VLDL are detectable and the HDL concentration is usually normal. Obligate heterozygotes demonstrate a 50% reduction in their lipoprotein concentration.

Treatment

Treatment is limited to supplementation of fat-soluble vitamins.

Familial High-Density Lipoprotein Deficiency (Tangier Disease)

Tangier disease is a rare abnormality of HDL deficiency presenting in childhood with large orange-colored tonsils. The first case of this condition, a 5-year-old boy, was discovered in Tangier Island of Chesapeake Bay in Virginia.[18] Few other cases have been reported.

Clinical Presentation

The enlarged, lobulated orange tonsils are the earliest recognizable findings. Splenomegaly and lymphadenopathy are invariably present. Thrombocytopenia and reticulocytosis may necessitate splenectomy. Hepatomegaly has been reported in about one-third of the cases. Neuropathy is usually mild, although it could become progressive. Typically, deep tendon reflexes are diminished and muscle atrophy and loss of pain and sensation are present. Corneal clouding may occur.

Diagnosis

The combination of low cholesterol and elevated triglycerides are characteristic of the disorder. HDL usually is absent, or present in trace quantities. Chylomicronemia is present for up to 12 hours in postabsorptive states. VLDL concentration is normal or moderately elevated. LDL in Tangier disease has an abnormal composition in that the triglyceride content is increased to 30% (6% in normal controls). Apolipoproteins A-I and A-II are markedly diminished. However, lipolytic enzyme activity, particularly that of LCAT, appears to be intact. Despite reduced HDL activity, CHD at an early age has not been observed. This is related to the low cholesterol and LDL concentrations that are usually present.[52]

Treatment

No effective treatment is available. Dietary modification of fats might be considered.

Familial Lecithin-Cholesterol Acyltransferase Deficiency

Familial LCAT deficiency is a genetic abnormality of lipoprotein metabolism resulting from deficiency of the LCAT enzyme. Patients present with ocular, hematologic, and renal abnormalities and early atherosclerosis. The primary lipoprotein abnormality involves HDL, although abnormalities of LDL and VLDL are often present.[46] Early death results from atherosclerotic heart disease or renal failure.

Clinical Presentation

Corneal opacities are present from early childhood. The opacities consist of numerous grayish dots scattered throughout the cornea, leading to the cloudly appearance. The increased number of these opacities near the limbal area produces a circular band resembling arcus senilis. A normochromic anemia is present. Erythrocytes are abnormal in appearance and lipid composition. Proteinuria of moderate amount is present and may persist for several years before renal insufficiency develops. Several patients have developed early atherosclerosis.

Lipoprotein Profile

Lipoprotein abnormalities involve all major classes of lipoproteins. Both composition and shape of the lipoproteins are affected. Cholesterol and triglyceride levels are usually increased. Concentrations of unesterified cholesterol and phosphatidylcholine are increased and those of cholesteryl esters and lysolecithin decreased.[47]

Treatment

The only form of therapy at present is repeated blood transfusions to replace enzyme activity. Dietary restriction of fat has been recommended. Kidney transplantation in patients with renal failure has been performed.

HYPERCHOLESTEROLEMIA AS A MAJOR RISK FACTOR FOR ADULT CORONARY HEART DISEASE

The hypothesis that cholesterol plays a major role in the development of adult CHD has gained increasing support in recent years. In addition to overwhelming evidence derived from epidemiologic, experimental, and interventional studies, longitudinal studies of blood lipids and cholesterol in children and young adults indicate that atherosclerotic CHD may have its origin in childhood.

Several population studies have revealed a direct correlation between blood cholesterol levels and the incidence of CHD. This correlation extends to the pediatric population.[39] In Western countries with a high incidence of CHD, such as the United States, a high level of cholesterol is found in children less than 10 years old. Conversely, in countries with a low incidence of CHD, the level of cholesterol in children is low.[4,34] Genetic studies provide the strongest evidence for the role of cholesterol in atherosclerotic CHD. Children who suffer from familial hypercholesterolemia develop atherosclerosis and CHD at very young ages in the absence of other risk factors.[35,54] In experimental animals, the process of atherosclerosis may be initiated by a high cholesterol diet and alleviated by reducing cholesterol intake.[50]

Pathologic studies of humans have indicated a progressive course for the development of atheromas and atherosclerotic CHD. The process begins with the appearance of fatty streaks in the aorta and evolves to the formation of raised plaques and atheromatous lesions in the wall of the arteries. Fatty streaks, the earliest lesion attributable to hypercholesterolemia, have been observed as early as the second decade of life.[29] In a population study of children in Bogalusa, Louisiana, aortic fatty streaks found at postmortem examination were strongly related to antemortem levels of blood cholesterol.[45]

Clinical and interventional studies support the contention that hypercholesterolemia is a major risk factor in CHD. The Lipid Research Clinics' coronary primary prevention trials evaluated the effect of lowering blood cholesterol on the incidence of CHD in hypercholesterolemic subjects. In the group on a low cholesterol diet receiving cholestyramine, the incidence of CHD was significantly lower than in the group given diet and placebo.[40] Similar studies from other countries have confirmed these observations.[19]

The National Institutes of Health Consensus Development Conference on lowering blood cholesterol to prevent heart disease, after considering the body of evidence, issued guidelines for identifying and treating hypercholesterolemia in the general population.[44] They recommend that children at high risk be identified primarily by a carefully obtained family history, rather than by routine screening. The history should include parents, grandparents, and all first-degree relatives. A positive family history of hypercholesterolemia or premature CHD, occurring at less than 50 years of age, would necessitate two blood cholesterol determinations. In those children whose blood cholesterol level falls outside the low-risk range, i.e., above the 75th percentile (Table 12–9), consideration should be given to diet therapy alone or diet in combination with a lipid-lowering agent.

The American Academy of Pediatrics has made similar recommendations.[11] These recommendations include regular elective testing of children older than 2 years who have a family history (parent, sibling, grandparent, uncle, aunt) of hyperlipidemia or early myocardial infarction (<50 years of age in men; <60 years of age in women); several determinations of fasting cholesterol, triglycerides, and HDL cholesterol in children with borderline or elevated levels of cholesterol; exclusion of secondary hyperlipidemias; dietary intervention for children with values persistently exceeding the 75th percentile (176 mg/dL); and pharmacotherapy for children with cholesterol levels above the 95th percentile (200 mg/dL) after failure of dietary intervention.

Since the publication of these guidelines several groups of investigators have examined the reliability of family history as the sole determinant of risk for CHD. The findings point to the fact that screening by family history alone does not identify all children with hypercholesterolemia at risk for CHD.[13,27] Since several longitudinal studies have tracked cholesterol beginning at a young age,[38] and it is well known that eating habits are established early in life, proponents of routine screening argue that early screening will identify most, if not all, children at risk, and will offer the opportunity of early intervention at a time when dietary habits have not been firmly established.[20]

MANAGEMENT OF HYPERCHOLESTEROLEMIA IN CHILDREN

Whether by routine screening or by family history, an elevated total cholesterol concentration (above the 75th percentile for age) should be repeated after fasting and complemented by measurement of triglycerides and HDL cholesterol. LDL cholesterol can be calculated by the formula LDL cholesterol = total cholesterol − (HDL + triglycerides/5). Secondary hypercholesterolemia, particularly in the presence of hypothyroidism, should be ruled out by appropriate studies. For cholesterol levels in the upper quartile of the normal range for age, dietary counseling may suffice. In children with a total cholesterol level greater than 200 mg/dL, a lipid profile of the parents should be obtained to establish the genetic basis of the hypercholesterolemia. Management of hypercholesterolemia in such families may be initiated by implementing an appropriate diet. Guidelines for dietary levels of cholesterol and saturated and unsaturated fatty acids have been published.[14] The principles of a low-fat diet are as follows:

TABLE 12–9.
Normal Values for Plasma Lipid and Lipoprotein Cholesterol Concentrations*†

Age	Plasma Cholesterol (mg/dL)					Plasma Triglycerides (mg/dL)			VLDL Cholesterol (mg/dL)			LDL Cholesterol (mg/dL)					HDL Cholesterol (mg/dL)				HDL/Cholesterol Ratio		
	10	25	50	75	90	10	50	90	10	50	90	10	25	50	75	90	10	25	50	90	10	50	90
Males																							
0–4	125	137	151	171	186	33	51	84	—	—	—	—	—	—	—	—	—	—	—	—	—	—	—
5–9	130	143	159	175	191	33	51	85	2	7	15	69	80	90	103	117	42	49	54	70	0.27	0.36	0.44
10–14	127	140	155	173	190	37	59	102	2	9	18	72	81	94	109	122	40	49	55	71	0.26	0.34	0.43
15–19	120	132	146	165	183	43	69	120	3	12	23	68	80	93	109	123	34	39	46	59	0.21	0.30	0.41
20–24	130	146	165	186	204	50	86	165	5	12	24	73	85	101	118	138	32	38	45	57	0.19	0.28	0.39
25–29	143	159	178	202	227	54	95	199	6	15	31	75	96	116	138	157	32	37	44	58	0.17	0.25	0.37
30–34	148	167	190	213	239	58	104	213	8	18	36	88	107	124	144	166	32	38	45	59	0.16	0.24	0.34
35–39	157	176	197	223	249	62	113	251	7	19	46	92	110	131	154	176	31	36	43	58	0.15	0.21	0.30
40–44	163	182	203	228	250	64	122	248	8	21	43	98	115	135	157	173	31	36	43	60	0.15	0.21	0.30
45–49	169	188	210	234	258	68	154	253	8	20	40	106	120	141	163	186	33	38	45	60	0.15	0.21	0.29
50–54	169	187	210	235	261	68	124	250	10	23	49	102	118	143	162	185	31	36	44	58	0.14	0.21	0.28
55–59	167	189	212	235	262	67	119	235	6	19	39	103	126	145	168	191	31	38	46	64	0.15	0.22	0.34
60–64	171	188	210	235	259	68	119	235	4	16	35	106	121	143	165	188	34	41	49	69	0.16	0.24	0.33
65–69	170	190	210	233	258	64	112	208	6	16	40	104	125	146	170	199	33	39	49	74	0.15	0.23	0.34
70+	162	182	205	229	252	67	111	212	3	15	31	100	119	142	164	182	33	40	48	70	0.16	0.24	0.34
Females																							
0–4	120	139	156	172	189	38	59	96	—	—	—	—	—	—	—	—	—	—	—	—	—	—	—
5–9	134	146	163	179	195	36	55	90	1	9	19	73	88	98	115	125	38	47	52	67	0.24	0.32	0.43
10–14	131	144	158	174	190	44	70	114	3	10	20	73	81	94	110	126	40	45	52	64	0.25	0.33	0.42
15–19	126	139	154	171	190	44	66	107	4	11	20	67	78	93	110	127	38	43	51	68	0.24	0.33	0.44
20–24	130	143	160	182	203	41	64	112	3	10	22	62	80	98	113	136	37	43	50	68	0.22	0.32	0.42
25–29	136	151	168	187	209	42	65	116	4	11	22	73	87	103	122	141	40	47	55	73	0.22	0.33	0.43
30–34	139	154	172	193	213	44	69	123	2	9	20	73	89	108	126	142	40	46	55	71	0.22	0.32	0.42
35–39	147	163	182	202	225	46	73	137	3	13	26	81	96	116	139	161	38	44	52	74	0.19	0.30	0.43
40–44	154	170	191	214	235	51	82	155	5	12	26	89	105	120	145	164	39	48	55	78	0.19	0.28	0.41
45–49	161	177	199	224	247	53	87	171	4	14	32	90	105	127	150	173	39	46	56	78	0.19	0.28	0.39
50–54	172	192	215	241	268	59	97	186	4	14	32	102	118	141	169	192	40	49	59	77	0.15	0.26	0.35
55–59	183	204	228	253	282	63	106	204	4	18	40	103	126	148	176	204	39	47	58	82	0.17	0.26	0.36
60–64	186	203	228	254	280	64	105	202	3	13	30	105	130	151	172	201	43	49	60	85	0.14	0.25	0.36
65–69	183	208	229	256	280	66	112	204	3	15	36	104	128	156	189	208	38	46	60	79	0.14	0.25	0.38
70+	180	200	226	256	278	69	111	204	0	13	34	107	126	146	170	189	37	48	60	82	0.16	0.26	0.37

*From JB Lippincott Co, *Principles and Practice of Endocrinology and Metabolism*, Becker KL (ed). Philadelphia, 1990, p 1231. Used by permission.
†Based on Lipid Research Clinics population studies in the United States and Canada for white males and females (non-sex hormone users) as derived from NHI publication No. 80-1527, 1980. All subjects were sampled in the fasting state.

1. Calories: Appropriate for age, rate of growth, and activities
2. Caloric distribution:
   a. 55% carbohydrates, mostly complex carbohydrates
   b. 30% fat
   c. 15% protein
3. Fat distribution:
   a. 10% saturated fatty acids
   b. 10% polyunsaturated fatty acids
   c. 10% monounsaturated fatty acids
4. Cholesterol: 100 mg/1,000 calories, not to exceed 300 mg/24 hr

Following implementation of a low fat diet, a reduction of 10% to 15% in the levels of cholesterol and LDL may be expected. This should be confirmed by repeat determination of the lipid profile after 3 months. If the desired reduction (10% to 15%) does not occur, an attempt should be made to increase intake of dietary fiber. This may be accomplished by increasing the consumption of foods high in fiber (e.g., whole wheat bread, bran cereal, leafy vegetables, fruits), or by supplementing the diet with commercially available preparations. Since hypertension, obesity, and cigarette smoking are considered additional risk factors for the development of CHD, appropriate preventive measures should be taken.

The question of drug intervention in the pediatric age group with nongenetic hypercholesterolemia at slight to moderately increased risk (cholesterol >175 and <250) has not been resolved. In children with heterozygous familial hypercholesterolemia, diet alone will not reduce cholesterol below the high-risk level (250 mg/dL), and therefore drug intervention must be implemented.

If dietary modification and increased dietary fiber does not produce the desired effect, then one of the lipid-lowering drugs should be administered (Table 12–10). Bile acid sequestrants have been used in children as the first drug of choice with success.[21] The dose of cholestyramine necessary to reduce cholesterol to normal levels is directly proportional to the pretreatment levels of cholesterol and may be given twice daily.[16] In children and young adults, a dose of 1 to 16 g/day (average 7 g/day) is necessary to effectively reduce cholesterol concentrations. Long-term studies in

TABLE 12–10.
Some Characteristics of Lipid-Lowering Drugs*

Drug	Mechanism of Action	Effects on Lipoproteins			Major Side Effects
		LDL	VLDL-TG	HDL	
Cholestyramine Colestipol	Bile acid sequestrants	↓	↑	↑	Nausea, constipation
Clofibrate Gemfibrazol	↑ Intravascular catabolism of VLDL, IDL	↑	↓	↑	Myalgia, gallstones
Niacin	↓ VLDL production	↓	↓	↑	Flushing, pruritus, ↑ liver enzymes, hyperglycemia
Lovastatin Pravastatin	Inhibition of cholesterol synthesis, ↑ LDL removal	↓	↓	↑	Myalgia, ↑ liver enzymes, nausea, diarrhea

*TG = triglycerides; ↓ = decreases; ↑ = increases.

hypercholesterolemic children have emphasized the need for strict dietary adherence in order for pharmacologic therapy to succeed.

Experience with the new antilipid drugs in the pediatric age group is limited. These drugs, lovastatin and its analogue pravastatin, act by inhibiting HMG-CoA reductase, the enzyme that catalyzes the rate-limiting step in intracellular cholesterol biosynthesis.[58] A critical factor in the long-term success of dietary and pharmacologic intervention in familial hypercholesterolemia is patient compliance. Dietary adherence might be difficult to enforce for an indefinite period and pharmacologic therapy is both expensive and not readily accepted by all families.

REFERENCES

1. Balfour JF, Kim R: Homozygous type II hyperlipoproteinemia treatment. Partial ileal bypass in two children. *JAMA* 1974; 227:1145.
2. Bierman EL, Glomset JA: Disorders of lipid metabolism, in Wilson JD, Foster DW (eds): *Textbook of Endocrinology*. Philadelphia, WB Saunders Co, 1985, p 1108.
3. Bilheimer DW, et al: Mevinolin and colestipol stimulate receptor-mediated clearance of low-density lipoprotein from plasma in familial hypercholesterolemia heterozygotes. *Proc Natl Acad Sci USA* 1983; 80:4124.
4. Blackburn H: Conference on the health effects of blood lipids: Optimal distribution for populations. *Prev Med* 1979; 8:612.
5. Bounik J, et al: Early effects of thyroidectomy and triiodothyonine administration on rat liver mitochondria. *Mol Cell Endocrinol* 1979; 15:1.
6. Bown MS, Goldstein JL: A receptor mediated pathway for cholesterol homeostasis. *Science* 1986; 233:34.
7. Breckenridge WC, et al: Hypertriglyceridemia associated with a deficiency of apolipoprotein C-II. *N Engl J Med* 1978; 298:1265.
8. Breslow JL: Human apolipoprotein molecular biology and genetic variation. *Annu Rev Biochem* 1985; 54:699.
9. Brown MS, Goldstein JL: Familial hypercholesterolemia: A genetic defect in the low-density lipoprotein receptor. *N Engl J Med* 1976; 294:1386.
10. Brown MS et al: Prenatal diagnosis of homozygous familial hypercholesterolemia. *Lancet* 1978; 1:526.
11. Committee on Nutrition: Indications for cholesterol testing in children. *Pediatrics* 1989; 83:141.
12. Cortner JA, Coats PM, Gallagher PR: Prevalence and expression of familial combined hyperlipidemia in childhood. *J Pediatr* 1990; 116:514.
13. Dennison BA, et al: Parental history of cardiovascular disease as an indication for screening for lipoprotein abnormalities in children. *J Pediatr* 1989; 115:186.
14. Dietary guidelines for Healthy Americans: A statement for physicians and health professionals by the Nutrition Committee, American Heart Association. *Arteriosclerosis* 1988; 8:218A.
15. Eckel RH: Lipoprotein lipase. A multifunctional enzyme relevant to common metabolic diseases. *N Engl J Med* 1989; 321:1060–1068.
16. Farah JR, Kwiterovich PO Jr, Neill CA: Dose-effect relation of cholesteryramine in children and young adults with familial hypercholesterolemia. *Lancet* 1977; 1:59.
17. Fielding CJ: Mechanism of action of lecithin-cholesterol acylatransferase. *Methods Enzymol* 1986; 129:783.

18. Frederickson S, et al: Tangier disease: Combined clinical staff conference at the NIH. *Ann Intern Med* 1961; 55:1016.

19. Frick MH, et al: Helsinky heart study: Primary-prevention trial with gemfibrozil in middle-aged men with dyslipidemia. *N Engl J Med* 1987; 317:1237.

20. Glueck CJ: Pediatric primary prevention of atherosclerosis. *N Engl J Med* 1986; 314:175.

21. Glueck CJ, et al: Therapy of familial hypercholesterolemia in childhood: Diet and cholestyramin resin for 24 to 36 months. *Pediatrics* 1977; 59:433.

22. Goldstein JL, Brown MS: Familial hypercholesterolemia, *The Metabolic Basis of Inherited Disease.* In Stanbury, et al (eds). New York, McGraw-Hill Book Co, Inc, 1983, p 627.

23. Goldstein JL, et al: Hyperlipidemia in coronary heart disease. II. Genetic analysis of lipid levels in 176 families and delineation of a new inherited disorder, familial combined hyperlipidemia. *J Clin Invest* 1973; 52:1544.

24. Gordon DJ, Rifkind BM: High density lipoprotein—the clinical implications of recent studies. *N Engl J Med* 1989; 321:1311–1316.

25. Gotto AM Jr, Powell HJ, Havel RJ: Introduction to the plasma lipoproteins. *Methods Enzymol* 1986; 128:3.

26. Granot E, Deckelbaum RJ: Hypocholesterolemia in childhood. *J Pediatr* 1989; 115:171.

27. Griffith TC, et al: Family history evaluation as a predictive screen for childhood hypercholesterolemia. *Pediatrics* 1989; 84:365.

28. Havel RJ: Origin, metabolic fate and metabolic function of plasma lipoproteins, in Steingerg D, Olefsky J (eds): *Contemporary issues in endocrinology and metabolism* vol 3, New York, Churchill Livingston Inc, 1987, p 117.

29. Holman RL, et al: The natural history of atherosclerosis: The early aortic lesions as seen in New Orleans in the middle of the 20th century. *Am J Pathol* 1968; 34:209.

30. Jackson RL: Lipoprotein lipase and hepatic lipase, in Boyer PD (ed): *The Enzymes*, vol 16, New York, Academic Press, 1984, p 141.

31. John D, Brunzell: Familial lipoprotein lipase deficiency and other causes of the chylomicronemia syndrome, in Scriver ER, et al (eds): *Metabolic Basis of Inherited Disease.* New York, McGraw-Hill Book Co, Inc, 1990, chap 45.

32. Kihara S, et al: Autoimmune hyperchylomicronemia. *N Engl J Med* 1989; 320:1255.

33. King ME, Breslow JL, Lees RS: Plasma exchange therapy of homozygous familial hypercholesterolemia. *N Engl J Med* 1980; 302:1457.

34. Knuiman JT, Hermus RJJ, Hautvast JGAJ: Serum total and high density lipoprotein cholesterol concentrations in rural and urban boys from 16 countries. *Atherosclerosis* 1980; 36:529.

35. Kwiterovich PO, Frederickson DS, Levy RI: Familial hypercholesterolemia (one form of familial type II hyperlipoproteinemia): A study of its biochemical, genetic, and clinical presentation in childhood. *J Clin Invest* 1974; 53:1237.

36. Kwiterovich PO Jr: Neonatal screening for hyperlipidemia. *Pediatrics* 1974; 53:455.

37. LaRosa JC: Effect of estrogen replacement therapy in lipids. *J Reprod Med* 1985; 30(suppl 10):811.

38. Lauer RM, Lee J, Clark WR: Factors affecting the relationship between childhood and adult cholesterol levels: The Muscatine study. *Pediatrics* 1988; 82:309.

39. Lee J, Lauer RM, Clark WR: Lipoprotein in the progeny of young men with coronory artery disease: Children with increased risk. *Pediatrics* 1986; 78:330.

40. Lipid Research Clinics Program: The lipid research clinic coronary primary prevention trial results. I. Reduction in incidence of coronary heart disease. *JAMA* 1984; 251:351.

41. Mabuchi H, et al: Reduction of serum cholesterol in heterozygous patients with familial

hypercholesterolemia. Additive effects of compactin and cholestyramine. *N Engl J Med* 1983; 208:609.

42. Muller DP, Lloyd JK, Bird AC: Long-term management of abetalipoproteinemia: Possible role for vitamin E. *Arch Dis Child* 1977; 52:209.
43. Muller DP, Lloyd JK, Wolff OH: The role of vitamin E in the treatment of neurological features of abetalipoproteinemia and other disorders of fat absorption. *J Inherit Metab Dis* 1985; 8(suppl 1): 88.
44. NIH Consensus Development Conference: Lower blood cholesterol to prevent heart disease. *JAMA* 1985; 253:2080.
45. Newman WP, et al: Serum lipoproteins and systolic blood pressure are related to atherosclerosis in early life: the Bogalusa Heart Study. *N Engl J Med* 1986; 314:138.
46. Norum KR, Gyone E: Familial plasma lecithin-acyltransferase deficiency: Biochemical study of a new inborn error of metabolism. *Scand J Clin Lab Invest* 1976; 20:231.
47. Norum KR, Gyone E, Glomset JA: Familial lecithin: cholesterol acyltransferase deficiency, including fish eye disease, in Scriver CR, et al (eds): *Metabolic Basis of Inherited Disease*. New York, McGraw-Hill Book Co, Inc, 1990, chap 46.
48. Oster P, et al: Effect of estrogens and progesterones on lipid metabolism. *Am J Obstet Gynecol* 1982; 142:773.
49. Reaven EP, Kilterman OG, Reaven GM: Ultrastructural and physiological evidence for corticosteroid-induced alterations in hepatic production of very low density lipoprotein particles. *J Lipid Res* 1974; 15:74.
50. Ross R: The pathogenesis of atherosclerosis—An update. *N Eng J Med* 1986; 314:488.
51. Schaffer EJ, Levy RI: Pathogenesis and management of lipoprotein disorders. *N Engl J Med* 1985; 312:1300–1310.
52. Schaffer EJ, et al: Metabolism of high-density lipoprotein apolipoproteins in Tangier disease. *N Engl J Med* 1978; 299:905.
53. Shepherd J, et al: Cholestyramine promotes receptor-mediated low-density lipoprotein catabolism. *N Engl J Med* 1980; 302:1219.
54. Sprecher DS, et al: Cardiovascular features of homozygous familial hypercholesterolemia: Analysis of sixteen patients. *Am J Cardiol* 1984; 54:20.
55. Starzl TE, et al: Heart-liver transplantation in a patient with familial hypercholesterolemia. *Lancet* 1984; 1:1382.
56. Stein EA: Familial hyperbetalipoproteinemia. *Am J Dis Child* 1977; 131:1363.
57. Stein EA, et al: Portacaval shunt in four patients with homozygous hypercholesterolemia. *Lancet* 1975; 1:832.
58. Tobert JA, et al: Rapid and sustained lowering of human serum cholesterol by an inhibition of hydroxymethylglutaryl coenzyme A reductase. *Atherosclerosis* 1981; 41:61.
59. Torvisk H, et al: Effects of intravenous hyperalimentation on plasma lipoproteins in severe familial hypercholesterolemia. *Lancet* 1975; 1:601.
60. West RJ, Lloyd JK: Hypercholesterolemia in childhood. *Adv Pediatr* 26:1.
61. Yamamoto A, Sudo H, Endo A: Therapeutic effects of ML-236B in primary hypercholesterolemia. *Atherosclerosis* 1980; 35:259.

Chapter 13

Psychologic Aspects of Pediatric Endocrine Disorders

W. Douglas Tynan

Specific psychologic aspects of endocrine disorders can be classified into three areas of concern. The first is the direct effect of the endocrine disorder and its treatment on the nervous system and cognitive ability. Second are the effects of the disorder and treatment on social, emotional, and gender-specific behaviors. Third is the issue of behavior problems and personality style. These problems include poor adherence to treatment regimen by the family and child and possible family conflicts, as well as emotional reactions to changes in body image, and other effects of the disorder.

DISORDERS OF GROWTH

The body of older research studies of growth disorders have indicated that there is a complex set of emotional, behavioral, and cognitive effects in children, regardless of the physiologic etiology of poor growth. These studies indicated that these difficulties included poor self-esteem, poor school performance, and somewhat lowered intelligence quotient (IQ) scores. Later studies indicated that children with growth hormone deficiency were retained more frequently in school, did poorer on neuropsychological tests, and suffered more emotional difficulties than controls.[19] Regardless of the specific hormonal etiology of children with short stature, a greater percentage of them fail one or more grades and are not promoted in school, even though, as a group, they tend to have average intellectual ability as measured by IQ scores.

Several studies indicate a higher rate of learning disabilities[7] overall. Those who do fail a grade and are not promoted in school suffer a very high rate of learning disabilities and emotional problems. School failure and retention, then, are strong indicators for a referral for mental health services. In particular, children with learning disabilities also are at high risk for attention deficit, conduct or oppositional disorders, and need appropriate psychological or psychiatric treatment.

Poor growth due to environmental factors, which includes the diagnoses of reversible hyposomatotropinism, psychosocial dwarfism, or failure to thrive, inevitably includes poor cognitive and social development as part of the syndrome. Following the diagnosis, medical and psychosocial intervention can result in dramatic improvement, but there are usually long-term cognitive and emotional sequelae that require ongoing monitoring and treatment.[1] For both physiologic and environmentally induced short stature, contrary to the common clinical lore, age and greater maturity do not improve the impulsivity and conduct problems that often co-occur. These problems require professional evaluation and appropriate psychotherapeutic treatment.

Obesity is one of the most common conditions referred to pediatricians. Current estimates are that 10% to 25% of all American children are obese, and it has been the subject of extensive and varied research. Indeed, the definition of obesity itself is not agreed upon. Possible measures include comparisons of weight for height, weight compared with others of the same age, total body mass, and percentages of body fat. The most serious risk is the tendency of obese children to remain obese throughout their life, and 80% of them become obese adults. Socially, they have a more difficult time, and have emotional problems related to body image and self-esteem. This is usually the result of teasing and being systematically excluded from games and activities with other children. In adolescence, they are less likely to date or become involved in activities outside of school.[4] It is often difficult to convince patients and their parents to enter treatment. Because of the high initial motivation of those families who finally decide to enter treatment, programs often result in initial weight loss. However, the major drawback of short-term weight loss programs is the high probability for relapse after the program has ended. Thus, any program should be planned with long-term maintenance and follow-up.[4]

Long-term studies in the treatment of obesity in children have been carried out by Epstein and colleagues.[6] Their outcome studies have demonstrated that successful treatment involves permanent change in family eating and activity patterns. Children with obese parents do not do well unless the parents also lose weight. The comprehensive treatment programs include diet information that is simple and direct,[5] behavioral management strategies to learn new eating habits, and the establishment of increased daily activity and exercise levels. Increased daily activity includes using stairs instead of elevators, walking more, and decreased television viewing. Programmed, planned exercise such as jogging works well during initial weight loss, but tends not to be maintained over several years. Psychotherapy is effective in managing the emotional upset related to obesity, including social withdrawal and depression, but has not been shown to be an effective method of weight reduction.[4] Thus a child who is both obese and has emotional difficulties often needs to have both areas of concern addressed.

Diabetes mellitus is the most common endocrinologic problem in children and its behavioral effects vary with age of onset, duration, and age of the child. Among children diagnosed before age 5 years, there is an increased risk of learning disability.[18] In the treatment of younger children, those less than 7 years old, there are relatively few behavior problems. The incidence rate of needle phobias or noncompliance is quite low, and the occurrence of such phobias is usually a behavior learned from a phobic individual in the home. The most frequent problems in this age range are recognition of hypoglycemic episodes and food refusals. Children less than 7 years old usually cannot reliably report symptoms of hypoglycemia and adults need to monitor their behavior and interpret it to the child. Food refusals or extremely slow eating patterns are the most disruptive behaviors in this age group. A very effective treatment for this is to establish a reward system[15] for eating quickly at mealtimes, and to teach parents to play with and pay attention to their child at other times of the day. Younger children should be allowed to participate in injections and blood tests, but they should not be forced to do these procedures. If they choose to do these procedures themselves, they should be done under strict observation and supervision. The parent should still do the procedures some of the time. Children under 8 years of age who do these procedures by themselves make a large number of critical errors.[9]

Children of ages 8 to 12 also manage quite well. However, learning disabilities or school behavior problems may now become evident. Parents often attribute these difficulties to the diabetes. Regardless of the cause, referral should be made for a psychological or psychiatric evaluation by a professional who is knowledgeable about diabetes, and who will actively consult with the physician. For learning disabilities secondary to the diabetes, standard psychoeducational evaluation and appropriate special education programs are indicated.

The major problems in diabetes usually occur in adolescence. Studies demonstrate that this is the most frequent time for readmissions,[8] increased family conflicts, and worsening metabolic control.[9] Although it is common practice to allow adolescents to take over full self-care of their diabetes, there are no empiric studies to support this strategy. Letting the patient take over briefly reduces family conflicts, but usually results in a worsened metabolic state. Therapeutic interventions should be family-oriented and address the specific goals of how the patient's diabetes care will be managed. The adolescent patient needs to understand that regardless of age, other family members will always be concerned about his or her health, and that true independence means knowing how and when to accept help and suggestions. Parents need to learn to supervise and help in their adolescent child's care without nagging or engaging in arguments. To encourage families to stay involved, some time should be given to making concrete suggestions on how to keep parents and adolescents involved in a mutual contract. These suggestions could include simple contracts[16] making privileges contingent upon good diabetes self-care. In addition, the parent should observe or do one injection per week, and closely monitor one or two blood tests. Affective reactions to diabetes can be particularly strong during adolescence. Depressive symptoms in both patients and parents, particularly mothers,[9] are common in this population. These emotional reactions are particularly damaging because the depressed affect may directly interfere with the motivation for self-care. This can result in physical symptoms and further depression. Psychotherapy can be useful to change the patient's mood, increase the activity level, and improve adherence to regimen.

DISORDERS OF SEX HORMONES AND CHROMOSOMES

Behavioral concerns of children and adolescents with sex chromosome and endocrine abnormalities that affect development of the genitalia cover three broad areas: intellectual capacity and school performance; gender identity and sexual functioning; psychopathology and personality characteristics. The two major classes of disorders are disorders of timing of the onset of puberty, either precocious or delayed; and disorders of sex chromosome or endocrine abnormalities that result in the child having an abnormal appearance.

Of the timing disorders, idiopathic precocious puberty (IPP) results in considerable distress and concern in parents. Untreated, these children quickly develop secondary sex characteristics and are physically larger than their same-age peers. However, they may be short as adults because of premature fusion of their epiphyses. Intellectually, studies of children with IPP after age 5 years have documented at least average intellectual ability. There is some evidence of increased lateralization marked by differences between verbal and nonverbal intellectual abilities. Onset of IPP before age 5 has been linked with lowered intellectual ability.[10]

Delayed puberty has been the subject of many studies of intellectual development, and results have been mixed. There is no obvious detrimental effect of later sexual maturity on the child's intellectual capacity. Behavioral expression, particularly sexual behavior and affective expression, are the major concerns of parents of children with these disorders. In boys, free testosterone levels, not pubertal status, predict sexual arousal and behaviors such as masturbation and intent to have intercourse.[13] In girls, androgen levels also predict sexual arousal and behavior, including masturbation. Thus children who are successfully medically treated to suppress androgen levels should have a decrease in the biologic drives of these behaviors.

Because of their physical development and increased sexual arousal, these children are at increased risk for sexual abuse and exploitation by others. If they display specific attempts at intercourse, or attempts at other sexual activity such as oral or anal sexual activity, an evaluation for possible sexual abuse should be carried out. If a child demonstrates knowledge of specific sexual acts, it is likely that he or she has been exposed to those acts in some fashion. Affectively, there has been no documented consistent association between negative, depressed affect, and mood lability and hormonal level in this population.[13] Aggressive behavior in males has long been linked to androgen levels and there is certainly a high probability of increased irritability and aggression in IPP, with the association stronger in boys than in girls. If the aggression remains problematic after treatment, families should be referred for mental health services that are specifically targeted toward helping parents manage these behaviors at home.

The most common etiology of pseudohermaphroditism in females is some form of congenital adrenal hyperplasia (CAH); males are phenotypically normal. In these female patients the external genitalia can range from clitoral enlargement to a male appearance. Sex assignment decisions need to be made as quickly as possible, but not until all of the essential information has been gathered. Genetic sex, potential fertility, and, most important, the functional anatomy of the adult, are the major factors to be considered. Most girls with CAH are raised as females, after having surgical correction. The psychological research on this population has focused on intellectual ability and gender identity issues. The studies of Money et al.[11] indicated that CAH patients had above-average intellectual capabilities compared to national norms. But later, more methodologically rigorous work showed that CAH patients were not different from their peers in general intellectual abilities, and may show enhanced spatial abilities, typically a male pattern.[3] There is no evidence of learning disabilities or intellectual impairment from CAH.

Psychosocial gender differentiation is usually of more concern for parents. Generally, CAH females develop normal female gender identity. Gender role behavior, i.e., the activities and interests of these children, does show some effect of their prenatal hormonal status. There is a preference for these girls to engage in more active play and with toys appropriate for boys, and to have less interest in dolls and other play that is more typical of girls. Along with this play pattern, there is also less concern for clothing and feminine appearance. This occurs in 50% to 70% of these children. In adolescents and adults, studies of the specific sexual preferences of these patients have yielded mixed results. To date, there has not yet been a thorough study of the outcome of children treated early in life. The review of Money et al.[11] indicated higher rates of homosexuality and bisexuality in a late-treated group, with the majority still maintaining a heterosexual preference. One study[12] found low rates, quite comparable to non-CAH women, of homosexuality. Further, this study found that heterosexual activity was related to adequacy of vaginal reconstruction, and emphasized the importance of surgical and medical treatment for development of later heterosexual behavior. Parents need to know that the well-documented masculine play behaviors in childhood are not directly related to eventual sexual orientation, and that the majority of these girls develop heterosexual preferences, with a minority developing homosexual or bisexual preferences. There is no reported personality style associated with CAH.[3]

Males with CAH are phenotypically normal and there is no change in their gender-related behaviors. They demonstrate some increased anxiety and poor self-esteem which appears to be related to their shorter stature. The short stature can result from either poor control of the CAH or from late diagnosis. Microphallus in males can have a number of possible causes. Regardless of etiology, this physical condition often results in anxiety, depression, and possible feelings of helplessness. Adolescent males as a group have a high rate of impulsive and risk-taking behaviors. Thus any patient with evidence of strong emotional response to this condition should be referred immediately to a psychiatrist or psychologist for evaluation and treatment.

Pseudohermaphroditism in males is rare and is caused by a prenatal defect in testosterone synthesis or action. As with the CAH females, determination of genetic sex, potential fertility, and, most important, functional anatomy as an adult, are all factors in the sex assignment. If a female sex assignment is made, these patients, with hormonal treatment, display distinctively feminine patterns of play and socialization. This is probably due to the fact that they are either insensitive to androgens or were never exposed to them, and thus there is no hormonal basis for male behavior patterns.[11] In adolescence, of course, some counseling by the physician or a therapist familiar with these disorders is essential to help these young women deal with their genetic status and their infertility.

Of the genetically linked disorders, Turner syndrome (45,X girls) has been the subject of the most research. A number of early studies suggested that mental retardation was common in this population, but later analysis indicated that the incidence of mental retardation was not as high as first suggested.[17] Specifically, this group is well within normal limits in verbal skills, but as a group show some deficits in spatial abilities, and thus are at some risk for learning disabilities. The group scores also tend to be highly variable which suggests that there is a wide range of ability among individuals, and it is impossible to predict intellectual outcome for any individual based only on this diagnosis.

Physically, this group is marked by short stature and delayed puberty. Studies of gender identity indicate that as a group there is a strong feminine identity with no confusion. Data on sexual functioning are less clear and suggest some lowered sex drive, and less satisfactory sexual relationships. Turner syndrome is not associated with severe psychopathology, or a particular personality style. However, there are several studies that indicate a high degree of immaturity and hyperactivity in latency-age girls.[2] Post-puberty, these girls have higher rates of anxious and depressive symptoms, as well as lowered self-esteem, and poor social adaptation.

Treatment with replacement hormones has yielded no known adverse side effects. It appears that hormonal replacement is best done to coincide with the usual age of onset of puberty, and that most problems occur in patients who are diagnosed late and have replacement therapy initiated much later in adolescence.

Unlike Turner syndrome, 47,XXX females do not have identifiable physical features other than tallness, and onset of puberty is not delayed. There is a higher rate of cognitive impairment and learning problems in this group, and it is likely that psychosocial problems can develop secondary to their cognitive difficulties. There is no evidence of a typical behavioral profile, but these girls tend to have difficulty developing good peer relationships. There is no evidence that this disorder is associated with severe psychopathology or thought disorder. Further, there are no known problems in gender identity.

The three genetic syndromes that involve one extra sex chromosome (47,XXY, 47,XYY, 47,XXX) and rarer disorders involving more than one extra chromosome are rarely identified at birth, because the affected infant appears normal. There is evidence of some cognitive impairment, increased rates of learning disability, and social difficulties for these children. As such, all should be screened for learning problems and when such problems occur, they should receive appropriate evaluations and school placement. In addition, the social problems should also be assessed and treated appropriately through individual or group psychotherapy. As with any physical disorder that makes a child different, these children have self-esteem problems that interfere with their forming good social relationships. Specific therapy groups designed to improve a child's social skills, as well as structured activities, can do much to improve social functioning, and prevent the isolation and depression that these children often experience.

Depressive disorders have a range of severity from mild dysthymia and moodiness to severe dysfunction and suicidal ideation. Medical evaluation and treatment is essential for all of these patients, and for those whose affective state does not improve with treatment, psychotherapy is an important addition to their care. Even if the depressive condition has an endocrinologic basis, psychotherapy may be indicated. These behaviors and thoughts will not automatically improve with medical treatment and will need to be addressed in therapy in a systematic fashion.

Finally, the critical behavioral concern that has a direct impact on the treatment of endocrine disorders is adherence to the prescribed regimen. Adherence to treatment is problematic in all populations of patients. It is estimated that up to 60% of all prescriptions are not filled and taken properly[14] in pediatric populations. Thus, when a patient is not responding well to treatment, or when blood levels are not at an expected therapeutic level, it is highly probable that poor adherence to treatment has occurred. An effective method of interview is to ask the patient or the parents quite specifically what they have done in the past 24 to 48 hours with regard to medication. This type of detailed structured interview has been shown to provide a better representative sample of the patient's adherence behavior. There is always a tendency for parents to only give medicine when a child is symptomatic, and it is difficult to maintain adherence when no symptoms are present.

REFERENCES

1. Annecillo C, Money J, Lobato C: Intelligence (IQ) lost and regained: The psychoneuroendocrinology of failure to thrive, catch up growth, the syndrome of abuse dwarfism and Munchausen's syndrome by proxy, in CS Holmes (ed): *Psychoneuroendocrinology, Brain, Behavior and Hormonal Interactions*. New York, Springer-Verlag, 1990.
2. Berch DB: Psychological aspects of Turner syndrome. *Adolesc Pediatr Gynecol* 1989; 2:175–180.
3. Berenbaum SA: Congenital adrenal hyperplasia: Intellectual and psychosexual functioning, in CS Holmes (ed): *Psychoneuroendocrinology, Brain, Behavior and Hormonal Interactions*. New York, Springer-Verlag, 1990.
4. Brownell K: Social and behavioral aspects of obesity in children, in Krasnegor NA, Arasteh JD, Cataldo MF (eds): *Child Health Behavior: A Behavioral Pediatrics Perspective*. New York, John Wiley & Sons, 1987.
5. Epstein LH, Squires S: The stop-light diet for children: An eight week program for parents and children. Boston, Little, Brown & Co, 1988.
6. Epstein LH, et al: Long term effects of family based treatment of childhood obesity. *J Consult Clin Psychol* 1987; 55:91–95.
7. Frisch H, et al: Psychological aspects in children and adolescents with hypopituitarism. *Acta Paediatr Scand* 1990; 79:644–651.
8. Glasgow A, Altieri ME: The epidemiology of readmissions of children with diabetes to a children's hospital, in Ahmed P, Ahmed N (eds): *Coping With Juvenile Diabetes*. Springfield, Ill, Charles Thomas, 1985.

9. Johnson SB: Diabetes mellitus, in DK Routh (ed): *Handbook of Pediatric Psychology*. New York, Guilford Press, 1988.

10. Karlsson JA: Time of puberty onset and intellectual and neuropsychological functioning, in Holmes CS ed: *Psychoneuroendocrinology, Brain, Behavior and Hormonal Interactions*. New York, Springer-Verlag, 1990.

11. Money J, Schwartz M, Lewis VG: Adult erotosexual status and fetal hormonal masculinization and demasculinization: 46,XX congenital virilizing adrenal hyperplasia and 46,XY androgen insensitivity syndrome compared. *Psychoneuroendocrinology* 1984; 9:405–414.

12. Mulaikal RM, Migeon CJ, Rock JA: Fertility rates in female patients with congenital adrenal hyperplasia due to 21-hydroxylase deficiency. *N Engl J Med* 1987; 316:178–182.

13. Paikoff RL, Brooks-Gunn J: Associations between pubertal hormones and behavioral and affective expression, in Holmes CS (ed): *Psychoneuroendocrinology, Brain, Behavior and Hormonal Interactions*. New York, Springer-Verlag, 1990.

14. Parrish JM: Parent compliance with medical and behavioral recommendations, in Krasnegor NA, Cataldo M (eds): *Child Health Behavior: A Behavioral Pediatrics Perspective*. New York, John Wiley, 1986.

15. Patterson GR: *Living with children: New methods for parents and teachers*. Chicago, Research Press, 1976.

16. Patterson GR, Forgatch M: *Parents and Adolescents Living Together. Part 1: The Basics*. Eugene, Ore, Castalia Publishing, 1987.

17. Rovet JF: The cognitive and neuropsychological characteristics of females with Turner syndrome, in Berch DB, Bender BG (eds): Boulder, Colo, AAAS/Westview Press, 1990.

18. Ryan C: Neurobehavioral disturbances associated with disorders of the pancreas, in Tarter RE, Van Thiel DH, Edwards K (eds): *Medical Neuropsychology*. New York, Plenum Press, 1988.

19. Siegel PT: Intellectual and academic functioning in children with growth delay, in Holmes CS (ed): *Psychoneuroendocrinology, Brain, Behavior and Hormonal Interactions*. New York, Springer-Verlag, 1990.

Index